SURGERY
SOURCEBOOK
FIFTH EDITION

Health Reference Series

SURGERY
SOURCEBOOK

FIFTH EDITION

Basic Consumer Health Information about Common Surgical Techniques and Procedures, Including Appendectomy, Breast Biopsy, Carotid Endarterectomy, Coronary Artery Bypass Grafting, Dilation and Curettage, Gallbladder Surgery, Hysterectomy, Tonsillectomy and Adenoidectomy, Cosmetic and Reconstructive Surgery, Gender Reassignment Surgery, and Weight-Loss (Bariatric) Surgery

Along with Facts about Emergency Surgery and Critical Care and Tips on Preparing for Surgery, Managing Pain and Surgical Complications, Recovery and Rehabilitation after Surgery, a Glossary of Related Terms, and a Directory of Resources for Additional Help and Information

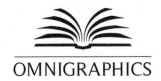

OMNIGRAPHICS

615 Griswold St., Ste. 520, Detroit, MI 48226

Bibliographic Note

Because this page cannot legibly accommodate all the copyright notices,
the Bibliographic Note portion of the Preface constitutes an extension
of the copyright notice.

* * *

OMNIGRAPHICS
Kevin Hayes, Managing Editor

* * *

Library of Congress Cataloging-in-Publication Data

Title: Surgery sourcebook: basic consumer health information about common surgical techniques and procedures, including appendectomy, breast biopsy, carotid endarterectomy, cataract removal, cesarean section, coronary artery bypass grafting surgery, cosmetic and reconstructive surgery, dilation and curettage (D&C), gallbladder removal surgery, Hemorrhoid surgery, hysterectomy, hernia surgery, spine surgery, mastectomy, prostatectomy, tonsillectomy, and weight-loss (Bariatric) surgery, along with Facts about emergency surgery and critical care and tips on preparing for surgery, getting a second opinion, managing pain and surgical complications, and recovering from surgery, a glossary of related terms, and a directory of resources for more information.

Description: Fifth edition. | Detroit, MI: Omnigraphics, 2020. | Series: Health reference series | Includes bibliographical references and index. | Summary: "Provides health information about an overview of surgical specialties, common types of surgery, surgical procedures, and the risks associated with surgery and how to manage pain along with the surgical complications. Includes glossary, index, and other resources"-- Provided by publisher.

Identifiers: LCCN 2020006699 (print) | LCCN 2020006700 (ebook) | ISBN 9780780817982 (library binding) | ISBN 9780780817999 (ebook)

Subjects: LCSH: Surgery--Popular works. | Consumer education--Popular works.

Classification: LCC RD31.3.S87 2020 (print) | LCC RD31.3 (ebook) | DDC 617--dc23

LC record available at https://lccn.loc.gov/2020006699
LC ebook record available at https://lccn.loc.gov/2020006700

Table of Contents

Part 4. Managing Pain and Surgical Complications

Part 5. Recovery and Rehabilitation after Surgery

Part 6. Additional Help and Information

Preface

ABOUT THIS BOOK

People undergo surgery for many reasons and it is sometimes considered to be an effective treatment option. Some surgeries are performed to ease the pain while some are done to treat a disease or help the body work better. According to the Agency for Healthcare Research and Quality (AHRQ), almost 15 million people in the United States undergo surgery each year at hospitals or at the same-day surgery centers. In most cases, surgeries save lives; however, they also carry significant risks such as bleeding, side effects to anesthesia, and infection. New developments in surgical techniques, such as lasers and laparoscopic surgery, have enabled surgeons to control surgical complications better and also minimize patient risks.

Surgery Sourcebook, Fifth Edition provides information about an overview of surgical specialties, common types of surgery, surgical procedures, and the risks associated with surgery and how to manage pain along with the surgical complications. It also discusses the recovery and rehabilitation after surgery. A glossary of related terms and directory of additional resources are also included.

HOW TO USE THIS BOOK

This book is divided into parts and chapters. Parts focus on broad areas of interest. Chapters are devoted to single topics within a part.

Part 1: Introduction to Surgery provides basic information about surgical specialties, including major types of surgeries such as emergency, exploratory, and cosmetic surgery. It also discusses surgical techniques including laser and robotic-assisted surgeries. The part concludes with statistics and the latest research on surgery.

Part 2: Preparing for Surgery offers patients information on finding a qualified surgeon, obtaining a second opinion, and preparing for surgery. Services provided by ambulatory surgical centers are also detailed. The part also discusses blood transfusion, anxiety before surgery, tips on ensuring patient safety and preventing medical errors, financial planning facts, and medical tourism.

Part 3: Common Types of Surgery and Surgical Procedures provides details about head and neck, eye, dental, breast, lung, heart and vascular, joint and spine, gastrointestinal, weight-loss (bariatric), gynecologic and obstetric, and urological surgeries. It also includes information on organ and tissue transplantation along with the plastic surgery procedures.

Part 4: Managing Pain and Surgical Complications focuses on the post-operative period and discusses methods for controlling pain, managing blood loss, and preventing surgical site and healthcare-associated infections such as catheter-associated urinary tract infections, *Clostridium difficile*, *Pseudomonas aeruginosa*, and methicillin-resistant *Staphylococcus aureus* (MRSA) infections. The part also identifies other complications that may affect surgical patients, including abdominal adhesions, deep vein thrombosis, and an overview of surgical adverse events.

Part 5: Recovery and Rehabilitation after Surgery offers insight into the process of recovering from surgery and what to expect after surgery, along with information on tube feeding, artificial airways and assisted ventilation, including hospital discharge planning, and disparities in surgical care.

Part 6: Additional Help and Information provides a glossary of important terms related to surgery and directory of organizations that offer information to people undergoing surgery or their caregivers.

BIBLIOGRAPHIC NOTE

This volume contains documents and excerpts from publications issued by the following U.S. government agencies: Agency for Healthcare Research and Quality (AHRQ); Centers for Disease Control and Prevention (CDC); Centers for Medicare & Medicaid Services (CMS); *Eunice Kennedy Shriver* National Institute of Child Health and Human Development (NICHD); Health Resources and Services Administration (HRSA); National Aeronautics and Space Administration (NASA); National Cancer Institute (NCI); National Eye Institute (NEI); National Heart, Lung, and Blood Institute (NHLBI); National Institute of Arthritis and Musculoskeletal and Skin Diseases (NIAMS); National Institute of Biomedical Imaging and Bioengineering (NIBIB); National Institute of Diabetes and Digestive and

Kidney Diseases (NIDDK); National Institute of General Medical Sciences (NIGMS); National Institute of Neurological Disorders and Stroke (NINDS); National Institute on Aging (NIA); National Institute on Deafness and Other Communication Disorders (NIDCD); National Institutes of Health (NIH); *NIH News in Health*; Office of Disease Prevention and Health Promotion (ODPHP); Office of Population Affairs (OPA); Office on Women's Health (OWH); U.S. Agency for International Development (USAID); U.S. Department of Justice (DOJ); U.S. Department of Veterans Affairs (VA); and U.S. Food and Drug Administration (FDA).

It may also contain original material produced by Omnigraphics and reviewed by medical consultants.

ABOUT THE *HEALTH REFERENCE SERIES*

The *Health Reference Series* is designed to provide basic medical information for patients, families, caregivers, and the general public. Each volume provides comprehensive coverage on a particular topic. This is especially important for people who may be dealing with a newly diagnosed disease or a chronic disorder in themselves or in a family member. People looking for preventive guidance, information about disease warning signs, medical statistics, and risk factors for health problems will also find answers to their questions in the *Health Reference Series*. The *Series*, however, is not intended to serve as a tool for diagnosing illness, in prescribing treatments, or as a substitute for the physician–patient relationship. All people concerned about medical symptoms or the possibility of disease are encouraged to seek professional care from an appropriate healthcare provider.

A NOTE ABOUT SPELLING AND STYLE

Health Reference Series editors use *Stedman's Medical Dictionary* as an authority for questions related to the spelling of medical terms and *The Chicago Manual of Style* for questions related to grammatical structures, punctuation, and other editorial concerns. Consistent adherence is not always possible, however, because the individual volumes within the *Series* include many documents from a wide variety of different producers, and the editor's primary goal is to present material from each source as accurately as is possible. This sometimes means that information in different chapters or sections may follow other guidelines and alternate spelling authorities. For example, occasionally a copyright holder may require that eponymous terms be shown in possessive forms (Crohn's disease vs. Crohn disease) or that British spelling norms be retained (leukaemia vs. leukemia).

MEDICAL REVIEW

Omnigraphics contracts with a team of qualified, senior medical professionals who serve as medical consultants for the *Health Reference Series*. As necessary, medical consultants review reprinted and originally written material for currency and accuracy. Citations including the phrase "Reviewed (month, year)" indicate material reviewed by this team. Medical consultation services are provided to the *Health Reference Series* editors by:

Dr. Vijayalakshmi, MBBS, DGO, MD
Dr. Senthil Selvan, MBBS, DCH, MD
Dr. K. Sivanandham, MBBS, DCH, MS (Research), PhD

OUR ADVISORY BOARD

We would like to thank the following board members for providing initial guidance on the development of this series:

- Dr. Lynda Baker, Associate Professor of Library and Information Science, Wayne State University, Detroit, MI
- Nancy Bulgarelli, William Beaumont Hospital Library, Royal Oak, MI
- Karen Imarisio, Bloomfield Township Public Library, Bloomfield Township, MI
- Karen Morgan, Mardigian Library, University of Michigan-Dearborn, Dearborn, MI
- Rosemary Orlando, St. Clair Shores Public Library, St. Clair Shores, MI

HEALTH REFERENCE SERIES UPDATE POLICY

The inaugural book in the *Health Reference Series* was the first edition of *Cancer Sourcebook* published in 1989. Since then, the *Series* has been enthusiastically received by librarians and in the medical community. In order to maintain the standard of providing high-quality health information for the layperson the editorial staff at Omnigraphics felt it was necessary to implement a policy of updating volumes when warranted.

Medical researchers have been making tremendous strides, and it is the purpose of the *Health Reference Series* to stay current with the most recent advances. Each decision to update a volume is made on an individual basis. Some of the considerations include how much new information is available and the feedback we receive from people who use the books. If there is a topic you would like to see added to the update list, or an area of medical concern you feel has not been adequately addressed, please write to:

Managing Editor
Health Reference Series
Omnigraphics
615 Griswold St., Ste. 520
Detroit, MI 48226

Part 1 | **Introduction to Surgery**

Chapter 1 | **Overview of Surgical Specialties**

There are various surgical specialties, and the 14 specialties that the American College of Surgeons (ACS) recognizes are explained in this chapter.

Besides the obvious differences in training that qualify surgeons to perform specific surgeries, these physicians are also specialist because they perform the same surgical procedures repeatedly. It is helpful for patients to know the various surgical specialties available to them so that they can choose the right surgeon for their condition.

WHO ARE SURGEONS?

In the United States, a minimum of five years of postmedical school experience in surgical residency training is required in order to qualify as a surgeon. For specialization in a particular field, physicians require even more years of training so that they can practice independently as a specialized surgeon for specific medical conditions. For example, if a patient has a broken leg, then an orthopedic surgeon who specializes in bone medical conditions performs that surgical procedure.

TRAINING OF SURGEONS

Both medical doctors (MDs) and doctors of osteopathic medicine (DOs) can pursue surgery specialization or subspecialization, but it is more common for MDs to do so. The career path for surgeons

"Overview of Surgical Specialties," © 2020 Omnigraphics. Reviewed April 2020.

in the United States is predictable; first, they complete medical school, then they complete five years of surgical residency training. Then they get trained in a surgical specialty of their choice. Following this, they can pursue a subspecialty with further training. For example, a surgeon who completes a general-surgery residency and specializes in cardiothoracic (heart/lung) surgery can subspecialize in pediatric heart-transplant surgery. The surgeon also may choose to specialize within their chosen specialty by focusing on performing heart bypass surgery, heart valve repair, or other heart surgeries.

TYPES OF SURGICAL SPECIALTIES

There are various surgical specialties, and many of them have subspecialties. Depending upon the medical problem, the requirement of a doctor with one or more of these specialties may be needed. The following are the 14 surgical specialties recognized by the American College of Surgeons:

General Surgery

A general surgeon specializes in the treatment of a broad category of problems. They provide preoperative, operative, and postoperative care of a patient. A general surgeon completes five years of postmedical school training, during which they acquire the knowledge and technical skills required to manage medical conditions related to the head and neck, breast, skin and soft tissues, abdominal wall, extremities, and the gastrointestinal, vascular, and endocrine systems.

Thoracic Surgery

Thoracic surgery involves preoperative, operative, postoperative, and critical care of patients with a chest disorder, specifically:
- Coronary artery disease
- Cancers of the lung, esophagus, and chest wall
- Abnormalities in the great vessels and heart valves
- Congenital anomalies

4

- Tumors of the mediastinum
- Diseases of the diaphragm

In addition to treating these conditions, thoracic surgeons also specialize in airway and chest injuries. A thoracic surgeon must have the knowledge, technical skills, and experience to accurately diagnose, safely operate, and manage the care of patients affected by intrathoracic abnormalities.

Colon and Rectal Surgery

The colorectal surgeons specialize in treating issues of the small and large intestines, the rectum, and the anus with surgery. Their extensive knowledge in the field qualifies them to surgically deal with other organs and tissues such as the liver, urinary tract, and female reproductive systems. Apart from that, they also perform surgeries for those affected with gastrointestinal tract diseases.

Obstetrics and Gynecology

Commonly known as "OBGYNs," these surgeons specialize in the medical and surgical care of pregnant women and treat conditions that affect the female reproductive system. Some OBGYN surgeons further specialize in urogynecology, pelviscopy, adolescent/pediatric gynecology, or infectious diseases.

Gynecologic Oncology

Gynecologic oncologist surgeons are trained in managing patients affected by gynecologic cancer that affects the female reproductive system. There may be some overlap between an OBGYN and a gynecologic oncologist. However, a gynecologic oncologist specializes in performing surgery as a treatment specifically for those affected with cancer.

Neurological Surgery

Neurosurgeons specialize in diagnosing, evaluating, and treating disorders related to the central nervous system (the brain and spinal cord) and perform brain surgery, back-pain correction surgery, and surgery for cancer of the nervous system and other neurological conditions.

Ophthalmic Surgery
An ophthalmologist specializes in the complete care of the eye and vision. These are the only medical practitioners who are medically trained to diagnose and treat all eye and vision problems. An ophthalmologist provides vision services (spectacles and contact lenses) and treats or performs surgery for eye disorders that may be present from birth or occur due to an accident or trauma, or that develop with age.

Oral and Maxillofacial Surgery
Oral and maxillofacial surgeons specialize in the care of a wide range of diseases related to the head, neck, face, jaws, and the hard and soft tissues of the oral and maxillofacial region (jaw and face). These professionals are also trained to administer anesthesia and to treat other dental and mouth-related problems such as misaligned jaws, removal of tumors and cysts of the jaw and mouth, dental-implant surgery, and extraction of wisdom teeth.

Orthopedic Surgery
Orthopedic surgeons specialize in treating issues related to bones, joints, ligaments, and tendons. Most of the orthopedic surgeon's practice involves surgery; however, many orthopedic conditions are also treated medically or physically by using braces, casts, splints, or physical therapy. The field of orthopedic surgery has become very broad and consists of various subspecialties such as:
- Hand surgery
- Sports medicine
- Foot and ankle orthopedics
- Joint replacement
- Orthopedic oncology
- Pediatric orthopedics

- Spine surgery
- Trauma surgery

Otolaryngology

Otolaryngologists provide medical and surgical care to those who have diseases or disorders related to the ear, nose, and throat (ENT). Additionally, they specialize in head and neck oncology, and in facial plastic and reconstructive surgeries. An otolaryngologist has basic knowledge and skill in the following:
- Audiology and speech-language pathology
- Chemical senses
- Allergy
- Endocrinology
- Neurology

Pediatric Surgery

Pediatric surgeons specialize in children's health issues and normally treat them with surgery. They operate on newborns and children up until their teenage years. However, some adults consult a pediatric surgeon too, if their medical issues have been present since birth or childhood. Some of the subspecialties of a pediatric surgeon are:
- Neonatal
- Prenatal
- Trauma
- Pediatric oncology

Plastic and Maxillofacial Surgery

Plastic and maxillofacial surgery is the repair, replacement, and reconstruction of defects in the forms and functions of the body. Usually, these surgical corrections are done to the craniofacial structures, the oropharynx, the upper and lower limbs, the breast, and the external genitalia. Plastic surgery also focuses on the aesthetic surgery of structures with undesirable forms. This type of plastic surgery has been gaining popularity for physical-enhancement purposes. After completing residency training in plastic surgery, a plastic surgeon can subspecialize in hand surgery.

Urology

Urologists specialize in the medical and surgical treatment of the urinary tract. They treat conditions ranging from an overactive bladder to minimally invasive procedures (MIS) for kidney stones. Some urologists also perform surgery to remove the prostate of a cancer patient, which can be a minor or major procedure.

Vascular Surgery

Vascular surgeons care for those affected by artery and vein diseases. Atherosclerosis is the hardening of the arteries and it is one of the most common medical conditions that a vascular surgeon treats. Additionally, these surgeons are trained to diagnose and treat strokes—which are caused by the blockage or narrowing of arteries in the neck—and aneurysms and blood clots within the arteries and veins.

The key to receiving the best surgical treatment is finding the right surgeon with the right experience in the fields in which they specialize. It is also advisable to consult two or more surgeons before making a choice because a significant part of patient-intervention management involves surgical specialties. This makes finding the right surgeon especially critical for the well-being of a patient.

References

1. "What Are the Surgical Specialties?" American College of Surgeons (ACS), February 1, 2001.
2. Jennifer, Whitlock. "An Overview of Surgical Specialties," Verywell Health, December 2, 2019.

Chapter 2 | **Major Types of Surgery**

Chapter Contents

Section 2.1 | Emergency Surgery

Emergency surgery is a nonelective surgery (urgent medical procedure) that is performed when the patient's life is in immediate danger. It is usually performed by surgeons specialized in emergency medicine. This surgery can be conducted for many reasons but is performed most often in critical cases such as response to trauma, brain injuries, mass casualties, cardiac events, poison episodes, and pediatric emergencies.

When a medical emergency occurs, immediate action is necessary to save a patient's life or to prevent further damage. An ambulance is usually called to transport a patient who is severely injured or not breathing. The patient is then assessed, and first aid is immediately administered by paramedics or other trained emergency medical personnel.

EMERGENCIES THAT REQUIRE SURGERY
Medical conditions that require emergency surgery are not planned or organized. A few common emergencies that require surgery include:
- Invasive resuscitation and surgery for acute respiratory failure, pulmonary embolism, and pulmonary obstructions
- Acute trauma to the head, chest, abdomen, or extremities
- Injuries resulting in the loss or amputation of body parts
- Severe burns
- Heart attacks, cardiac shock, and cardiac arrhythmia
- Aneurysms
- Neurological conditions (brain injuries)
- Complications of pregnancy
- Abdominal emergencies, including perforated ulcer, appendicitis, cholecystitis (gallbladder infection), or bowel blockage.

STEPS IN AN EMERGENCY SURGERY PROCEDURE

There are various steps involved in an emergency surgical procedure as detailed below.

The Intake Assessment Process

A physical assessment of the patient's overall condition is performed by the emergency medical staff. This involves checking symptoms; taking vitals; and reviewing medical history, including past and present illnesses, allergies, and current medications or illicit drugs the patient may have consumed. If the patient is in a critical condition, treatment will begin immediately, and some of these assessments will be done simultaneously.

Emergency room (ER) patients often need to be stabilized, so an intravenous therapy (IV) is inserted into a vein to allow for quick delivery of medications, transfusions, or intravenous fluids based on the emergency physician's directions.

Presurgery Diagnostic Testing

After the patient has been stabilized and the intake assessment is confirmed, diagnostic tests may be ordered, depending on the condition. Common diagnostic tests include:
- X-rays and blood tests
- Computed tomography (CT) scans
- Magnetic resonance imaging (MRI) scans
- Electrocardiograms (ECGs) for heart problems
- Electroencephalograms (EEGs) for brain injury

Once the diagnostic testing is done, a trauma or general surgeon will be brought in immediately to perform their own assessment of the condition.

Facilitating an Emergency Transfer

Large hospitals are accustomed to high volumes of traffic, and hence they have trauma or general surgeons on staff 24 hours a day. In contrast, small or rural hospitals may not have the technical capabilities or the staff required to perform a surgery. In such cases, the smaller facility will stabilize the patient and then coordinate a patient transfer to a spacious and well equipped facility.

Transfers can happen through an ambulance or air service with trained staff onboard to ensure the patient's safety. Transfers are typically done within an hour so that the patient gets the proper treatment immediately and has the necessary specialists to take care of them.

Preparing for Emergency Surgery
A patient undergoing emergency surgery will be fully sedated with general anesthesia, administered through an IV. The anesthesia helps to relax the muscles, allowing a physician to place an endotracheal tube into the windpipe. This is connected to a ventilator, and it takes over the breathing during the surgical procedure. An anesthesiologist remains present throughout the procedure, ready to administer other medications if required to keep the patient unconscious and prevent them from moving during the surgery.

Undergoing Surgery
During surgery, fluids are administered intravenously to balance the loss of blood and other bodily fluids. In addition, transfusions may be required to further stabilize the patient. The nature of the surgery and any postsurgical complications that may arise will determine the length of the procedure. When the surgery is complete, patients are stitched up or stapled, and once stabilized, they are moved to a postanesthesia care unit (PACU).

Postemergency Surgery Recovery
During the recovery phase, the patient's vital signs are closely watched and pain medications and any other prescriptions will be administered as required. Some patients may need to remain on a ventilator and others may need additional surgeries. However, in general, once the effects of anesthesia have fully worn off, stable patients are moved to a hospital room to begin the healing process;

while those who are unstable will be transported to an intensive care unit (ICU).

References

1. "What to Expect during Emergency Surgery," BandGrip, April 18, 2019.
2. "When You Are Undergoing Emergency Surgery," VeryWellHealth, November 12, 2019.
3. "Emergency Surgery," Encyclopedia, March 14, 2020.
4. "Emergency Surgery," MaineHealth, May 20, 2017.

Section 2.2 | Elective Surgery

Elective surgery is a nonemergency surgical procedure that an individual may choose to have. Optional or elective surgery is planned in advance and not considered a necessity for a person to stay alive and functioning. Cosmetic surgeries, such as breast implants or nose jobs are elective surgeries. Women sometimes opt to have elective cesarean births. Other surgeries such as organ donation, scoliosis surgery, tonsillectomies, and a few other minor surgeries, can also be considered elective.

The majority of medical procedures performed in the United States are elective surgeries. Since a person can decide whether or not to have elective surgery, there is a misconception that medical insurance will not cover these types of procedures. Many elective surgeries are usually covered in full or in part by medical insurance.

ELECTIVE SURGERY PROCEDURES

There is a wide range of elective surgeries spanning all the systems of the body in modern medical practice.

The major categories of common elective procedures include:

- **Plastic surgery.** Reconstructive or cosmetic surgery that enhances appearance and, in some cases, physical function of the body.
- **Refractive surgery.** Laser surgery for vision correction.
- **Gynecological surgery.** Either medically necessary or optional surgery based on the patient's condition. It includes hysterectomy and tubal ligation.
- **Exploratory or diagnostic surgery.** Surgery to determine the origin and extent of a medical problem, such as cancer, or to obtain biopsy tissue samples.
- **Cardiovascular surgery.** Usually considered medically necessary; however, there are few nonemergency procedures to improve blood flow or heart function, such as angioplasty or the implantation of a stent or pacemaker.
- **Musculoskeletal system surgery.** Certain cases of orthopedic surgical procedures, including joint or hip replacement and anterior cruciate ligament (ACL) reconstruction (knee surgery).

TYPES OF ELECTIVE SURGERY

Elective surgery can be classified into two different types, based on their importance.

Elective and Medically Necessary

A medically necessary elective surgical procedure:

- Treats or diagnoses an injury, deformity, disease, or significant symptoms, such as severe pain.
- May be required for the body to function properly and to enhance the quality of life.

These types of surgeries are recommended when all other forms of treatment are no longer effective. For example, if someone has knee arthritis and is unable to get relief from injections, medications, or therapy, a knee replacement becomes the best option to improve the quality of life. Medical insurance will usually cover all or part of the cost for these surgeries.

Elective but Not Medically Necessary

The other type of elective surgery is one that is not medically necessary. These are procedures that a person may desire, but that does not fulfill a medical need. For example, cosmetic surgeries, such as a facelift is not considered medically necessary since the face functions properly even without a surgery. Most insurance plans will not cover these types of surgeries. However, there are few exceptions like reconstructive surgery after a mastectomy (breast cancer surgery).

ELECTIVE SURGERY METHODS

Although surgery is performed for a specific purpose, there are different options available for the method of operation. Traditional surgeries are those where an incision is made to open up an area of the body for a procedure. However, most procedures are usually performed with the noninvasive approach known as "laparoscopy" (one or more small incisions where a small scope and surgical tools are inserted to perform the procedure). Laparoscopic surgery can also be performed with a robotic device that assists the surgeon. Most surgeons will outline the options for each patient and explain the risks and benefits of each option. If an individual is unsure about the options provided, getting a second opinion from another surgeon can help with the decision process.

RISKS OF ELECTIVE SURGERY

The risks of elective surgery will vary based on the type of procedure performed. Typically, any form of surgery involves a risk of infection, hemorrhage (bleeding), and circulatory problems, including shock or thrombosis (clotting within the circulatory system). The anesthesia used may also cause certain complications, such as anaphylactic shock (allergic reaction).

References
1. "What Is Elective Surgery," Whitehall of Deerfield healthcare, February 15, 2020.
2. "Different Types of Surgery," OakBend Medical Center, September 23, 2017.
3. Davis, Elizabeth "Will Your Health Insurance Pay for an Elective Surgery," Verywell Health, March 2, 2020.
4. "Elective Surgery," The Encyclopedia of Surgery, October 24, 2005.

Section 2.3 | Exploratory Surgery

"Exploratory Surgery," © 2020 Omnigraphics. Reviewed April 2020.

Exploratory surgery is a surgery that is performed for diagnostic purposes when physicians fail to obtain an accurate diagnosis using typical imaging techniques. It can be used to diagnose suspected cancers that cannot be identified using other diagnostic methods, such as medical imaging studies.

The primary goal of exploratory surgery is to examine the internal organs and to use the information gained to arrive at a diagnosis, or to present a differential diagnosis. Sometimes, a surgical procedure turns exploratory when the surgeon realizes that the patient's condition is more complicated than it was initially diagnosed, requiring an updated assessment and a better approach for an effective treatment.

REASONS FOR EXPLORATORY SURGERY
Exploratory surgery is performed on patients with injuries that result in internal bleeding or a hematoma. It can also be used to check for the recurrence of cancerous tumors even after the patient has received radiation treatment. In some cases, exploratory surgery is performed on a fetus if a deformity or other life-threatening condition is suspected.

There are certain rare cases where magnetic resonance imaging (MRI) may fail to detect certain tumors or other problems. Individuals who have suffered from knee injuries undergo exploratory surgery when an MRI is not able to detect tears that could be causing pain or immobility. Surgeons often perform exploratory surgery to identify problems involving joints, muscles, tendons, and tissue in the elbows, wrists, and knees, which are the common areas of injury for professional athletes.

When a child swallows a foreign object and it gets lodged in the digestive tract, severe complications may occur. An exploratory operation is performed on the child to check for obstructions in the intestines. The surgery is usually treated as a last resort when an ultrasound fails to provide a definitive diagnosis.

THE PROCEDURE

The patient is thoroughly examined before the surgery for any signs of potential surgical complications, and once the patient has been cleared for surgery, anesthesia is administered.

In a typical exploratory surgery, the surgeon makes an incision at the diagnostic site, uses retractors to hold the incision open, and examines the organs and tissues for signs of disease, such as an infection or inflammation. Surgical tools may be used to move organs, fat, and muscles around for better visibility. Once the surgeon reaches a final diagnosis, the incision will be stitched up or stapled, and the patient will be taken off the anesthesia machine and sent to the recovery room.

The two most common types of exploratory surgeries are:
- Laparotomy
- Laparoscopy

Laparotomy

When the source of an abdominal problem is not obvious, an exploratory laparotomy (open abdominal surgery) is used to inspect the organs and tissues of the abdomen. Laparotomy can be used to diagnose cancer, gallstones, gastrointestinal perforation, endometriosis (uterus disorder), appendicitis, diverticulitis (bladder condition), liver abscess, ectopic pregnancy, and other conditions involving abdominal organs. During exploratory laparotomy, tissue samples may also be obtained through a procedure known as a "biopsy."

Laparoscopy

Exploratory laparoscopy is a minimally invasive approach that is used more frequently than laparotomy. Laparoscopic surgery is done by making small incisions in the skin to insert tubes that hold cameras, along with the surgical tools. The cameras are used to visualize the surgical field, allowing the surgeon to clearly see the internal organs, and the objects in the surgical field can be manipulated with clamps and probes inserted through the incisions. Recovery from laparoscopic surgery is quicker and less painful when compared to laparotomy.

RISKS AND COMPLICATIONS OF EXPLORATORY SURGERY

Both laparoscopy and laparotomy have certain complications associated with them, along with the general risks of surgery and the risks of anesthesia. The risks may vary depending on the underlying problem or disease that makes the procedure necessary, but the risks specific to the procedure are:

- Infection
- Incisional hernia
- Bleeding from the surgery site
- Damage to organs in the abdomen

References

1. "What Are the Different Types of Exploratory Surgery?" wiseGEEK, March 6, 2020.
2. Whitlock Jennifer "Understanding Laparotomy and Laparoscopy Procedures," Verywell Health, January 8, 2020.
3. "Abdominal Exploration," A.D.A.M. Inc, URAC, January 7, 2018.

Section 2.4 | **Cosmetic Surgery**

Cosmetic surgery is done to change the appearance of a person and restructure the body's contour and shape, smoothen the wrinkles, or eliminate balding areas, as well as to treat varicose veins and breast augmentation. The most performed cosmetic surgeries include breast augmentation, nose reshaping, liposuction, tummy tuck, eyelid surgery, and facelift. The cost of cosmetic procedures is often not covered under the health insurance.

A neck lift, forehead lift, mid-face lift, eyelid surgery, or chin surgery can reduce the effects of aging and present a youthful appearance. However, a surgeon may refer a patient for counseling before surgery if they believe there is an underlying problem that cannot be solved by the operation, or if the patient shows indications of body dysmorphic disorder (BDD). BDD is a psychological disorder that causes a person to think that there is something seriously wrong with their appearance when objective evidence suggests otherwise.

TYPES OF COSMETIC SURGERY

Cosmetic surgery procedures that require general anesthesia or intravenous (IV) sedation are performed in the hospital under the care of an anesthesiologist. In contrast, procedures, such as facial filler injections may be performed in an outpatient setting or the physician's office under local anesthesia.

Several cosmetic procedures are available to create an image to feel more confident and comfortable with one's appearance. Cosmetic surgeries are classified into two basic types:

Invasive Cosmetic Procedures

An invasive procedure is any type of surgery that breaks the skin. In the case of cosmetic procedures, this may include implants or procedures in which a tiny incision is made in a part of the body.

Invasive cosmetic procedures can include:
- Facelifts
- Fat reductions
- Breast augmentation
- Brow lift
- Body lift

Invasive cosmetic procedures also include liposuction (fat reduction), breast augmentation or reduction, and abdominoplasty (tummy tuck).

Minimally Invasive Cosmetic Surgery

For many surgical procedures including cosmetic surgery, the preferred method has moved on from traditional open surgery to the use of less invasive techniques. These minimally invasive procedures usually result in less pain, reduced scarring, and a quicker recovery for the patient. In cosmetic surgery, minimally invasive procedures use newer technologies, including lasers, to perform procedures that previously required extensive surgery and longer recovery time.

Depending upon the procedure, recovery times may vary, but the general healing period is between one and two weeks for facial cosmetic surgery. Most patients resume normal activities within two weeks after the surgery.

COMPLICATIONS OF COSMETIC SURGERY

Possible complications for a cosmetic surgical procedure include:
- Complications linked to anesthesia such as blood clots, pneumonia, and, rarely, death
- Infection at the incision site
- Accumulation of fluid beneath the skin
- Bleeding, which may require another surgical procedure or even a transfusion
- Visible scarring or skin breakdown, which must be surgically removed
- Numbness and tingling due to the nerve damage, which may be permanent

- Abnormal pain at the surgical site
- White pigmentation in the skin near the incision site

References
1. "Cosmetic Surgery," Mayo Foundation for Medical Education and Research (MFMER), July 19, 2017.
2. "Cosmetic Surgery: What You Should Know," Healthline, March 10, 2017.
3. "Cosmetic Surgery Options," WebMD, February 6, 2019.
4. "Invasive Cosmetic Procedures versus Non-Invasive Cosmetic Procedures," Kessel Dermatology, December 9, 2017.

Section 2.5 | By Type of Procedure

"By Type of Procedure," © 2020 Omnigraphics. Reviewed April 2020.

Surgical procedures are typically categorized by urgency, type of procedure, body system involved, the level of invasiveness, and special instrumentation.

Based on the type of procedure, they can be classified into the following types:
- Amputation
- Resection
- Excision
- Extirpation
- Reconstructive surgery
- Replantation
- Transplant surgery

AMPUTATION
Amputation is defined as the surgical removal of all or part of a limb or extremity (toe or finger). Castration is also an example

of amputation surgery. Currently, there are about 1.8 million Americans who have undergone amputations. The most common amputation surgery is the amputation of the leg, either above or below the knee.

Amputation may be required due to many medical reasons. The most common reason being poor blood circulation caused by damage or narrowing of the arteries, known as "peripheral arterial disease." Without adequate blood flow, the cells do not get oxygen and nutrients they require from the bloodstream. As a result, the affected tissue begins to die and lead to infection.

RESECTION

Resection is surgically removing part or all of a tissue, structure, or organ. This form of surgery involves the complete removal of an internal organ or a vital part (lung lobe or liver quadrant) of such an organ. It may be performed for various reasons, including removing a tissue that is known to be cancerous or diseased. Resection surgery can be performed either using the open surgery method or a laparoscopy (inserting a scope through a small incision or a natural entry point, such as the urethra or cervix). The most common type of resection is the small bowel resection, where one or more part of the small intestine is removed. This is done when colon problems are experienced in a specific area of the intestine.

EXCISION

Excision (meaning "surgical removal") is the removal of only a part of an organ, tissue, or other body parts. It involves removing a mass of tissue using a scalpel, laser, or other surgical tools. "Excision" refers to completely removing the tissue in a particular area of the body, instead of a sample of the tissue, as is done in a biopsy. For example, an appendix is excised during an appendectomy as the entire appendix is cut away from the healthy tissue.

EXTIRPATION

"Extirpation" refers to the surgical destruction of a body part, usually done to prevent the spread of a disease or infection. It is the complete removal or eradication of an organ or tissue, and is used in cancer treatment, as well as in the treatment of diseased or infected organs. The primary aim of extirpation in cancer treatment is to remove all cancerous tissue, which involves removing the visible tumor along with the adjacent tissue that may contain microscopic extensions of the tumor. If complete removal of a tumor is not possible, palliative surgery (surgery to make symptoms less severe) is done to relieve pain or pressure on the adjacent parts of the body.

RECONSTRUCTIVE SURGERY

Reconstructive surgeries are performed to reconstruct a mutilated, injured, or deformed part of the body. It is done when a significant amount of tissue is missing due to trauma or surgical removal. A skin graft may be required if the wound cannot be directly closed. If a large surface area of the body is involved, a thin split-thickness skin graft (consisting of the epidermis) is used. In case of a small defect, particularly one involving the face or hand, a full-thickness skin graft (consisting of epidermis and dermis), is used, and skin is usually taken from the ear, neck, or groin. In some cases, biomaterials (plastic implants) are used to fix or replace the damaged body parts.

REPLANTATION

Replantation is done to reattach a severed body part, most commonly a thumb, finger, hand, or arm. Replantation of other body parts such as the scalp, ear, face, penis, leg, foot, and toes are also possible. A surgeon will only perform a replantation procedure if the limb is still expected to function without any pain. In some cases, the body part is severely damaged for a replant to be considered.

This procedure is done by carefully removing the damaged tissue, after which the bone ends are shortened and rejoined with pins, wires, or plates and screws. This holds the detached part in place while the rest of the tissues are being restored. Muscles, tendons, arteries, nerves, and veins are then repaired, and, sometimes, grafts or artificial spacers (fasteners) of bone, skin, tendons, and blood vessels may be required.

TRANSPLANT SURGERY

Transplantation is the transfer (engraftment) of cells, tissues, or organs from one part of the body to another or from a donor to a recipient with the aim of restoring function in the body. The two types of donors available are living and deceased donors (cadaveric transplantation). In the latter case, the organ to be transplanted is removed and kept in a cold storage until the surgery. The removal of an organ or body part from a live human or animal for use in transplant is also a type of surgery.

Most organs cannot be stored outside the body for longer than 12 hours. The most common form of transplant surgery is a kidney transplant surgery. Heart and heart-lung organs can be preserved for 4 to 6 hours. In order to minimize the risk of rejection, an extensive matching of blood groups and tissue types is done.

References

1. "Surgical Therapy," Encyclopaedia Britannica, February 1, 2001.
2. "Amputation Overview," WebMD, February 5, 2020.
3. Whitlock, Jennifer "Reasons for a Resection Surgery," Verywell Health, November 11, 2019.
4. Whitlock, Jennifer "How and Why Excisions Are Performed during a Surgery," Verywell Health, November 11, 2019.
5. "What Is Replantation," Handcare, November 17, 2017.

Chapter 3 | **Cryosurgery**

WHAT IS CRYOSURGERY?

Cryosurgery (also called "cryotherapy") is the use of extreme cold produced by liquid nitrogen (or argon gas) to destroy abnormal tissue. Cryosurgery is used to treat external tumors, such as those on the skin. For external tumors, liquid nitrogen is applied directly to the cancer cells with a cotton swab or spraying device.

Cryosurgery is also used to treat tumors inside the body (internal tumors and tumors in the bone). For internal tumors, liquid nitrogen or argon gas is circulated through a hollow instrument called "cryoprobe," which is placed in contact with the tumor. The doctor uses ultrasound or magnetic resonance imaging (MRI) to guide the cryoprobe and monitor the freezing of the cells, thus limiting damage to nearby healthy tissue. (In ultrasound, sound waves are bounced off organs and other tissues to create a picture called a "sonogram.") A ball of ice crystals forms around the probe, freezing nearby cells. Sometimes more than one probe is used to deliver the liquid nitrogen to various parts of the tumor. The probes may be put into the tumor during surgery or through the skin (percutaneously). After cryosurgery, the frozen tissue thaws and is either naturally absorbed by the body (for internal tumors), or it dissolves and forms a scab (for external tumors).

WHAT TYPES OF CANCER CAN BE TREATED WITH CRYOSURGERY?

Cryosurgery is used to treat several types of cancer, and some precancerous or noncancerous conditions. In addition to prostate

This chapter includes text excerpted from "Cryosurgery in Cancer Treatment," National Cancer Institute (NCI), September 10, 2003. Reviewed April 2020.

and liver tumors, cryosurgery can be an effective treatment for the following:

- Retinoblastoma (a childhood cancer that affects the retina of the eye). Doctors have found that cryosurgery is most effective when the tumor is small and only in certain parts of the retina.
- Early-stage skin cancers (both basal cell and squamous cell carcinomas).
- Precancerous skin growths known as "actinic keratosis."
- Precancerous conditions of the cervix known as "cervical intraepithelial neoplasia." (abnormal cell changes in the cervix that can develop into cervical cancer).
- Cryosurgery is also used to treat some types of low-grade cancerous and noncancerous tumors of the bone. It may reduce the risk of joint damage when compared with more extensive surgery, and help lessen the need for amputation. The treatment is also used to treat acquired immunodeficiency syndrome (AIDS)-related Kaposi sarcoma when the skin lesions are small and localized.
- Researchers are evaluating cryosurgery as a treatment for a number of cancers, including breast, colon, and kidney cancer. They are also exploring cryotherapy in combination with other cancer treatments such as hormone therapy, chemotherapy, radiation therapy, or surgery.

IN WHAT SITUATIONS CAN CRYOSURGERY BE USED TO TREAT PROSTATE CANCER? WHAT ARE THE SIDE EFFECTS?

Cryosurgery can be used to treat men who have early-stage prostate cancer that is confined to the prostate gland. It is less well established than standard prostatectomy and various types of radiation therapy. Long-term outcomes are not known. Because it is effective only in small areas, cryosurgery is not used to treat prostate cancer that has spread outside the gland, or to distant parts of the body.

Some advantages of cryosurgery are that the procedure can be repeated, and it can be used to treat men who cannot have surgery or radiation therapy because of their age or other medical problems.

Cryosurgery for the prostate gland can cause side effects. These side effects may occur more often in men who have had radiation to the prostate.

- Cryosurgery may obstruct urine flow or cause urinary incontinence (lack of control over urine flow); often, these side effects are temporary.
- Many men become impotent (loss of sexual function).
- In some cases, the surgery has caused injury to the rectum.

IN WHAT SITUATIONS CAN CRYOSURGERY BE USED TO TREAT PRIMARY LIVER CANCER OR LIVER METASTASES (CANCER THAT HAS SPREAD TO THE LIVER FROM ANOTHER PART OF THE BODY)? WHAT ARE THE SIDE EFFECTS?

Cryosurgery may be used to treat primary liver cancer that has not spread. It is used especially if surgery is not possible due to factors, such as other medical conditions. The treatment also may be used for cancer that has spread to the liver from another site (such as the colon or rectum). In some cases, chemotherapy and/ or radiation therapy may be given before or after cryosurgery. Cryosurgery in the liver may cause damage to the bile ducts and/ or major blood vessels, which can lead to hemorrhage (heavy bleeding) or infection.

DOES CRYOSURGERY HAVE ANY COMPLICATIONS OR SIDE EFFECTS?

Cryosurgery does have side effects, although they may be less severe than those associated with surgery or radiation therapy. The effects depend on the location of the tumor. Cryosurgery for cervical intraepithelial neoplasia has not been shown to affect a woman's fertility, but it can cause cramping, pain, or bleeding. When used to treat skin cancer (including Kaposi sarcoma), cryosurgery may cause scarring and swelling; if nerves are damaged, loss of sensation may occur, and, rarely, it may cause a loss of pigmentation and loss of hair in the treated area. When used to treat tumors of the bone, cryosurgery may lead to the destruction of nearby bone tissue and result in fractures, but these effects may not be seen for some time after the initial treatment and can often be delayed with other treatments. In rare cases, cryosurgery may interact badly with certain types of chemotherapy. Although the side effects of cryosurgery may be less severe than those associated with conventional surgery or radiation, more studies are needed to determine the long-term effects.

WHAT ARE THE ADVANTAGES OF CRYOSURGERY?

Cryosurgery offers advantages over other methods of cancer treatment. It is less invasive than surgery, involving only a small incision or insertion of the cryoprobe through the skin. Consequently, pain, bleeding, and other complications of surgery are minimized. Cryosurgery is less expensive than other treatments and requires shorter recovery time and a shorter hospital stay, or no hospital stay at all. Sometimes cryosurgery can be done using only local anesthesia.

Because physicians can focus cryosurgical treatment on a limited area, they can avoid the destruction of nearby healthy tissue. The treatment can be safely repeated and may be used along with standard treatments such as surgery, chemotherapy, hormone therapy, and radiation. Cryosurgery may offer an option for treating cancers that are considered inoperable or that do not respond to standard treatments. Furthermore, it can be used for patients who are not good candidates for conventional surgery because of their age or other medical conditions.

WHAT ARE THE DISADVANTAGES OF CRYOSURGERY?

The major disadvantage of cryosurgery is the uncertainty surrounding its long-term effectiveness. While cryosurgery may be effective in treating tumors the physician can see by using imaging tests (tests that produce pictures of areas inside the body), it can miss microscopic cancer spread. Furthermore, because the effectiveness of the technique is still being assessed, insurance coverage issues may arise.

WHAT DOES THE FUTURE HOLD FOR CRYOSURGERY?

Additional studies are needed to determine the effectiveness of cryosurgery in controlling cancer and improving survival. Data from these studies will allow physicians to compare cryosurgery with standard treatment options such as surgery, chemotherapy, and radiation. Moreover, physicians continue to examine the possibility of using cryosurgery in combination with other treatments.

WHERE IS CRYOSURGERY CURRENTLY AVAILABLE?

Cryosurgery is widely available in gynecologists' offices for the treatment of cervical neoplasias. A limited number of hospitals and cancer centers throughout the country currently have skilled doctors and the necessary technology to perform cryosurgery for other noncancerous, precancerous, and cancerous conditions.

Individuals can consult with their doctors or contact hospitals and cancer centers in their area to find out where cryosurgery is being used.

Chapter 4 | Computer-Assisted and Robotic Surgery

Chapter Contents

Section 4.1 | **Computer-Assisted Surgery**

This section includes text excerpted from "Computer-Assisted Surgical Systems," U.S. Food and Drug Administration (FDA), March 13, 2019.

WHAT ARE COMPUTER-ASSISTED SURGICAL SYSTEMS?

Different types of computer-assisted surgical systems can be used for preoperative planning, surgical navigation and to assist in performing surgical procedures. The robotically-assisted surgical (RAS) devices are one type of computer-assisted surgical system. Sometimes referred to as "robotic surgery," the RAS devices enable the surgeon to use computer and software technology to control and move surgical instruments through one or more tiny incisions in the patient's body (minimally invasive) for a variety of surgical procedures.

The benefits of the RAS device may include its ability to facilitate minimally invasive surgery and assist with complex tasks in confined areas of the body. The device is not actually a robot because it cannot perform surgery without direct human control.

The RAS devices generally have several components, which may include:

- A console, where the surgeon sits during surgery. The console is the control center of the device and allows the surgeon to view the surgical field through a 3D endoscope and control movement of the surgical instruments;
- The bedside cart that includes three or four hinged mechanical arms, camera (endoscope) and surgical instruments that the surgeon controls during surgical procedures; and
- A separate cart that contains supporting hardware and software components such as an electrosurgical unit (ESU), suction/irrigation pumps, and light source for the endoscope.

Most surgeons use multiple surgical instruments and accessories with the RAS device such as scalpels, forceps, graspers, dissectors, cautery, scissors, retractors, and suction irrigators.

COMMON USES OF ROBOTICALLY-ASSISTED SURGICAL DEVICES

The U.S. Food and Drug Administration (FDA) has cleared the RAS devices for use by trained physicians in an operating room environment for laparoscopic surgical procedures in general surgery, cardiac, colorectal, gynecologic, head and neck, thoracic, and urologic surgical procedures. Some common procedures that may involve the RAS devices are gall-bladder removal, hysterectomy, and prostatectomy (removal of the prostate).

RECOMMENDATIONS FOR PATIENTS AND HEALTHCARE PROVIDERS ABOUT ROBOTICALLY-ASSISTED SURGERY
Healthcare Providers

The RAS is an important treatment option that is safe and effective when used appropriately and with proper training. The FDA does not regulate the practice of medicine and, therefore, does not supervise or provide accreditation for physician training nor does it oversee training and education related to legally marketed medical devices. Instead, training development and implementation is the responsibility of the manufacturer, physicians, and healthcare facilities. In some cases, professional societies and specialty board certification organizations may also develop and support training for their specialty physicians. Specialty boards also maintain certification status of their specialty physicians.

Physicians, hospitals, and facilities that use the RAS devices should ensure that proper training is completed and that surgeons have appropriate credentials to perform surgical procedures with these devices. Device users should ensure they maintain their credentialing. Hospitals and facilities should also ensure that other surgical staff that use these devices complete proper training.

Users of the device should realize that there are several different models of robotically-assisted surgical devices. Each model may operate differently and may not have the same functions. Users should know the differences between the models and make sure to get appropriate training on each model.

If you suspect a problem or complications associated with the use of the RAS devices, the FDA encourages you to file a voluntary report through MedWatch, the FDA Safety Information and Adverse Event Reporting program. Healthcare personnel employed by facilities that are subject to the FDA's user facility reporting requirements should follow the reporting procedures established by their facilities. Prompt reporting of adverse events can help the FDA identify and better understand the risks associated with medical devices.

Patients

Robotically-assisted surgery is an important treatment option, but may not be appropriate in all situations. Talk to your physician about the risks and benefits of robotically-assisted surgeries, as well as the risks and benefits of other treatment options.

Patients who are considering treatment with robotically-assisted surgeries should discuss the options for these devices with their healthcare provider, and feel free to inquire about their surgeon's training and experience with these devices.

THE U.S. FOOD AND DRUG ADMINISTRATION ACTIVITIES

- The FDA is aware of an increase in the number of medical device reports (MDRs) related to robotically-assisted surgical devices. The majority of the medical device reports the FDA received were of device malfunctions such as component breakage, mechanical problems, and image/display issues. However, the FDA has also received reports of injuries and deaths related to the device. This increase in reports may be due to a number of factors, including an increase in the number of devices being used or surgeries being conducted, better awareness of how to report device issues to the FDA, increased publicity resulting from product recalls, media coverage, and litigation, as well as other influences. In addition, because reports submitted to the FDA can contain incomplete, inaccurate, duplicative, and unverified information, confirming whether a device actually caused a specific event can be difficult based solely on information provided in a given report. For these reasons, the FDA also evaluates other information to make decisions about a device's safety and effectiveness, relying on a variety of postmarket surveillance data sources to monitor the safety and effectiveness of medical devices. MDRs of suspected device-associated deaths, serious injuries, and malfunctions are one of these sources, but submission of a report to the FDA does not necessarily indicate a faulty or defective medical device.

- To obtain additional information, the FDA conducted a small sample Medical Product Safety Network (MedSun) survey of experienced surgeons who use robotically-assisted surgical devices in a variety of procedures. The goal was to better understand the user's perspectives and the different challenges identified when using this type of system to perform surgery compared to conventional surgical procedures.

- The FDA is working with professional societies to encourage training and education associated with the use of these devices.

- The FDA routinely monitors postmarket performance of marketed devices and inspects manufacturing facilities that make the medical devices, and will continue to collect and analyze all available information regarding robotically-assisted surgical devices to better understand the risks and benefits. The FDA will keep the public informed if new information becomes available.

Section 4.2 | **Robotic Surgery**

This section includes text excerpted from "Robotic Surgery: Risks versus Rewards," Effective Health Care Program, Agency for Healthcare Research and Quality (AHRQ), February 2016. Reviewed April 2020.

BACKGROUND AND PREVALENCE OF ROBOTICS IN SURGERY

The use of robotic assistance in surgery has expanded exponentially since it was first approved in 2000. It is estimated that, worldwide, more than 570,000 procedures were performed with the da Vinci robotic surgical system in 2014, with this figure growing almost 10 percent each year. The robotic-assisted surgery (RAS) has found its way into almost every surgical subspecialty and now has approved uses in urology, gynecology, cardiothoracic surgery, general surgery, and otolaryngology. The RAS is most commonly used in urology and gynecology; more than 75 percent of robotic procedures performed are within these two specialties. Robotic surgical systems have the potential to improve surgical technique and outcomes, but they also create a unique set of risks and patient safety concerns.

The RAS is a derivative of standard laparoscopic surgery and was developed to overcome the limitations of standard laparoscopy. Like traditional laparoscopy, the RAS uses small incisions and insufflation of the anatomical operative space with carbon dioxide. The robotic camera and various instruments are placed through the ports into the body and can be manipulated by the surgeon performing the operation. In the case of the RAS, though, the surgeon, seated at a computer console in the operating room, uses robot assistance to utilize the tools (instead of doing it herself or himself directly at the bedside). In the RAS, a bedside assistant exchanges the instruments and performs manual tasks, such as retraction and suction. The da Vinci robotic surgical system, made by Intuitive Surgical, Inc., is the only robotic system on the market. There are three major components of the system including:

- The robot, which is a mobile tower with four arms, including a camera arm and three instrument arms.
- The bedside cart, consisting of the image processing equipment and light source, which is transmitted to

monitors in the operating suite and sends the image to the surgeon console.

- The console, at which the surgeon sits to operate; there are two binocular lenses that magnify and create a three-dimensional image for the surgeon. Two handpieces transmit the surgeon's hand movements to the instruments within the patient, manipulating the surgical instruments to perform the operation. A built-in motion filtration system minimizes tremor, and foot pedals at the console control different types of energy and also allow for movement of the different robotic components within the patient.

BENEFITS OF ROBOTIC-ASSISTED SURGERY

In theory, the RAS marries the benefits of laparoscopic surgery with that of open techniques by combining a minimally invasive approach with the additional benefit of a three-dimensional, magnified image. In addition, the RAS offers improved ergonomics and dexterity compared to traditional laparoscopy, and these advantages may lead to a shorter learning curve for surgeons. The purported benefits of RAS also include smaller incisions, decreased blood loss, shorter hospital stays, faster return to work, improved cosmesis, and lower incidence of some surgical complications.

While these advantages of RAS have been appreciated, most of these benefits are short term and limited to the acute perioperative period. In fact, there is little evidence demonstrating that robotic surgery provides any long-term benefits over open techniques. Taking the above case as an example, robotic-assisted laparoscopic prostatectomy (RALP) has been one of the most commonly adopted robotic procedures; more than 85 percent of all prostatectomies are now performed with robotic assistance in the United States. Multiple, well-validated studies have shown that (RALP) has significantly less blood loss, with much lower transfusion rates, and shorter hospital stays than with open approaches. In addition, the rates of some complications—deep vein thrombosis, wound infections, lymphoceles and hematomas, anastomotic leaks, and ureteral injuries—appear to be slightly lower than with open approaches.

The RALP appears to have similar advantages over laparoscopic prostatectomy, although the difference is less pronounced. When compared to standard laparoscopic prostatectomy, robotic assistance has been shown to have decreased blood loss, lower rates of blood transfusion, and slightly shorter hospital stays. Like with robotic assistance, pure laparoscopic techniques share a significant learning curve. While some studies have also suggested that robotic surgery may be more effective at total removal of cancerous tissue in prostate surgery (i.e., lower positive surgical margin rates) than with open and pure laparoscopic procedures, large systematic reviews and well-validated meta-analyses have shown similar rates of oncologic control.

Interestingly, the proponents of the RALP frequently boast improved urinary continence and sexual function after surgery (or at least equivalent rates) when compared to open prostatectomy. The data has generally been equivocal in this area; standardized, comparable, long term data are lacking. A study using surveillance, epidemiology, and end results Medicare claims data compared open to minimally invasive prostatectomy (laparoscopic and robotic). Their results supported previous findings of lower transfusion rates, shorter hospital stays, similar oncologic control, and fewer miscellaneous complications. On the other hand, they discovered that men who had undergone robotic prostatectomy had higher rates of postprostatectomy incontinence and erectile dysfunction than men who had an open procedure. It may be a matter of experience: many of the RALP proponents have performed thousands of procedures, which may lead to improved outcomes in their hands, but may not be generalized to other, less experienced, urologists.

RISKS OF ROBOTIC-ASSISTED SURGERY

The RAS shares the same risks of open and laparoscopic surgery, including the potential for infection, bleeding, and the cardiopulmonary risks of anesthesia. On top of that, there are additional risks that are unique to the robotic system. Not only is there potential for human error in operating the robotic technology, but an added risk of mechanical failure is also introduced. Multiple components of the system can malfunction, including the camera, binocular lenses, robotic tower, robotic arms, and instruments. The energy source, which is prone to electric arcing, can cause unintended internal burn injuries from the cautery device. Arcing occurs when electrical current from the robotic instrument leaves the robotic arm and is misdirected to surrounding tissue. This can cause sparks and burns leading to tissue damage which may not always be immediately recognized. There is a small risk of temporary, and even permanent, nerve palsies from the extreme body positioning needed to dock the robot and access the pelvis adequate to perform the RALP. Direct nerve compression from the robotic arms can also lead to nerve palsies. The RAS has also been shown to take significantly longer than nonrobotic procedures when performed at centers with lower robotic volume and by surgeons with less experience, and, overall, it is more expensive than open surgery.

As mentioned earlier, the outcomes in the RAS seem to correlate with individual surgeon experience. For example, in cancer surgery, surgeons with more experience are more likely to have clean margins. Other studies have documented lower complication rates with an increasing number of procedures. These findings of practice make perfect are not specific to robotic surgery; such findings have been seen in many procedures. There are varying reports of exactly how many cases are required to master the robotic learning curve, and the number varies by surgical procedure. For the RALP, range has been reported from as low as 40 to as many as 250. For hysterectomies, the literature reports a range of 20 to 50 cases to master the operation and reports that less experienced surgeons have significantly longer operative times.

Notwithstanding the concerns, RAS has been accepted as generally safe. The RALP has reported complication rates (including all grades of perioperative complications, from minor to life-threatening) of around 10 percent. Multiple risk factors can increase the possibility of complications and errors: patient factors (i.e., obesity or underlying comorbidities), surgeon factors (training and experience), and robotic factors (i.e., mechanical malfunction). The reported complication rate related directly to robotic malfunction is very low (approximately 0.1%–0.5%). However, when robotic errors do occur, the rates of permanent injury have been reported anywhere from 4.8 percent to 46.6 percent, and this literature may suffer from underreporting. Although fewer than 800 complications directly attributable to the robotic operating system have been reported to the U.S. Food and Drug Administration (FDA) over the past 10 years, in a web-based survey among urologists performing the RALP, almost 57 percent of respondents had experienced an irrecoverable intraoperative malfunction of the robot. The most common areas of complications were malfunction of the robotic arms, joint setup and camera, followed by power error, instrument malfunction, and breakage of the handpiece.

PREVENTING COMPLICATIONS OF ROBOTIC-ASSISTED SURGERY
Standardized Credentialing and Training

There are no universal standard guidelines on appropriate training or credentialing for robotic surgery. Some organizations have made progress in this area. The American Urological Association (AUA) has made recommendations for training and credentialing procedures consisting of specific online curriculum, testing, caseload requirements, and also recommendations that all physicians complete the da Vinci online robotic safety training course on set up, draping, specific safety features, and troubleshooting. Training in robotics is still a relatively new field, and there is not a strong body of evidence to support a specific training and credentialing model. Various authors have developed different curriculums and simulation models, but an ideal model has yet to be found, as this is a new and developing field. Until well-validated credentialing and training models can be developed, hospitals should require a basic robotic safety curriculum, such as provided by the AUA, for any surgeons using the surgical robot, and require case logs be supplied or case proctoring prior to granting robotic privileges.

Stricter Reporting Guidelines

Developing a more uniform system of error reporting and tougher penalties for noncompliance may potentially help capture a more accurate representation of the true incidence of adverse events. It is important to determine the true incidence of different complications and the surrounding circumstances. The goal should be to identify key risk factors for errors and complications with a focus on those that are modifiable. This ideally would lead to improved outcomes and fewer complications. There are clearly gaps with the FDA device tracking system, as many more robotic errors are experienced than are ever reported to the FDA. There needs to be a more rigorous reporting effort by individual hospitals to capture the true incidence of robotic malfunction. These institutional reports can be submitted to the FDA so that recurrent mechanical problems can be more easily and rapidly recognized and addressed by the manufacturer.

Appropriate Risk Disclosure to Patients

The idea of robotic surgery is very enticing to patients and has influenced the growth of robotics in the United States. However, Schroeck and colleagues found that men undergoing robotic prostatectomy were more likely to express "regret" and "dissatisfaction" than men undergoing open surgery, which was attributed to unrealistic patient expectations associated with the robot. Kaushik and colleagues found that less than 70 percent of patients were appropriately counseled preoperatively on the potential risks specific to robotic surgery, including possible robotic malfunction or potential conversion to an open procedure. The direct-to-consumer marketing phenomenon could be used to improve safety in robotics by appropriately educating patients. Institutions should ensure appropriate patient counseling and informed consent for the RAS is happening consistently. This tracking could be accomplished through auditing of informed consent materials as well as intermittent patient interviews.

While the RAS has many potential benefits for patients and providers, the case above clearly demonstrates that the technology itself may place patients at risk. National organizations and individual institutions should ensure appropriate training and credentialing, accurate and timely error reporting, and consistent informed consent for patients. Discussions about robotic surgery—both with individual patients and at the policy level—should appropriately balance the advantages and potential with the real risks and limited evidence of major advantages in terms of long-term outcomes.

Take-Home Points

- Robotic surgery is a rapidly expanding technology that has found a niche in multiple different surgical specialties worldwide.
- Although robotic-assisted surgery shows some short-term benefits surrounding the direct perioperative period, it has fairly equivalent long-term outcomes when compared to open surgery.
- Robotic surgery is generally safe with low overall complication rates, but adding the robot to the surgical equation inserts another potential entry point for error into an already complex and risk-fraught arena.
- In general, surgical outcomes are ultimately a direct manifestation of the skill and experience of the surgeon, not the technology or approach used.
- Potential areas for improvement and reduction of error in robotic surgery include more standardized training and credentialing practices, improved reporting systems for robotic-associated adverse events, and enhanced patient education.

Chapter 5 | Laser Surgery

Medical lasers are medical devices that use precisely focused light sources to treat or remove tissues.

The term "laser" stands for light amplification by stimulated emission of radiation. Ordinary light, such as that from a light bulb, has many wavelengths and spreads in all directions. Laser light, on the other hand, has a specific wavelength. It is focused in a narrow beam and creates a very high-intensity light. Because lasers can focus very accurately on tiny areas, they can be used for very precise surgical work or for cutting through tissue (in place of a scalpel).

PROCEDURES

Lasers are used in many types of surgical procedures. Some examples include:
- Cosmetic surgery (to remove tattoos, scars, stretch marks, sunspots, wrinkles, birthmarks, spider veins, or hair)
- Refractive eye surgery (to reshape the cornea in order to correct or improve vision as in laser-assisted in situ keratomileusis (LASIK) or photorefractive keratectomy (PRK))
- Dental procedures (such as endodontic/periodontic procedures, tooth whitening, and oral surgery)
- General surgery (such as tumor removal, cataract removal, breast surgery, plastic surgery, and most other surgical procedures)

This chapter includes text excerpted from "Medical Lasers," U.S. Food and Drug Administration (FDA), May 14, 2018.

RISKS AND BENEFITS

With proper use, lasers allow the surgeon to accomplish more complex tasks, reduce blood loss, decrease postoperative discomfort, reduce the chance of wound infection, and achieve better wound healing.

As with any type of surgery, laser surgery has potential risks. Risks of laser surgery include incomplete treatment of the problem, pain, infection, bleeding, scarring, and skin color changes.

Laser surgery uses nonionizing radiation, so it does not have the same long-term risks as x-rays or other types of ionizing radiation.

LAWS, REGULATIONS, AND PERFORMANCE STANDARDS

Manufacturers of electronic radiation-emitting products sold in the United States are responsible for compliance with the Federal Food, Drug, and Cosmetic Act (FFDCA), Chapter V, Subchapter C—Electronic Product Radiation Control.

Manufacturers of surgical laser products are responsible for compliance with all applicable requirements of Title 21 Code of Federal Regulations (Subchapter J, Radiological Health) Parts 1000 through 1005:

1000—General
1002—Records and Reports
1003—Notification of defects or failure to comply
1004—Repurchase, repairs, or replacement of electronic products
1005—Importation of electronic products

In addition, surgical lasers must comply with radiation safety performance standards in Title 21 Code of Federal Regulations (Subchapter J, Radiological Health) Parts 1010, 1040.10, and 1040.11:

1010—Performance standards for electronic products: general
1040.10—Lasers and Products Incorporating Lasers
1040.11—Specific Purpose Laser Products

Because they are medical devices, surgical laser products must also comply with the medical device regulations.

Chapter 6 | **Understanding Pediatric Surgery**

Nearly 82 years ago, the understanding that children are not merely small adults paved way for the evolution of pediatric surgery as a specialty. Children need a different approach for their medical treatment. They cannot always clearly explain their symptoms and are generally incapable of answering medical questions. Medical examination of children can also be difficult due to their inability or refusal to cooperate.

WHO IS A PEDIATRIC SURGEON?

A pediatric surgeon is a specialist who is trained to perform surgical procedures on newborns, children, and adolescents. They have the proficiency to treat a range of congenital, oncologic, gastrointestinal, thoracic, vascular, infectious, and traumatic disorders specific to children, and they are skilled in negotiating with sick children and their anxious parents. Offices for pediatric surgical practices often have interiors decorated and designed specifically for children. The waiting and examination rooms may have toys, books, and videos to make the atmosphere conducive and nonthreatening.

WHAT ROLE DOES A PEDIATRIC SURGEON PLAY IN TREATING CHILDREN?

Pediatric surgeons are involved in the diagnosis and management of all operative stages during surgery for children. They often consult with neonatologists, pediatricians, and other specialists

"Understanding Pediatric Surgery," © 2017 Omnigraphics. Reviewed April 2020.

to determine if surgery can improve the quality of life (QOL) for a child. Pediatric surgeons also play a major role in treating congenital deformities that will hamper a child's QOL if not surgically corrected.

WHAT EXPERTISE DO PEDIATRIC SURGEONS POSSESS?

Pediatric surgery can be subdivided into several different specialties:

Neonatal. It focuses on treating life-threatening birth defects and conditions in newborns such as tracheoesophageal fistula, imperforate anus, etc.

Pediatric oncology. It is the diagnosis and surgery of malignant tumors and benign growths in children.

Prenatal. Prenatal pediatric surgeons consult radiologists and use diagnostic techniques, such as ultrasound to detect and correct developmental anomalies in fetuses.

Trauma. Pediatric trauma surgeons attend to a large number of children who have sustained traumatic injuries that require surgical intervention, such as gunshot wounds or injuries sustained in a car accident. Pediatric surgeons play an important role in preventing traumatic injuries in children by participating in community prevention programs.

WHAT ARE THE SURGERIES DONE BY PEDIATRIC SURGEONS?

Pediatric surgeons perform many of the same procedures as general surgeons, including:

- Surgery for congenital abdominal wall defects
- Surgical care for abnormalities of the groin which include undescended testes, hernias, hydroceles, and varicoceles
- Surgical removal of congenital obstructions of the gastrointestinal tract
- Surgical repair of birth defects
- Surgical treatment of injuries such as like gunshot wounds, knife cuts, and lacerations in the liver
- Cancer surgeries
- Transplantations

- Appendectomy
- Endoscopic procedures, such as bronchoscopy and colonoscopy

WHAT KIND OF TRAINING DO PEDIATRIC SURGEONS UNDERGO?

Pediatric surgeons complete regular medical school and have at least 5 years of experience in general surgery in an accredited residency program. They have to practice pediatric surgery for two more years in a fellowship program to ensure the highest level of surgical knowledge for treating infants and children before becoming certified by the American Board of Surgery (ABS). The certificate is renewable every 10 years to ensure competency and requires up to date knowledge in pediatric surgery.

References

1. "What Is a Pediatric Surgeon?" American Pediatric Surgical Association (APSA), n.d.
2. "What Is a Pediatric Surgeon?" American Academy of Pediatrics (AAP), November 21, 2015.
3. "Pediatric Surgery," Association of Women Surgeons (AWS), n.d.
4. "What Is a Pediatric Surgeon?" Actforlibraries.org, n.d.

Chapter 7 | **Surgery in Older Adults**

ASK ABOUT DIFFERENT TREATMENT OPTIONS

You will benefit most from a treatment when you know what is happening and are involved in making decisions. Make sure you understand what your treatment involves and what it will or will not do. Have the doctor give you directions in writing and feel free to ask questions. For example: "What are the pros and cons of having surgery at this stage?" or "Do I have any other choices?"

If your doctor suggests a treatment that makes you uncomfortable, ask if there are other treatments that might work. If cost is a concern, ask the doctor if less expensive choices are available. The doctor can work with you to develop a treatment plan that meets your needs.

Here are some things to remember when deciding on a treatment:

- **Discuss different treatment choices.** There are different ways to manage many health conditions, especially chronic conditions such as high blood pressure and cholesterol. Ask what your options are.
- **Discuss risks and benefits of treatment options.** Once you know your options, ask about the pros and cons of each one. Find out what side effects might occur, how long the treatment would continue, and how likely it is that the treatment will work for you.

This chapter includes text excerpted from "Discussing Health Decisions with Your Doctor," National Institute on Aging (NIA), National Institutes of Health (NIH), February 3, 2020.

- **Consider how a treatment may affect your life.**
  When thinking about the pros and cons of a treatment,
  do not forget to consider its impact on your overall
  life. For instance, will one of the side effects interfere
  with a regular activity that means a lot to you? Is one
  treatment choice expensive and not covered by your
  insurance? Doctors need to know about these practical
  matters so they can work with you to develop a
  treatment plan that meets your needs.

Questions to Ask about Treatment Options

- Are there any risks associated with the treatment?
- How soon should treatment start? How long will it last?
- Are there other treatments available?
- How much will the treatment cost? Will my insurance
  cover it?

TALKING WITH MEDICAL SPECIALISTS

Your doctor may send you to a specialist for further evaluation, or
you may request to see a specialist yourself. Your insurance plan
may require you to have a referral from your primary doctor. A visit
to the specialist may be short. Often, the specialist already has seen
your medical records or test results and is familiar with your case.
If you are unclear about what the specialist tells you, ask questions.

For example, if the specialist says you have a medical condition
that you are not familiar with, you may want to say something such
as: "I do not know much about that condition. Could you explain
what it is and how it might affect me?" or "I have heard that is a
painful problem. What can be done to prevent or manage the pain?"

You also may ask for written materials to read, or you can call
your primary doctor to clarify anything you have not understood.

Ask the specialist to send information about any diagnosis or
treatment to your primary doctor. This allows your primary doctor
to keep track of your medical care. You also should let your primary doctor know at your next visit how well any treatments or
medications the specialist recommended are working.

Questions to Ask Your Specialist

- What is the diagnosis?
- What treatment do you recommend? How soon do I need to begin the new treatment?
- Will you discuss my care with my primary doctor?

IF YOU NEED SURGERY

In some cases, surgery may be the best treatment for your condition. If so, your doctor will refer you to a surgeon. Knowing more about the operation will help you make an informed decision about how to proceed. It also will help you get ready for the surgery, which makes for a better recovery.

Ask the surgeon to explain what will be done during the operation and what reading material, videos, or websites you can look at before the operation.

Find out if you will have to stay overnight in the hospital or if the surgery can be done on an outpatient basis, if you will need someone to drive you home. Minor surgeries that do not require an overnight stay can sometimes be done at medical centers called "ambulatory surgical centers."

Questions to Ask Your Surgeon

- What is the success rate of the operation? How many of these operations have you done successfully?
- What problems occur with this surgery? What kind of pain or discomfort can I expect?
- What kind of anesthesia will I have? Are there any risks associated with its use in older people?
- Will I have to stay in the hospital overnight? How long is recovery expected to take? What does it involve? When can I get back to my normal routine?

GETTING A SECOND OPINION

When patients are diagnosed with a serious illness or surgery is recommended, patients often seek a second opinion. Hearing the views of two different doctors can help you decide what is best for you. In fact, your insurance plan may require it. Doctors are used to this practice, and most will not be insulted by your request for a second opinion. Your doctor may even be able to suggest other doctors who can review your case.

Always remember to check with your insurance provider in advance to find out if a second opinion is covered under your policy, if there are restrictions to which doctors you can see, and if you need a referral form from your primary doctor.

DISCUSS HOW PREVENTION CAN IMPROVE YOUR HEALTH

Doctors and other health professionals may suggest you change your diet, activity level, or other aspects of your life to help you deal with medical conditions. Research has shown that these changes, particularly an increase in exercise, have positive effects on overall health.

Until recently, preventing disease in older people received little attention. But, things are changing. We now know that it is never too late to stop smoking, improve your diet, or start exercising. Getting regular checkups and seeing other healthcare professionals, such as dentists and eye specialists, helps promote good health. Even people who have chronic diseases, like arthritis or diabetes, can prevent further disability and, in some cases, control the progress of the disease.

If a certain disease or health condition runs in your family, ask your doctor if there are steps you can take to help prevent it. If you have a chronic condition, ask how you can manage it and if there are things you can do to keep it from getting worse. If you want to discuss health and disease prevention with your doctor, say so when you make your next appointment. This lets the doctor plan to spend more time with you.

It is just as important to talk with your doctor about lifestyle changes as it is to talk about treatment. For example: "I know that you have told me to eat more dairy products, but they really disagree with me. Is there something else I could eat instead?" or "Maybe an exercise class would help, but I have no way to get to the senior center. Is there something else you could suggest?"

As with treatments, consider all the alternatives, look at pros and cons, and remember to take into account your own point of view. Tell your doctor if you feel her or his suggestions won't work for you and explain why. Keep talking with your doctor to come up with a plan that works.

Many doctors now recommend that older people try to make physical activity a part of everyday life. When you are making your list of things to talk about with your doctor, add exercise. Ask how exercise would benefit you, if there are any activities you should avoid, and whether your doctor can recommend any specific kinds of exercise.

Questions to Ask Your Doctor about Prevention

- Is there any way to prevent a condition that runs in my family—before it affects me?
- Are there ways to keep my condition from getting worse?
- How will making a change in my habits help me?
- Are there any risks in making this change?
- Are there support groups or community services that might help me?

Chapter 8 | Surgery Statistics

Chapter Contents

Section 8.1 | Ambulatory Surgery

This section includes text excerpted from "National Health Statistics Reports," Centers for Disease Control and Prevention (CDC), February 28, 2017.

Ambulatory surgery also called "outpatient surgery," refers to surgical and nonsurgical procedures that are nonemergency, scheduled in advance, and generally do not result in an overnight hospital stay.

Ambulatory surgery has increased in the United States since the early 1980s. Two factors that contributed to this increase were medical and technological advancements, including improvements in anesthesia and in analgesics for the relief of pain, and the development and expansion of minimally invasive and noninvasive procedures (such as laser surgery, laparoscopy, and endoscopy). Before these advances, almost all surgery was performed in inpatient settings. Any outpatient surgery was likely to have been minor, performed in physicians' offices, and paid for by Medicare and insurers as part of the physician's office visit reimbursement.

The above advances and concerns about rising healthcare costs led to changes in the Medicare program in the early 1980s that encouraged growth in ambulatory surgery. Medicare expanded coverage to include surgery performed in ambulatory surgery centers (ASCs) (both hospital based and freestanding). In addition, a prospective payment system for hospitals based on diagnosis-related groups was adopted, and that created strong financial incentives for hospitals to shift some surgery out of the hospital. Ambulatory surgery proved to be popular among both physicians and patients, and the number of Medicare-certified ASCs increased steadily, in 1983 to 5,316 in 2010.

AMBULATORY SURGERY PROCEDURE AND VISIT OVERVIEW

- In 2010, 28.6 million ambulatory surgery visits to hospitals and ASCs occurred. During these visits, an estimated 48.3 million surgical and nonsurgical

Table 8.1. Ambulatory Surgery Procedures and Visits to Hospitals and Ambulatory Surgery Centers: United States, 2010

Ambulatory Surgery Utilization	Estimate	Standard Error
Procedures (millions)	48.3	4.3
In hospitals	25.7	2.6
In ASCs	22.5	3.3
Visits (millions)	28.6	2.4
In hospitals	15.7	1.6
In ASCs	12.9	1.8

Note: ASC is an ambulatory surgery center. (Source: National Center for Health Statistics (NCHS), National Hospital Ambulatory Medical Care Survey (NHAMCS), 2010)

Table 8.2. Percent Distribution of Ambulatory Surgery Visits in Hospitals and Ambulatory Surgery Centers, by Discharge Disposition: United States, 2010

Discharge Disposition	Percent of Visits
Routine discharge	95
Observation status	2
Admission to hospital as inpatient	2
Other	1
Total	100

[1]Discharge to customary residence, generally home.
[2]Discharge for further observation without being admitted to a hospital.
[3]Includes discharge to postsurgical or recovery care facility, referral to emergency department, surgery terminated, and other
options.
[4]Excludes 1.2 million of the 28.6 million total visits with an unknown discharge disposition.
(Source: National Center for Health Statistics (NCHS), National Hospital Ambulatory Medical Care Survey (NHAMCS), 2010)

procedures were performed. An estimated 25.7 million (53%) ambulatory surgery procedures were performed in hospitals and 22.5 million (47%) were performed in ASCs.

- An estimated 25.7 million (53%) ambulatory surgery procedures were performed in hospitals and 22.5 million (47%) were performed in ASCs.
- Private insurance was the expected payment source for 51 percent of the visits for ambulatory surgery, Medicare payment was expected for 31 percent, and Medicaid for 8 percent. Only 4 percent were self-pay.
- Ninety-five percent of the visits with a specified discharge disposition had a routine discharge, generally to the patient's home. Patients were admitted to the hospital as inpatients during only 2 percent of these visits.

AMBULATORY SURGERY PROCEDURES, BY SEX AND AGE

- For both males and females, 39 percent of procedures were performed on those 45 to 64 years of age (Figure 8.2)
- For females, about 24 percent of procedures were performed on those 15 to 44 years of age compared with 18 percent for males, whereas the percentage of procedures performed on those under 15 years of age was lower for females than for males (4% compared with 9%).
- About 19 percent of procedures were performed on those 65 to 74 years of age, with about 14 percent performed on those 75 years of age and over.

TYPES OF PROCEDURES

Seventy percent of the 48.3 million ambulatory surgery procedures were included in the following clinical categories: operations on the digestive system (10 million or 21%), operations on the eye (7.9 million or 16%), operations on the musculoskeletal system (7.1 million or 15%), operations on the integumentary system (4.3 million or 9%), and operations on the nervous system (4.2 million or 9%). These procedure categories made up 72 percent of procedures performed on females and 67 percent of those performed on

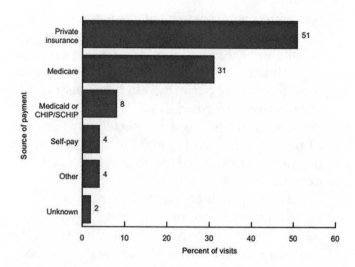

Figure 8.1. Percent Distribution of Ambulatory Surgery Visits in Hospitals and Ambulatory Surgery Centers, by Principal Expected Source of Payment: United States, 2010 *(Source: National Center for Health Statistics (NCHS), National Hospital Ambulatory Medical Care Survey (NHAMCS), 2010)*

Note: CHIP is Children's Health Insurance Program and SCHIP is State Children's Health Insurance Program.

males. Within the above-mentioned categories, data on procedures performed more than 1 million times are presented below.

Under operations on the digestive system, endoscopy of large intestine—which included colonoscopies—was performed 4.0 million times, and endoscopy of small intestine was performed 2.2 million times. Endoscopic polypectomy of the large intestine was performed an estimated 1.1 million times.

Eye operations included extraction of lens, performed 2.9 million times; insertion of lens, performed 2.6 million times for cataracts; and operations on eyelids, performed 1.0 million times.

Musculoskeletal procedures included operations on muscle, tendon, fascia, and bursa (1.3 million).

Operations on the integumentary system included excision or destruction of lesion or tissue of skin, and subcutaneous tissue (1.2 million).

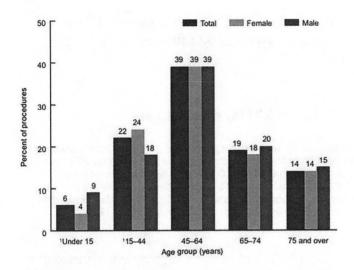

Figure 8.2. Percent Distribution of Ambulatory Surgery Procedures in Hospitals and Ambulatory Surgery Centers, by Age and Sex: United States, 2010 *(Source: National Center for Health Statistics (NCHS), National Hospital Ambulatory Medical Care Survey (NHAMCS), 2010)*

Notes: Numbers may not add to totals because of rounding.

Operations on the nervous system included injection of agent into spinal canal (2.9 million), including injections for pain relief.

DURATION OF SURGERY

The average time in the operating room for ambulatory surgery was almost 1 hour (57 minutes). On average, about one-half of this time (33 minutes) was spent in surgery. Postoperative care averaged 70 minutes. Time spent in the operating room, surgery, and receiving postoperative care were all significantly longer for ambulatory surgery performed in hospitals compared with ASCs.

Endoscopies averaged 14 minutes, while endoscopic polypectomy of the large intestine averaged 21 minutes. For cataract surgery, extraction or insertion of lens (often done together) averaged

10 minutes, and operations on the eyelids averaged 23 minutes. Arthroscopy of the knee averaged 32 minutes.

Section 8.2 | Inpatient Surgery

This section contains text excerpted from the following sources: Text in this section begins with excerpts from "Surgeries in Hospital-Based Ambulatory Surgery and Hospital Inpatient Settings, 2014," Agency for Healthcare Research and Quality (AHRQ), U.S. Department of Health and Human Services (HHS), February 5, 2018; Text under the heading "Inpatient Settings" is excerpted from "Overview of Operating Room Procedures during Inpatient Stays in U.S. Hospitals, 2014," Agency for Healthcare Research and Quality (AHRQ), U.S. Department of Health and Human Services (HHS), December 19, 2017.

Ambulatory surgery (AS), or outpatient surgery, is a planned operation for which the patient is not expected to be admitted to the hospital. Comparison of ambulatory surgery with inpatient surgery is essential for understanding utilization patterns for specific surgical procedures, including changing trends and estimates of total surgical volumes. As the number of surgical procedures capable of being safely performed in an ambulatory setting increases, comparisons of ambulatory surgery with inpatient surgery can also be useful in the evaluation of postsurgical complications, hospital cost savings, and patient experience of care surveys.

Self-reported facility estimates from the American Hospital Association (AHA) suggest that a growing share of all surgeries at community hospitals in the United States are performed in the AS setting (66% in 2014, up from 57% in 1994), although an ambiguous definition for AS introduces variation across facility volume estimates. The reports on specific surgical procedure trends in a subset of States also point to a shift from the inpatient surgical setting to the AS setting. Nationally representative AS estimates for a broad group of surgical procedures do not yet exist.

The Healthcare Cost and Utilization Project (HCUP) Statistical Brief presents national data on surgeries performed in two hospital settings: hospital inpatient and hospital-based AS settings. The findings in this Statistical Brief represent an update and expansion of 2012 statistics previously reported. Procedures performed in freestanding (nonhospital-owned) AS centers were not included because many State AS data sources do not include these types of centers.

The analysis was limited to visits for an invasive surgery commonly performed for therapeutic purposes (i.e., to treat disease or injury); excluded were noninvasive surgeries and surgeries typically used for diagnostic or exploratory purposes (e.g., colonoscopy). The HCUP Surgery Flag software was used to identify invasive, therapeutic surgeries based on a narrow and targeted definition.

This report presents characteristics of outpatient surgery visits and hospital inpatient stays for invasive, therapeutic surgical procedures. All references to surgeries, outpatient surgeries, or ambulatory surgeries refer to this subset of surgeries. The distribution of outpatient surgeries compared with inpatient surgical procedures by payer, body system, and the most common surgical procedures performed in an outpatient setting overall and by payer. In addition, ambulatory and inpatient volume and procedure rates are compared for each procedure. Unless otherwise noted, volumes and rates are based on all-listed procedure codes.

Figure 8.3 of this Statistical Brief was revised to include secondary inpatient surgical procedures that were not included in the original version. This only affected Figure 8.3 and resulted in an increase in the percentage of surgical visits or stays that occurred in the inpatient setting.

FINDINGS
Table 8.3 presents characteristics of community hospital visits for invasive, therapeutic surgeries performed in the ambulatory (outpatient) surgery setting versus the hospital inpatient setting (admitted to the hospital) in 2014.

- **In 2014, 17.2 million ambulatory hospital visits or inpatient stays included an invasive, therapeutic surgery; more than half of these visits occurred in the AS setting.**
  A total of 17.2 million hospital visits (AS visits or inpatient stays) in the United States included at least one surgery in 2014. Just over half of these visits

67

Table 8.3. Characteristics of Hospital Visits or Stays for Invasive, Therapeutic Surgery Performed in Hospital-Based Ambulatory and Inpatient Settings, 2014

Characteristic	Ambulatory Setting	Inpatient Setting
Total visits or stays for surgeries		
Total number, N	9,942,200	7,247,600
Percent of total visits or stays for surgeries, %	57.8	42.2
Total surgeries		
Total number, N	11,493,100	10,303,000
Percent of total surgeries, %	52.7	47.3
Number of surgeries per visit or stay, mean	1.2	1.4
Length of stay, mean, days	0.2	6
Visits or stays by type of community hospital, %		
By hospital bed size		
Large	53.9	58.3
Medium	26.1	26.3
Small	20	15.4
By hospital location, teaching status		
Rural	15.2	6.6
Urban nonteaching	27.1	24.6
Urban teaching	57.8	68.8
By control/ownership of hospital		
Nonfederal government	12	11.5
Private not-for-profit	77.2	73.7
Private for-profit	8	14.7

Note: Only invasive, therapeutic surgeries that are performed and reliably reported in the hospital-based ambulatory surgery setting were included.
(Source: Agency for Healthcare Research and Quality (AHRQ), Center for Delivery, Organization, and Markets, Healthcare Cost and Utilization Project (HCUP), National Inpatient Sample (NIS) and nationwide ambulatory surgery analytic file created from the State Ambulatory Surgery and Services Databases (SASD), weighted for national estimates, 2014)

(57.8%) occurred in a hospital-owned AS setting, and the remaining visits (42.2%) occurred in the hospital inpatient setting. These visits included nearly 22 million total surgeries, over half of which (52.7%) were performed in an outpatient setting. The average number of surgeries performed per visit was slightly higher in the inpatient than in the outpatient setting (1.4 versus 1.2).

- **The majority of ambulatory and inpatient invasive, therapeutic surgeries were performed at large, urban teaching, and private not-for-profit hospitals.**
  Most AS visits and most hospital inpatient surgical stays occurred in large, urban teaching, and private not-for-profit hospitals. However, compared with inpatient surgeries, outpatient surgeries were more likely to be performed in small hospitals (20.0 versus 15.4%) and less likely to be performed in private for-profit hospitals (8.0 versus 14.7%) and in urban teaching settings (57.8 versus 68.8%).
  Figure 8.3 presents the distribution of hospital visits or stays involving invasive, therapeutic surgeries performed in the ambulatory (outpatient) surgery setting versus the hospital inpatient setting (admitted to the hospital) by expected primary payer in 2014.
- **In 2014, private insurance accounted for the largest proportion of AS visits and Medicare accounted for the largest proportion of inpatient invasive, therapeutic surgeries.**
  Patients with primary private insurance coverage accounted for 48.6 percent of all AS visits in 2014. Medicare was the second most common payer, accounting for 30.8 percent of AS visits, followed by Medicaid with 14.0 percent of visits. Uninsured patients represented 2.0 percent of AS visits in 2014. Among surgeries in the inpatient setting, Medicare was the primary expected payer for 43.4 percent of stays, followed by private insurance (35.3%) and

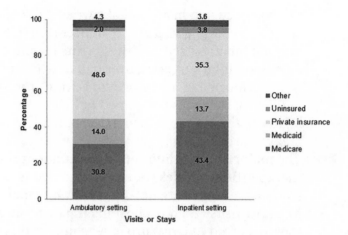

Figure 8.3. Hospital Visits or Stays with Invasive, Therapeutic Surgeries by Expected Primary Payer, 2014 *(Source: Agency for Healthcare Research and Quality (AHRQ), Center for Delivery, Organization, and Markets, Healthcare Cost and Utilization Project (HCUP), National Inpatient Sample (NIS) and nationwide ambulatory surgery analytic file created from the State Ambulatory Surgery and Services Databases (SASD), weighted for national estimates, 2014)*

Notes: Only invasive, therapeutic surgeries that are performed and reliably reported in the hospital-based ambulatory surgery setting were included. "Other" payer include Workers Compensation, TRICARE/CHAMPUS, CHAMPVA, Title V, and other government programs.

Medicaid (13.7%). Uninsured patients represented 3.8 percent of all inpatient surgical stays in 2014. *Comparison of invasive, therapeutic surgeries by body system in hospital-based ambulatory surgery versus inpatient settings, 2014.*

Figure 8.4 shows the distribution of invasive, therapeutic surgeries by body system that were performed in the AS and hospital inpatient settings in 2014.

The majority of invasive, therapeutic surgeries on the eye, ear, and nose/mouth/pharynx were performed in an outpatient setting.

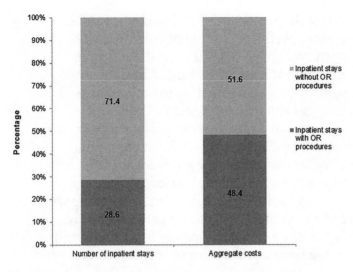

Figure 8.4. Ambulatory versus Inpatient Invasive, Therapeutic Surgeries in the United States by Body System, 2014 *(Source: Agency for Healthcare Research and Quality (AHRQ), Center for Delivery, Organization, and Markets, Healthcare Cost and Utilization Project (HCUP), National Inpatient Sample (NIS) and nationwide ambulatory surgery analytic file created from the State Ambulatory Surgery and Services Databases (SASD), weighted for national estimates, 2014)*

Notes: Only invasive, therapeutic surgeries that are performed and reliably reported in the hospital-based ambulatory surgery setting were included. Body systems are based on Clinical Classifications Software (CCS) and Clinical Classifications Software for Services and Procedures. Gastric bypass and volume reduction, which is not classified by the CCS, has been included with the digestive body system. The percentage of surgical visits or stays is calculated using unrounded data.

Nearly all surgeries performed on the eye occurred in the AS setting (99.5%). The outpatient setting also represented at least 80 percent of hospital visits involving surgeries performed on the ear (93.4%) and nose/mouth/pharynx (86.9%).

- **The majority of invasive, therapeutic surgeries on the cardiovascular, respiratory, and urinary systems were performed in the inpatient setting.**

Compared with the AS setting, more cardiovascular surgeries were performed in the inpatient setting (73.8 versus 26.2%). In 2014, the inpatient setting also represented at least 70 percent of hospital visits involving surgeries performed on the respiratory system (73.2%) and urinary system (71.3%).

The most common ambulatory invasive, therapeutic surgeries performed, 2014 the 25 most common, invasive, therapeutic clinically grouped surgeries that were performed in the hospital-based ambulatory surgery setting in the United States in 2014, along with the percentage of these types of surgeries that were performed in the ambulatory versus inpatient setting. Surgeries are ranked from most to least common in the AS setting.

A comprehensive list of the distribution between outpatient and inpatient settings for all specific, invasive, therapeutic surgeries by body system is presented in the appendix.

- **Lens and cataract procedures were the most common invasive, therapeutic type of surgery performed in an outpatient setting.**

  Lens and cataract procedures were the most common type of surgery performed in the AS setting, accounting for 12.4 percent of all outpatient surgeries performed. Nearly all lens and cataract procedures (99.9%) were performed in an outpatient setting.

- **Muscle, tendon, and soft tissue operating room (OR) procedures and incision or fusion of joint, destruction of joint lesion were the second and third most common types of outpatient invasive, therapeutic surgery.**

  Muscle, tendon, and soft tissue OR procedures (mostly rotator cuff repair and trigger finger surgery) were the second most common type of surgery performed in the AS setting, accounting for 6.6 percent of all outpatient surgeries. Incision or fusion of joint, destruction of joint lesion (mostly knee and shoulder arthroscopies) were ranked third, accounting for 5.3 percent of all outpatient surgeries. The majority of both types of procedures were performed in the outpatient setting (71.9 and 80.4%, respectively). Four other musculoskeletal system procedures were also commonly performed in the outpatient setting: excision of semilunar cartilage of knee (4.4%), nonfracture, nonarthroplasty OR procedures on the bone (2.4%), partial excision bone (2.2%), and bunionectomy or repair of toe deformities (1.6%).

- **Operations on the digestive system accounted for 4 of the 25 most common ambulatory invasive, therapeutic surgeries and constituted 13.9 percent of all outpatient surgeries.**
  Operations on the digestive system accounted for 4 of the 25 most common types of AS and constituted 13.9 percent of all outpatient surgeries: cholecystectomy and common duct exploration (5.0%), inguinal and femoral hernia repair (3.8%), repair of diaphragmatic, incisional, and umbilical hernia (3.3%), and appendectomy (1.8%). Approximately 61 percent of all cholecystectomy and all repair of diaphragmatic, incisional, and umbilical hernia surgeries, 92 percent of inguinal and femoral hernia repair surgeries, and 47 percent of appendectomy surgeries were performed in the outpatient setting.

- **Four of the 25 most common outpatient ambulatory invasive, therapeutic surgeries were performed predominantly on women.**
  Four of the 25 most common outpatient surgeries were procedures that are performed primarily on women: OR procedures of skin and breast, including plastic procedures on breast (2.8%); lumpectomy, quadrantectomy of breast (2.6%); hysterectomy, abdominal and vaginal (2.4%); and vaginal, vulvar, and female pelvic OR procedures (1.6%). The majority of these surgeries were performed in the outpatient setting.

The most common ambulatory invasive, therapeutic surgeries performed by payer, 2014

The five most common, invasive, therapeutic surgeries that were performed in the hospital-based AS setting by payer in 2014, along with the percentage of these types of surgeries that were performed in the ambulatory versus inpatient setting are mentioned below. Surgeries are ranked from most to least common in the AS setting for patients with expected primary payers of Medicare, Medicaid, private insurance, and uninsured.

- **Both lens and cataract procedures and muscle, tendon, and soft tissue OR procedures were among the five most common invasive, therapeutic types of surgery performed in an outpatient setting for all payers.**

  Lens and cataract procedures were the most common type of surgery performed in the AS setting among Medicare patients in 2014, with 987,600 surgeries. More lens and cataract procedures were performed during AS visits than the other four most-frequently-performed procedure categories for Medicare patients combined. Lens and cataract procedures also were among the five most common types of surgery performed among the other payers.

  Muscle, tendon, and soft tissue OR procedures were the most common type of surgery performed in the AS setting for privately insured patients in 2014, with 405,300 surgeries, although they were still common ambulatory surgeries among other payers as well.

- **Cholecystectomy and common duct exploration surgeries were in the five most common invasive, therapeutic types of surgery performed in an outpatient setting for Medicaid, private insurance, and uninsured.**

  Cholecystectomy and common duct exploration were common AS procedures for Medicaid (108,200 surgeries), privately insured (328,700 surgeries), and uninsured (14,500 surgeries). The majority of cholecystectomy surgeries were performed in the AS setting among procedures covered by Medicaid and private insurance (61.2 and 71.1%, respectively). In contrast, only 32.5 percent of all cholecystectomy surgeries were performed in the AS setting among uninsured individuals.

INPATIENT SETTINGS

The majority of patients admitted to the hospital undergo at least one type of procedure during their stay. Many diagnostic and therapeutic procedures, such as x-rays and blood transfusions, are performed outside of the operating room (OR), whereas surgical procedures, such as Cesarean sections and hip replacements, take place in the OR. On average, hospital costs for stays with OR procedures are more than double the costs for inpatient stays without OR procedures.

Identifying the characteristics, costs, and volume of OR procedures can guide healthcare improvement efforts. Such information can also provide baseline data for assessing the potential impact of advances in medical practice and technology and changes in healthcare provider arrangements.

This Healthcare Cost and Utilization Project (HCUP) Statistical Brief updates previous HCUP reports focused on OR procedures in the inpatient setting, presenting data from U.S. hospitals in 2014, the last full year that procedures were coded using ICD-9-CM. In this Statistical Brief, OR procedures are defined using diagnosis-related group (DRG) algorithms, which were based on reviews by clinical panels. The percentage of all inpatient stays involving operating room (OR) procedures and the percentage of aggregate costs attributed to inpatient stays involving OR procedures are presented. Patient characteristics, resource use, and outcomes are provided for inpatient stays with OR procedures. The most frequent and most costly OR procedures are also presented.

Findings

Characteristics of inpatient stays involving operating room procedures, 2014

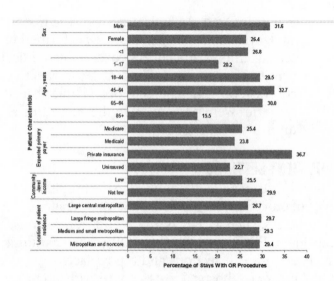

Figure 8.5. Percentage of Inpatient Stays and Aggregate Costs for Inpatient Stays with and without Operating Room (or) Procedures, 2014 *(Source: Agency for Healthcare Research and Quality (AHRQ), Center for Delivery, Organization, and Markets, Healthcare Cost and Utilization Project (HCUP) National Inpatient Sample (NIS), 2014)*

Figure 8.5 shows the percentage of all inpatient stays with operating room (OR) procedures and the percentage of aggregate hospital costs attributed to stays involving OR procedures.

- **Inpatient stays with OR procedures accounted for more than one-fourth of all hospitalizations and almost half of all aggregate hospital costs in 2014.** In 2014, 28.6 percent of all inpatient stays involved at least one OR procedure, but costs for stays with OR procedures constituted 48.4 percent of all aggregate hospital costs.

Table 8.4 presents select utilization characteristics and outcomes for inpatient stays with and without OR procedures in 2014. The unit of analysis is the inpatient stay; stays that listed an OR procedure in any procedure field are compared with those that did not involve any OR procedures.

Table 8.4. Utilization and Outcomes for Inpatient Hospital Stays with and without Operating Room (or) Procedures, 2014

Characteristic or Outcome	Stays with One or More Operating Room Procedures	Stays without Any Operating Room Procedures
Number of stays	10,115,800	25,243,000
All hospital stays, %	28.6	71.4
Rate of stays per 100,000 population3,172.5	7,916.70	
Aggregate costs, $ billions	187.1	199.1
Aggregate costs, %	48.4	51.6
Mean cost per stay, $	18,500	7,900
Mean length of stay, days	5.1	4.4
Mean cost per day, $	4,800	2,100
Admitted from emergency department, %	27.7	58.7
Discharge status, %		
Discharged to self-care (routine discharge) or home healthcare	83	80.3
Transferred to short-term hospital	0.8	2.5
Transferred to other type of facility, including long-term care	14.8	13.5
Died in hospital	1.2	2.2
Other[a]	0.2	1.5

Notes: Number of stays, mean cost per stay, and mean cost per day are rounded to the nearest hundred.
[a]Other discharges include alive/destination unknown, against medical advice, and missing.
(Source: Agency for Healthcare Research and Quality (AHRQ), Center for Delivery, Organization, and Markets, Healthcare Cost and Utilization Project (HCUP) National Inpatient Sample (NIS), 2014)

- **On average, inpatient stays involving OR procedures were longer and more than twice as expensive as stays without OR procedures.**
  In 2014, inpatient stays involving OR procedures averaged 5.1 days in length with an average cost of $18,500, compared with 4.4 days and $7,900 for stays without OR procedures.
- **Compared with inpatient stays without OR procedures, a lower percentage of stays involving OR procedures began in the emergency department or ended with in-hospital death.**
  In 2014, only 27.7 percent of inpatient stays involving OR procedures were admitted from the emergency department, compared with nearly 60 percent of stays without OR procedures.
  The percentage of stays that resulted in in-hospital death was lower among stays that involved OR procedures than stays without OR procedures (1.2 versus 2.2%). Similarly, the percentage of stays transferred to a short-term hospital was lower among stays that involved OR procedures than those that did not (0.8 versus 2.5%).
- **Females accounted for more than half of inpatient stays with and without OR procedures.**
  In 2014, 52.8 percent of hospital stays involving OR procedures were among females, and 47.2 percent of OR-related stays were among males. Females constituted an even larger proportion of inpatient stays that did not involve an OR procedure—59.1 percent.
- **In 2014, the youngest and the oldest age groups accounted for the fewest hospital stays involving OR procedures.**
  Although age distributions were similar among stays with and without OR procedures, the youngest and oldest age groups accounted for a smaller proportion of stays with OR procedures than stays without OR procedures (11.2 versus 12.3% for patients younger than 1 year, 2.7 versus 4.3% for patients 1 to 17 years of age, and 4.4 versus

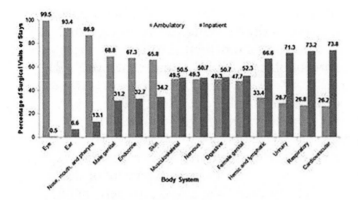

Figure 8.6. Percentage of Inpatient Stays That Involved Operating Room (or) Procedures, by Patient Characteristic, 2014 *(Source: Agency for Healthcare Research and Quality (AHRQ), Center for Delivery, Organization, and Markets (CDOM), Healthcare Cost and Utilization Project (HCUP), National Inpatient Sample (NIS), 2014)*

9.5% for patients 85 years of age and older). Conversely, patients 45 to 64 years of age accounted for a larger proportion of stays with OR procedures (28.1%) than stays without OR procedures (23.2%).

- **Private insurance and Medicare were the most common expected primary payers for inpatient stays with OR procedures in 2014.**
  Among inpatient stays involving OR procedures, the most common payers were private insurance (39.3% of stays with OR procedures) and Medicare (34.7%). For stays that did not involve OR procedures, Medicare was the most common payer (40.8% of stays) and privately insured stays made up only 27.2 percent.
  Figure 8.6 shows the percentage of inpatient stays that involved OR procedures for select patient subgroups in 2014. Whereas the distribution of all stays with OR procedures, this figure simply reports the percentage of each patient subgroup that underwent one or more OR procedures.

- **OR procedures were more common during inpatient stays among males than during stays among females.** In 2014, 31.6 percent of inpatient stays among males and 26.4 percent of stays among females involved OR procedures.
- **In 2014, nearly one-third of inpatient stays for patients 18 to 84 years of age involved OR procedures.** OR procedures were involved in 29.5 percent of stays for patients 18 to 44 years of age, 32.7 percent of stays for patients 45 to 64 years of age, and 30.0 percent of stays for patients 65 to 84 years of age.

  OR procedures were less common among the youngest and oldest age groups. Only 26.8 percent of inpatient stays for patients younger than 1 year and 20.2 percent of stays for patients 1 to 17 years of age involved OR procedures. Among inpatients 85 years of age and older, only 15.5 percent of stays involved OR procedures.
- **OR procedures were more common among inpatient stays covered by private insurance than among stays covered by other payers.** More than one-third (36.7%) of inpatient stays covered by private insurance involved OR procedures, compared with only 25.4 percent of stays for Medicare patients, 23.8 percent of stays for Medicaid patients, and 22.7 percent of stays for uninsured patients.
- **OR procedures were less common among inpatient stays for patients in the lowest income quartile and for patients living in large central metropolitan areas.** OR procedures were involved in 25.5 percent of hospital stays for patients in the lowest income quartile compared with 29.9 percent of stays for patients in the upper three income quartiles.

  Approximately 27 percent of inpatient stays for patients living in large central metropolitan areas involved OR procedures, compared with 29 to 30 percent of stays for patients living in less populated areas.

- **More than 14 million OR procedures were performed during inpatient hospital stays in 2014—a rate of 4,453.1 OR procedures per 100,000 population.**
  Overall, the highest rates were for one of two childbirth—and infant-related procedures— Cesarean section (389.8 per 100,000 population) and male circumcision (337.2 per 100,000 population).

- **The 20 most common OR procedures accounted for more than half of all OR procedures.**
  Six musculoskeletal procedures—knee arthroplasty, hip replacement, spinal fusion, treatment of hip and femur fracture or dislocation, treatment of fracture or dislocation of other lower extremity, and amputation of lower extremity—constituted 16.6 percent of all OR procedures.
  Four obstetric/gynecologic procedures—Cesarean section, ligation of fallopian tubes, hysterectomy, and oophorectomy—together made up 13.5 percent of all OR procedures, whereas male circumcision alone constituted 7.6 percent of all OR procedures.
  Three digestive procedures—cholecystectomy, colorectal resection, and appendectomy—together accounted for 6.4 percent of all OR procedures. Three cardiovascular procedures—percutaneous coronary angioplasty, coronary artery bypass graft, and heart valve procedures—accounted for 5.7 percent.
  Table 8.5 presents the five most common operating room procedures by age group in 2014.

- **Childbirth—and delivery-related procedures and appendectomies were the most common OR procedures among younger patients in 2014.**
  Of all OR procedures performed on patients younger than 1 year, 90.3 percent were male circumcisions. Other procedures among infants demonstrate how infrequently this age group undergoes surgery.

Table 8.5. Top Five Most Frequent All-Listed Operating Room (or) Procedures by Age Group, 2014

Rank	Operating Room Procedure	Number of Operating Room Procedures	Percent of Operating Room Procedures in This Age Group
Age <1 year		**1,186,700**	**100**
1	Circumcision	1,071,200	90.3
2	Inguinal and femoral hernia repair	4,600	0.4
3	Insertion, replacement, or removal of extracranial ventricular shunt	3,400	0.3
4	Colorectal resection	3,000	0.3
5	Small bowel resection	2,800	0.2
Ages 1–17 years		**384,100**	**100**
1	Appendectomy	54,400	14.2
2	Cesarean section	13,000	3.4
3	Spinal fusion	12,500	3.2
4	Treatment, fracture or dislocation of hip and femur	12,400	3.2
5	Tonsillectomy and/or adenoidectomy	10,500	2.7
Ages 18–44 years		**3,585,700**	**100**
1	Cesarean section	1,225,500	34.2
2	Ligation of fallopian tubes	253,600	7.1
3	Cholecystectomy and common duct exploration	122,800	3.4

Table 8.5. Continued

Rank	Operating Room Procedure	Number of Operating Room Procedures	Percent of Operating Room Procedures in This Age Group
4	Hysterectomy, abdominal and vaginal	89,700	2.5
5	Appendectomy	88,800	2.5
Ages 45–64 years		**4,382,700**	**100**
1	Arthroplasty of knee	314,800	7.2
2	Spinal fusion	216,500	4.9
3	Percutaneous coronary angioplasty (PTCA)	207,500	4.7
4	Laminectomy, excision of intervertebral disc	199,200	4.5
5	Hip replacement, total and partial	188,000	4.3
Ages 65–84 years		**4,094,500**	**100**
1	Arthroplasty of knee	402,500	9.8
2	Hip replacement, total and partial	253,700	6.2
3	Percutaneous coronary angioplasty (PTCA)	205,200	5
4	Spinal fusion	155,900	3.8
5	Laminectomy, excision of intervertebral disc	149,000	3.6
Age 85+ years		**561,700**	**100**
1	Treatment, fracture or dislocation of hip and femur	85,800	15.3

Table 8.5. Continued

Rank	Operating Room Procedure	Number of Operating Room Procedures	Percent of Operating Room Procedures in This Age Group
2	Hip replacement, total and partial	61,700	11
3	Percutaneous coronary angioplasty (PTCA)	26,700	4.8
4	Colorectal resection	18,700	3.3
5	Arthroplasty of knee	18,200	3.2

Notes: The number of procedures is rounded to the nearest hundred. Percentage is based on unrounded data values. Procedures are grouped using the Agency for Healthcare Research and Quality (AHRQ) Clinical Classifications Software (CCS). CCS categories identified as "Other" and procedure categories that are nonspecific or likely to be adjuncts to other procedures were not reported. Procedure totals include only one occurrence of a CCS category per hospitalization because multiple codes may be used for related procedures performed during a single operation. The overall number of procedures for each age group represents the sum of all CCS category totals for that age group.
(Source: Agency for Healthcare Research and Quality (AHRQ), Center for Delivery, Organization, and Markets (CDOM), Healthcare Cost and Utilization Project (HCUP))

Appendectomy was the most common OR procedure among patients 1 to 17 years of age, accounting for 14.2 percent of OR procedures for this age group. Orthopedic procedures and tonsillectomy were also in the top five procedures for children and adolescents. Cesarean section accounted for about 13,000 procedures among adolescents (teen pregnancy).

- **Among the top five procedures for 18- to 44-year-olds, three are performed only on females.**
Cesarean section was the most common procedure among 18 to 44-year-olds, accounting for more than

one-third of OR procedures in this age group. Two gynecologic procedures were also among the top five OR procedures for this age group. Among all patients 18 to 44 years of age, fallopian tube ligation accounted for 7.1 percent and hysterectomy accounted for 2.5 percent of all OR procedures. Cholecystectomy and appendectomy are the only top five procedures in this age group that are performed for both males and females.

- **Musculoskeletal and cardiovascular procedures were most common among older patients in 2014.**
  Knee arthroplasty was the most common OR procedure among older patients, accounting for 7.2 percent of OR procedures among patients 45 to 64 years of age, 9.8 percent of procedures among patients 65 to 84 years of age, and 3.2 percent of procedures among patients 85 years of age and older.
  Hip replacement was also one of the top five OR procedures among these three older age groups, accounting for 4 to 11 percent of OR procedures for patients 45 years of age and older.
  Percutaneous coronary angioplasty was the third most common OR procedure among the three oldest age groups, accounting for approximately 5 percent of OR procedures for patients 45 years of age and older. The 20 OR procedures with the highest aggregate costs for the entire hospital stay during which the procedure was the first-listed procedure on the record. Procedures are ranked by aggregate hospital costs. Rankings are based on first-listed procedure to avoid double-counting costs of inpatient stays involving more than one type of OR procedure. (The unit of analysis is the inpatient stay. Numbers of stays vary from all-listed analyses presented earlier because of the focus on first-listed procedures.) Aggregate costs, mean cost per stay, and number of stays are provided.

- **Inpatient stays for the 20 most costly OR procedures accounted for nearly 60 percent of aggregate costs for all inpatient stays with a first-listed OR procedure.**
  In 2014, there were 9,204,100 inpatient stays with a first-listed OR procedure. The aggregate costs for these stays totaled $163.8 billion. Stays for the 20 most costly OR procedures accounted for 58.6 percent of this total, or $96.0 billion.
- **Inpatient stays for six musculoskeletal procedures accounted for one-quarter of aggregate costs for all stays with a first-listed OR procedure.**
  Six musculoskeletal procedures combined accounted for $41.2 billion in hospital costs, or 25 percent of aggregate costs for stays with a first-listed OR procedure: spinal fusion (7.3% of aggregate costs), knee arthroplasty (7.2%), hip replacement (5.1%), treatment of hip and femur fracture or dislocation (2.6%), amputation of lower extremity (1.5%), and treatment of fracture or dislocation of other lower extremity (1.4%).
  Costs associated with four cardiovascular procedures—percutaneous coronary angioplasty, coronary artery bypass graft, heart valve procedures, and procedures related to pacemakers/defibrillators—constituted about 14 percent of aggregate costs for inpatient stays with a first-listed OR procedure, or $23.4 billion in aggregate hospital costs.
  Four digestive procedures—colorectal resection, cholecystectomy, appendectomy, and small bowel resection—together accounted for roughly 8 percent of aggregate costs associated with a first-listed OR procedure, or $13.2 billion in aggregate costs.
- **Although they were not among the 20 most common all-listed OR procedures, procedures related to pacemakers/defibrillators and small bowel resection were among the 20 most expensive OR procedures in 2014.**

Procedures related to pacemakers/defibrillators and small bowel resection were less common than other costly procedures. Still, these procedures were associated with high aggregate costs because of their relatively high mean costs per stay—$35,000 for procedures related to pacemakers/ defibrillators and $34,300 for small bowel resection. Among the 20 most expensive OR procedures overall, the only procedures with higher or equivalent average hospital costs were heart valve procedures (mean cost, $52,000), coronary artery bypass graft ($41,900), and incision and excision of the central nervous system ($34,600).

Section 8.3 | Cesarean Delivery

This section includes text excerpted from "Cesarean Delivery," Health Resources and Services Administration (HRSA), October 25, 2013. Reviewed April 2020.

Cesarean delivery represents a potentially life-saving procedure for both mother and infant in cases of labor complications and health conditions that require early or immediate delivery. However, in the absence of medical indications, cesarean sections can pose avoidable risks, including longer maternal recovery, neonatal respiratory problems, and potentially severe complications in subsequent pregnancies. After increasing every year from 1996 to 2009, the U.S. cesarean delivery rate declined slightly between 2009 and 2010 from 32.9 percent to 32.8 percent and remained unchanged through preliminary data for 2012. Though no longer increasing, the current rate of about one in three births far exceeds the upper limit of 15 percent advised by the World Health Organization.

Healthy People 2020 has set national objectives to reduce the cesarean delivery rate by ten percent among low-risk women giving birth for the first time and among low-risk women with a prior cesarean section. Low-risk is defined as nonbreech, singleton

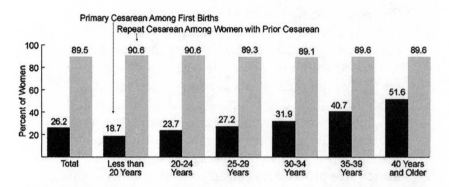

Figure 8.7. Primary and Repeat Cesarean Delivery Rates among Low-Risk Women* by Age *(Source: Centers for Disease Control and Prevention (CDC), National Center for Health Statistics (NCHS). 2011 Natality File. Analysis conducted by the Maternal and Child Health Bureau (MCHB))*

Low risk is defined as nonbreech, singleton deliveries at 37 weeks or more gestation; Data are from 36 states and the District of Columbia that implemented the 2003 revision of the birth certificate as of January 1, 2011, representing 83 percent of all U.S. births.

deliveries at 37 weeks or more gestation. In 2011, among the 36 states and the District of Columbia that had implemented the 2003 revision to the standard birth certificate as of January 1st, 26.2 percent of low-risk women giving birth for the first time and 89.5 percent of low-risk women with a prior cesarean section delivered by cesarean. Cesarean delivery among low-risk, first births increased greatly with maternal age from 18.7 percent of women less than 20 years of age to 51.6 percent of women 40 years of age and older. This pattern may partly reflect age-related increases in medical indications for cesarean delivery. However, the repeat cesarean rate among low-risk women was about 90 percent, regardless of maternal age.

Recently, cesarean delivery rates among low-risk pregnancies were found to vary fifteen-fold across U.S. hospitals from 2.4 percent to 36.5 percent, highlighting the importance of quality improvement and standardization in maternity care. To reduce cesarean delivery rates, there have been calls to expand public and provider education, to tie payments to quality improvement, and to publicly report hospital-level data.

Table 8.6. Primary and Repeat Cesarean Delivery Rates among Low-Risk Women* by Age

Age of Mother	Percent of Women with Primary Cesarean Among First Births	Percent with Repeat Cesarean Among Women with Prior Cesarean
Less than 20 years	18.7	90.6
20–24 Years	23.7	90.6
25–29 Years	27.2	89.3
30–34 Years	31.9	89.1
35–39 Years	40.7	89.6
40 years and older	51.6	89.6
Total	26.2	89.5

*Low-risk is defined as nonbreech, singleton deliveries at 37 weeks or more gestation. Data are from 36 states and the District of Columbia that implemented the 2003 revision of the birth certificate as of January 1, 2011, representing 83 percent of all U.S. births.

(Source: Centers for Disease Control and Prevention, National Center for Health Statistics. 2011 Natality File. Analysis conducted by the Maternal and Child Health Bureau (MCHB))

Section 8.4 | Statistics of Knee Replacement Surgery

This section includes text excerpted from "Hospitalization for Total Knee Replacement among Inpatients Aged 45 and Over: United States, 2000–2010," Centers for Disease Control and Prevention (CDC), November 6, 2015. Reviewed April 2020.

In 2010, total knee replacement was the most frequently performed inpatient procedure on adults 45 years of age and over. In the 11-year period from 2000 through 2010, an estimated 5.2 million total knee replacements were performed. Adults 45 years of age and over comprised 98.1 percent of those surgeries. The report uses data from the National Hospital Discharge Survey (NHDS) to present trends in the rate of hospitalizations for total knee replacement,

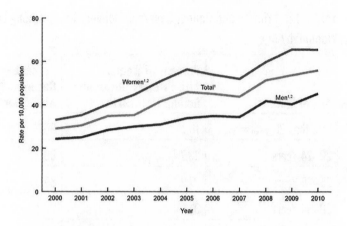

Figure 8.8. Total Knee Replacement among Inpatients Aged 45 and Over, by Sex: United States, 2000–2010 *(Source: Centers for Disease Control and Prevention (CDC)/National Center for Health Statistics (NCHS), National Hospital Discharge Survey (NHDS), 2000–2010)*

[1]Significant linear trend from 2000 through 2010 ($p < 0.05$).
[2]Significant difference in rates between men and women in each year
Notes: Total knee replacement is defined as code 81.54 of the International Classification of Diseases, Ninth Revision, Clinical Modification (ICD-9-CM) for any of four collected procedures. Rates were calculated using U.S. Census Bureau 2000-based postcensal civilian population estimates.

mean age at hospitalization, and discharge status for inpatients 45 years of age and over from 2000 through 2010.

HOSPITALIZATION FOR TOTAL KNEE REPLACEMENT AMONG INPATIENTS 45 YEARS OF AGE AND OVER: UNITED STATES, 2000–2010
Did the Rate of Total Knee Replacement in the Population 45 Year of Age and Over Vary by Sex from 2000 through 2010?

- The rate of total knee replacement increased for both men and women. Among men, the rate increased from 24.3 per 10,000 population in 2000 to 45.3 per 10,000 in 2010 (an 86 increase) (Figure 8.8). Among women, the rate almost doubled from 33.0 per 10,000 in 2000 to 65.5 per 10,000 in 2010 (a 99% increase).

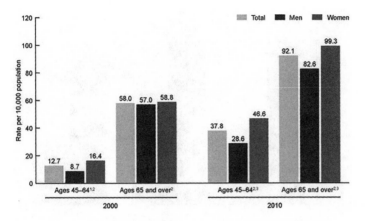

Figure 8.9. Total Knee Replacement among Inpatients Aged 45 and Over, by Sex and Age Group: United States, 2000 and 2010 *(Source: Centers for Disease Control and Prevention (CDC)/ National Center for Health Statistics (NCHS), National Hospital Discharge Survey (NHDS), 2000 and 2010)*

[1]*Significant difference in 2000 between men and women within age group (p < 0.05).*
[2]*Significant difference between 2000 and 2010 within sex and age group (p < 0.05).*
[3]*Significant difference in 2010 between men and women within age group (p < 0.05).*
NOTES: Total knee replacement is defined as code 81.54 of the International Classification of Diseases, Ninth Revision, Clinical Modification (ICD-9-CM) for any of four collected procedures. Rates were calculated using U.S. Census Bureau 2000-based postcensal civilian population estimates.

- The rate of total knee replacement was higher for women compared with men for each year of the 11-year period. In 2000, the rate of total knee replacement for women was 35.8 percent higher than for men (33.0 and 24.3, respectively). In 2010, the rate of total knee replacement for women was 45.6 higher than for men (65.5 and 45.3, respectively).

Did the Rate of Total Knee Replacement Vary by Sex and Age in 2000 and 2010?

Women 45 to 64 years of age had higher rates (16.4 and 46.6) than men 45 to 64 years of age (8.7 and 28.6) in both 2000 and 2010 (Figure 8.9).

In 2000, there was no difference in the rate of total knee replacement between men and women 65 years of age and over, while in 2010, women had a higher rate (99.3) than men (82.6).

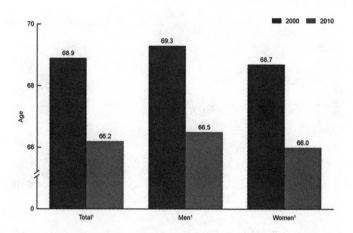

Figure 8.10. Mean Age at Total Knee Replacement among Inpatients Aged 45 and Over, by Sex: United States, 2000 and 2010 *(Source: Centers for Disease Control and Prevention (CDC)/National Center for Health Statistics (NCHS), National Hospital Discharge Survey (NHDS), 2000 and 2010)*

[1]Significant difference in mean age between 2000 and 2010 (p < 0.05). NOTES: Total knee replacement is defined as code 81.54 of the International Classification of Diseases, Ninth Revision, Clinical Modification (ICD-9-CM) for any of four collected procedures. Percentages are calculated only for inpatients 45 years of age and over.

Those 65 years of age and over had higher rates of total knee replacement than those 45 to 64 years of age in both 2000 and 2010 (58.0 and 92.1, respectively for those 65 years of age and over compared with 12.7 and 37.8 for those 45 to 64 years of age).

Higher rates of total knee replacement were found for both men and women aged 65 and over compared with those 45 to 64 years of age in both 2000 and 2010.

Has the Mean Age at Which Inpatients 45 Years of Age and Over Have Total Knee Replacement Changed from 2000 through 2010?

- Overall, the mean age for having a total knee replacement was lower in 2010 compared with 2000, by 3.9 percent, decreasing from 68.9 in 2000 to 66.2 in 2010 (Figure 8.10).

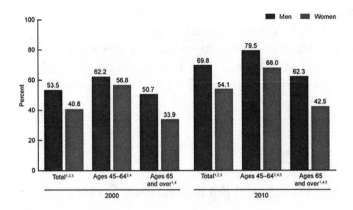

Figure 8.11. Inpatients Aged 45 and Over with Total Knee Replacement Discharged Home, by Sex and Age Group: United States, 2000 and 2010 *(Source: Centers for Disease Control and Prevention (CDC)/National Center for Health Statistics (NCHS), National Hospital Discharge Survey (NHDS), 2000 and 2010)*

[1]Significant difference between men and women (p < 0.05).
[2]Significant difference between 2000 and 2010 for men (p < 0.05).
[3]Significant difference between 2000 and 2010 for women (p < 0.05).
[4]Significant difference between age groups for women (p < 0.05).
[5]Significant difference between age groups for men (p < 0.05).
Notes: Total knee replacement is defined as code 81.54 of the International Classification of Diseases, Ninth Revision, Clinical Modification (ICD-9-CM) for any of four collected procedures. Percentages are calculated only for inpatients 45 years of age and over.

- Among men, the mean age decreased from 69.3 to 66.5, and among women, the mean age decreased from 68.7 to 66.0.
- Significant difference in mean age between 2000 and 2010 ($p < 0.05$).

Did Being Discharged Home after a Total Knee Replacement Vary by Age and Sex?

- The percentages of men and women 45 years of age and over-discharged home after hospitalization for total knee replacement were higher in 2010 (69.8% and 54.1 percent, respectively) than in 2000 (53.5% and 40.8%, respectively) (Figure 8.11).

- In both 2000 and 2010, lower percentages of women than men were discharged home after total knee replacement.
- In 2010, nearly two-thirds of men 65 years of age and over (62.3%) were discharged home, while less than one-half of women 65 years of age and over (42.5%) were discharged home.

Section 8.5 | Statistics of Hip Replacement Surgery

This section includes text excerpted from "Hospitalization for Total Hip Replacement among Inpatients Aged 45 and Over: United States, 2000–2010," Centers for Disease Control and Prevention (CDC), November 6, 2015. Reviewed April 2020.

HOSPITALIZATION FOR TOTAL HIP REPLACEMENT AMONG INPATIENTS 45 YEARS OF AGE AND OVER

Total hip replacement, in which both the head of the femur and its socket are replaced, is done to restore movement to hips damaged by osteoarthritis, late-stage degenerative bone and cartilage disease, or other injuries and disease. The number of total hip replacements is expected to increase over the next few decades. National Hospital Discharge Survey (NHDS) data show trends and estimates of the number and rate of total hip replacements and average length of stay among inpatients 45 years of age and over.

Has the Number of Total Hip Replacements Changed since 2000?

- In 2010, 326,100 total hip replacements were performed among inpatients of all ages. Inpatients 45 years of age and over accounted for 95 percent (310,800) of all total hip replacements (data not shown).
- The annual number of total hip replacements among inpatients 45 years of age and over more than doubled between 2000 and 2010, from 138,700 in 2000 to 310,800 in 2010 (Figure 8.12).

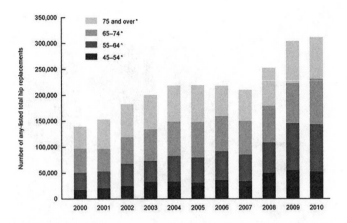

Figure 8.12. Number of Total Hip Replacements among Inpatients Aged 45 and Over, by Age Group and Year: United States, 2000–2010 *(Source: Centers for Disease Control and Prevention (CDC)/National Center for Health Statistics (NCHS), National Hospital Discharge Survey (NHDS), 2000–2010)*

Significant linear trend from 2000 through 2010 among all age groups and total number.

Notes: Total hip replacement is defined as code 81.51 of the International Classification of Diseases, Ninth Revision, Clinical Modification (ICD-9-CM) for any of the four collected procedures. Although data on eight procedures were collected in 2010, data from only four procedure codes were collected in 2000–2009. For consistency across years, only the first four listed procedures were included in the analysis for this figure.

- Similarly, the percentage increase in the number of total hip replacements among inpatients 45 years of age and over by age ranged from 92 percent for those 75 and over (from 41,600 in 2000 to 80,000 in 2010) to 205 percent for those 45 to 54 years of age (from 17,000 to 51,900).

Has the Age Distribution of Total Hip Replacement among Inpatients 45 Years of Age and Over Changed between 2000 and 2010?

- In 2000, 12 percent of all inpatient total hip replacements were performed on those 45 to 54 years of age; this

95

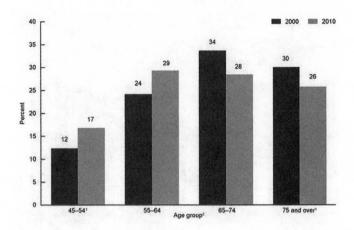

Figure 8.13. Percent Distribution of Total Hip Replacements among Inpatients Aged 45 and Over: United States, 2000 and 2010 *(Source: Centers for Disease Control and Prevention (CDC)/National Center for Health Statistics (NCHS), National Hospital Discharge Survey (NHDS), 2000 and 2010)*

[1]*Significantly different from age groups 55 to 64 and 65 to 74 in both 2000 and 2010.*
[2]*Significant differences between 2000 and 2010 for each age group.*
Notes: Total hip replacement is defined as code 81.51 of the International Classification of Diseases, Ninth Revision, Clinical Modification (ICD-9-CM) for any of the four collected procedures. Percentages are calculated only for ages 45 and over. Although data on eight procedures were collected in 2010, data from only four procedure codes were collected in 2000–2009. For consistency across years, only the first four listed procedures were included in the analysis for this figure.

percentage increased to 17 percent in 2010. The percentage of total hip replacements performed on those 55 to 64 years of age also increased (from 24% to 29%) (Figure 8.13).

- The percentage of all inpatient hip replacements decreased for age groups 65 to 74 (from 34% in 2000 to 28% in 2010) and 75 and over (from 30% to 26%).
- In 2000, the percentage of total hip replacement among inpatients 55 to 64 years of age was 24 percent, which was significantly lower than the percentage in the 75 years of age and over group (30%). In contrast, by 2010, more total hip replacements were performed on inpatients 55 to 64 years of age (29%) than on inpatients 75 years of age and over (26%).

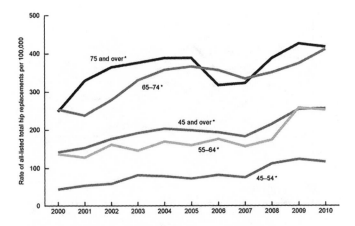

Figure 8.14. Rate of Hospitalization for Total Hip Replacement among Ages 45 and Over: United States, 2000–2010 *(Source: Centers for Disease Control and Prevention (CDC)/National Center for Health Statistics (NCHS), National Hospital Discharge Survey (NHDS), 2000–2010)*

*Significant linear trend from 2000 through 2010 for each age group.
Notes: Total hip replacement is defined as code 81.51 of the International Classification of Diseases, Ninth Revision, Clinical Modification (ICD-9-CM) for any of the four collected procedures. Although data on eight procedures were collected in 2010, data from only four procedure codes were collected for 2000–2009. For consistency across years, only the first four listed procedures were included in the analysis for this figure. The rate was calculated by dividing the number of discharges with any-listed total hip replacement procedure for each age group by the population of that group. The rates per 100,000 population were calculated using U.S. Census Bureau 2000-based postcensal civilian population estimates.*

Has the Rate of Total Hip Replacements in the Population 45 Years of Age and Over Changed since 2000?

- Between 2000 and 2010, the rate of total hip replacements in the population 45 years of age and over increased for each age group (Figure 8.14).
- The rate of total hip replacement more than doubled for those 45 to 54 years of age over the 11 years from 2000 through 2010, from 45 to 117 total hip replacements per 100,000 population. However, this rate was still lower than the rates for older age groups.
- The rate of total hip replacement increased among older age groups as well from 2000 to 2010: by 85 percent

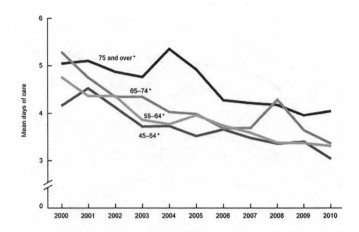

Figure 8.15. Average Length of Stay among Inpatients Aged 45 and Over with Total Hip Replacement: United States, 2000–2010 *(Source: Centers for Disease Control and Prevention (CDC)/National Center for Health Statistics (NCHS), National Hospital Discharge Survey (NHDS), 2000–2010)*

*Significant linear trend from 2000 through 2010.
Notes: Total hip replacement is defined as code 81.51 of the International Classification of Diseases, Ninth Revision, Clinical Modification (ICD-9-CM) for any of the four collected procedures. Although data on eight procedures were collected in 2010, data from only four procedure codes were collected during 2000–2009. For consistency across years, only the first four listed procedures were included in the analysis for this figure.

for those 55 to 64 years of age (from 137 to 253), by 62 percent for those 65 to 74 years of age (from 254 to 412), and by 68 percent for those 75 years of age and over (from 249 to 418).

Has the Average Length of Stay after Total Hip Replacement among Inpatients 45 Years of Age and Over Changed since 2000?

- The average length of stay following total hip replacement decreased approximately 1 day for inpatients among all age groups 45 and over from 2000 through 2010 (Figure 8.15).

Surgery Statistics

- In 2010, inpatients 45 to 54 years of age with total hip replacement stayed an average of 3 days, which was lower than all other age groups.
- Inpatients 75 years of age and over with total hip replacement stayed an average of 4 days in 2010, which was higher than all other age groups.

Chapter 9 | The Future of Surgery

Chapter Contents

Section 9.1 | **Artificial Kidney**

This section includes text excerpted from "Bionic Man," National Institute of Biomedical Imaging and Bioengineering (NIBIB), May 6, 2014. Reviewed April 2020.

An artificial kidney could be used in place of kidney dialysis for treatment of end-stage kidney disease. The researchers are developing an artificial kidney that could perform many of the functions of the natural kidney for patients suffering from kidney failure. It would be surgically implantable, require no tethers to machines outside the body, and not need pumps or electrical power to operate. The hope is that the self-regulating artificial kidney would be able to filter toxins from the blood through a silicon membrane and could be driven by a patient's normal blood flow. Human renal tubule cells will be used in the device to mimic the endocrine and metabolic functions of the kidney.

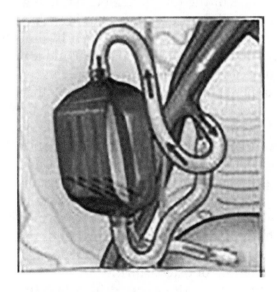

Figure 9.1. Artificial Kidney

This section includes text excerpted from "New Cartilage Grows, Helps Repair Damaged Joints Thanks to Novel Engineering," National Institute of Biomedical Imaging and Bioengineering (NIBIB), March 5, 2013. Reviewed April 2020.

Patients with cartilage damage were successful in regenerating new cartilage tissue. This technique creates a scaffold by combining the use of a biogel that solidifies when exposed to light and a strong biological adhesive. It was tested in a small clinical trial in patients undergoing microfracture surgery—a first-line therapy for cartilage repair. Patients who received the gel and adhesive experienced enhanced cartilage regeneration and decreased pain at six months postsurgery. The technique has the potential to transform the field of cartilage repair, which is notorious for poor clinical outcomes.

CURRENT APPROACHES TO CARTILAGE REPAIR

"Hyaline cartilage" is the name of the tough, flexible tissue that serves as a cushion for bones at joints, preventing them from rubbing against each other during physical activity. When hyaline cartilage is damaged as a result of trauma or gradual wear and tear normal movement of the joint can become limited and patients can experience severe pain as bones begin to grind against each other. Both can lead to disability over time.

Unfortunately, damage to cartilage is not readily repaired by the body. That is because cartilage unlike most tissues in the body does not have its own blood supply to bathe damaged tissue and provide factors promoting regeneration. Consequently, surgeons currently employ a technique called "microfracture" surgery to facilitate new cartilage growth. The surgery is generally performed in young adults who have a tear in the cartilage that surrounds the knee as a result of sports injury and is not effective in patients with widespread cartilage degeneration, or osteoarthritis.

During microfracture surgery, tiny holes are drilled into the bone located directly below missing cartilage in order to release blood and stem cells into the damaged space. The resulting "super clot" provides an enriched environment that promotes the production of new cartilage.

However, only 50 percent of microfracture surgeries are deemed successful in the long-term. A main issue is that the resulting clot produces a new type of cartilage called "fibrocartilage" a mixture of smooth hyaline cartilage and fibrous scar-like tissue. This fibrocartilage is tough and dense and does not function as well as hyaline cartilage as a cushion between joints. Additionally, microfractures can stimulate the production of bone tissue which can infiltrate regenerating cartilage and similarly disrupt its function.

LIGHTING THE WAY TOWARDS CARTILAGE REGENERATION

Though cartilage does a poor job of regenerating inside the body, researchers have been successfully building human cartilage outside of the body for decades. The process involves planting cartilage-producing cells or chondrocytes into a biological scaffold and then incubating them in conditions similar to those found in the human body.

Jennifer Elisseeff, Ph.D. director of the Cell and Tissue Engineering Program at Johns Hopkins University and inventor of the novel biogel and adhesive says scaffolds are key influencers of cartilage production. In her lab, she uses a specific type of scaffold called a "hydrogel."

"As we've been learning more about biomaterials and how cells respond to them, we've learned that chondrocytes prefer to be in a softer material," Elisseeff said. "The hydrogel environment provides a better mimic of the soft environment that is present when a tissue initially develops in a fetus."

Not only do hydrogels encourage the production of cartilage, but they also deter the development of unwanted tissue. "We want to reduce scar formation and bone formation and these types of hydrogel scaffolds do that," Elisseeff said.

After several years of growing high-quality cartilage in the lab, Elisseeff predicted that if she could introduce a hydrogel scaffold into a patient following microfracture surgery, she might be able to influence the quality of the cartilage regenerated. Perhaps she could deter stem cells from producing fibrous and bony tissue, and, instead encourage them to produce smoother, hyaline-like cartilage.

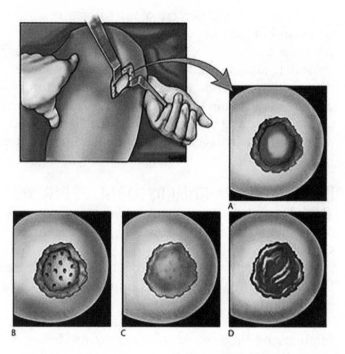

Figure 9.2. Cartilage Repair

But, implanting a scaffold into a cartilage defect—which is an irregular space where cartilage has broken off or deteriorated—is no easy task. That is because cartilage is slippery and any attempt to adhere a smooth gel scaffold to the walls of a cartilage defect is a losing battle. Adherence, however, is crucial. Without it, new tissue would not integrate into a patient's existing tissue, and thus would not become functional.

It was with these barriers in mind that Elisseeff began to develop two novel technologies. The first was a gel made up of special molecules that polymerize or form chains when exposed to light, causing the gel to harden, forming a scaffold. The second was a biological adhesive that could bond to both her gel and to specific proteins found on the surface of cartilage tissue. Not only does the adhesive help to secure the hydrogel in place, but the type of material used chondroitin sulfate also promotes tissue growth at the interface of the hydrogel and cartilage tissue.

Elisseeff's end goal was for a surgeon to be able to inject her gel into a cartilage defect directly following microfracture surgery whereupon it could mix with blood and stem cells released from the underlying bone and then make it harden with exposure to light. The biological adhesive would be applied to the cartilage walls surrounding the defect as well as the underlying bone prior to the surgery to ensure integration of the new tissue.

Section 9.3 | Image-Guided Robotic Interventions

This section includes text excerpted from "Image-Guided Robotic Interventions," National Institute of Biomedical Imaging and Bioengineering (NIBIB), July 2016. Reviewed April 2020.

WHAT ARE IMAGE-GUIDED ROBOTIC INTERVENTIONS?

Image-guided robotic interventions are medical procedures that integrate sophisticated robotic and imaging technologies, primarily to perform minimally invasive surgery. This integrated technology approach offers distinct advantages for both patients and physicians.

Imaging: In image-guided procedures, the surgeon is guided by images from various techniques, including magnetic resonance (MR) and ultrasound. Images can also be obtained using tiny cameras attached to probes that are small enough to fit into a minimal incision. The camera allows the surgery to be performed using a much smaller incision than in traditional surgery.

Robotics: The surgeon's hands and traditional surgical tools are too large for small incisions. Instead, thin, finger-like robotic tools are used to perform the surgery. As the surgeon watches the image on the screen, she or he uses a telemanipulation to transmit and direct hand and finger movements to a robot, which can be controlled by hydraulic, electronic, or mechanical means.

Robotic tools can also be controlled by computer. One advantage of a computerized system is that a surgeon could potentially perform the surgery from anywhere in the world. This type of

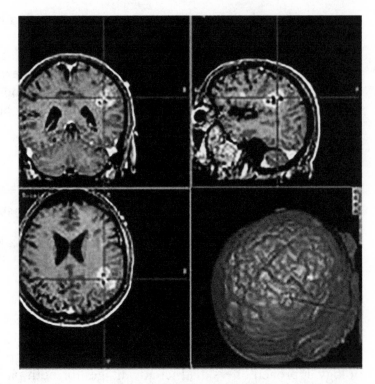

Figure 9.3. Image-Guided Robotic Interventions

long-distance surgery is currently in the experimental phase. The experiments illustrate the life-saving potential for such surgeries when a delicate operation requires a specially trained surgeon who is in a distant location.

Additionally, doctors can use image-guided robotic interventions to more accurately target tumors when performing biopsies and radiation treatments.

WHAT ARE THE ADVANTAGES OF MINIMALLY INVASIVE PROCEDURES?

Minimally invasive surgery can reduce the damage to surrounding healthy tissues, thus decreasing the need for pain medication and reducing patient's recovery time. For surgeons, image-guided interventions using robots also have the advantage of reducing fatigue during long operations, allowing the surgeon to perform the procedure while seated.

WHAT ARE SOME EXAMPLES OF IMAGE-GUIDED ROBOTIC INTERVENTIONS AND HOW ARE THEY USED?

Robotic prostatectomy. Complete prostate removal is performed through a series of small incisions, compared with a single large incision of four to five inches in traditional surgery. The small incisions result in a shorter postoperative recovery, less scarring, and a faster return to normal activities.

Ablation techniques for early cancers. Patients with early kidney cancer can be treated with minimally invasive procedures to destroy small tumors. Cryoablation uses cold energy to destroy the tumors. Doctors use computed tomography (CT) and ultrasound imaging to position a needle-like probe within each kidney tumor. Once in position, the tip of the probe is supercooled to encase the tumor in a ball of ice. Alternate freeze/thaw cycles kill the tumor cells. Other minimally invasive methods of destroying early kidney cancers include heating the tumor cells, and surgical removal using a robotic device. Many patients can go home the same day and are able to perform regular activities in several days.

Orthopedics. Image-guided robotic procedures are improving the precision and outcome of a number of orthopedic procedures. For example, partial knee resurfacing surgeries aim to target only the damaged sections of the knee joint. Orthopedic surgeons are combining the use of a robotic surgical arm and fiber optic cameras in such procedures, which results in patients retaining more of their normal healthy tissue. Image-guided robotic procedures also improve total knee replacements, allowing precise alignment and positioning of knee implants. The result is more natural knee function, better range of motion, and improved balance for patients.

WHAT ARE NIBIB-FUNDED RESEARCHERS DEVELOPING IN THE AREA OF IMAGE-GUIDED ROBOTIC INTERVENTIONS TO IMPROVE MEDICAL CARE?

Portable Robot Uses 3D Near-Infrared Imaging to Guide Needle Insertion into Veins

Drawing blood and inserting intravenous (IV) lines are the most commonly performed medical procedures in hospitals and clinics. However, for many patients it can be difficult to find veins and accurately insert the needle, resulting in patient injury. The National Institute of Biomedical Imaging and Bioengineering (NIBIB)-funded scientists are developing a portable, lightweight medical robot to help perform these procedures. The device uses 3D near-infrared imaging to identify an appropriate vein for the robot to insert the needle. The current goal is to integrate the imaging system and software into a miniaturized version of the prototype robot. The outcome will be a compact, low-cost system that will greatly improve the safety and accuracy of accessing veins.

Robot-Assisted Needle Guidance Aids Removal of Liver Tumors

Radiofrequency ablation (RFA) is a minimally invasive treatment that kills tumors with heat and can be a life-saving option for patients who are not eligible for surgery. However, broad use of RFA has been limited because the straight paths taken by the needles that carry tumor-killing electrodes may damage lung or other sensitive organs. Also, large tumors require multiple needle insertions, which increases bleeding risk. To address the problem of tissue damage using straight needles, NIBIB-funded scientists are developing highly flexible needles that can be guided along controlled, curved paths through tissue, allowing the removal of tumors that are not accessible by a straight-line path. The technology combines needle flexibility with a 3D ultrasound guidance system that allows the doctor to correct the path of the needle to avoid unexpected obstacles as the needle advances toward the tumor. The device will ultimately increase the accuracy and reduce the damage to healthy tissue during tumor removal resulting in wider use of the technology for better patient outcomes.

Swallowable Capsule Identifies and Biopsies Abnormal Tissue in the Esophagus

Barrett's esophagus is a precancerous condition that requires repeated biopsies to monitor abnormal tissue. NIBIB-funded researchers are developing a swallowable, pill-sized device to improve the management and treatment of this condition. The unsedated patient can easily swallow the pill, which is attached to a thin tether made of cable and optic fiber. The device detects microscopic areas of the esophagus that may show evidence of disease, and uses a laser to collect samples from the suspicious tissue—a technology known as "laser capture microdissection." The physician then retrieves the device from the patient without discomfort and the collected micro-samples are examined for visual evidence of disease, as well as genetic analysis. This minimally invasive device improves patient comfort and provides a precise molecular profile of the biopsied regions, which helps the physician to better monitor and treat the disorder.

Section 9.4 | neuroArm

This section includes text excerpted from "Robotic Arms Lend a Healing Touch," National Aeronautics and Space Administration (NASA), August 7, 2017.

The delicate touch that successfully removed an egg-shaped tumor from Paige Nickason's brain got a helping hand from a world-renowned arm—a robotic arm, that is. The technology that went into developing neuroArm—the world's first robot capable of performing surgery inside magnetic resonance machines—was born of the Canadarm (developed in collaboration with engineers MacDonald, Dettwiler, and Associates, Ltd. [MDA] for the United States Space Shuttle Program) as well as Canadarm2 and Dextre, the Canadian Space Agency's family of space robots performing the heavy lifting and maintenance aboard the International Space Station.

The development of neuroArm began with the search for a solution to a surgical dilemma: how to make difficult surgeries easier or impossible surgeries possible. MDA worked with a team led by Dr. Garnette Sutherland at the University of Calgary to develop a highly precise robotic arm that works in conjunction with the advanced imaging capabilities of magnetic resonance imaging (MRI) systems. Surgeons wanted to be able to perform surgeries while a patient was inside an MRI machine, which meant designing a robot that was as dexterous as the human hand but even more precise and tremor-free. Operating inside the MRI also meant it had to be made entirely from safe, MRI compatible materials (for instance, ceramic motors) so that it would not be affected by the MRI's magnetic field or, conversely, disrupt the MRI's images. The project team developed novel ways to control the robot's movements and give the robot's operator a sense of touch via an intuitive, haptic hand-controller located at a remote work station—essential so that the surgeon can precisely control the robot and can feel the tool-tissue interface during the surgery.

Since Paige Nickason's surgery in 2008, neuroArm has been used in initial clinical experience with 35 patients who were otherwise inoperable. In 2010, the neuroArm technology was licensed to IMRIS Inc., a private, publicly-traded medical device manufacturer based in Winnipeg, Manitoba, Canada, for development of the next-generation platform and for wide distribution under the name "SYMBIS Surgical System."

IMRIS is advancing the design to commercialize minimally invasive brain tumor resection procedures, which allow surgeons to see detailed, 3D images of the brain as well as use surgical tools and hand controllers that allow the surgeon to feel tissue and apply pressure when she or he operates. SYMBIS has been undergoing calibration, testing and validation at Dr. Sutherland's research facility since March 2015. SYMBIS is expected to be able to perform microsurgery and stereotactic biopsy within the bore of the magnet while real-time MR images are being acquired. The system is more compact, with improved haptics, safety no-go zones, motion scaling and tremor filters. SYMBIS is currently being reviewed by the U.S. Food and Drug Administration (FDA), and once approved, the system will be made available commercially for other centers worldwide to establish its clinical efficacy through clinical trials.

MDA is also continuing to apply its space technologies and know-how to medical solutions for life on Earth. The company has partnered with the Hospital for Sick Children (SickKids) in Toronto, Ontario, to collaborate on the design and development of an advanced technology solution for pediatric surgery. Dubbed KidsArm, the sophisticated, teleoperated surgical system is being designed specifically to operate on small children and babies. KidsArm is intended for use by surgeons in conjunction with a high-precision, real-time imaging technology to reconnect delicate vessels such as veins, arteries, or intestines.

In collaboration with the Centre for Surgical Invention and Innovation (CSII) in Hamilton, Ontario, MDA is also developing an advanced platform to provide a more accurate and less invasive identification and treatment of breast tumors in the MRI. The image-guided autonomous robot (IGAR) will provide increased access, precision and dexterity, resulting in more accurate and less invasive procedures. IGAR is currently in the second phase of clinical trials in Hamilton, Ontario, Canada, and Quebec City, Quebec, Canada.

Section 9.5 | Technologies Enhance Tumor Surgery

This section includes text excerpted from "Technologies Enhance Tumor Surgery," *NIH News in Health*, National Institutes of Health (NIH), February 2016. Reviewed April 2020.

HELPING SURGEONS SPOT AND REMOVE CANCER

For surgeons, removing a tumor is a balancing act. Cut out too much and you risk removing healthy tissues that have important functions. Remove too little and you may leave behind cancer cells that could grow back into a tumor over time.

The National Institutes of Health (NIH)-funded researchers are developing new technologies to help surgeons determine exactly where tumors end and healthy tissue begins. Their ultimate goal is to make surgery for cancer patients safer and more effective.

"Currently, surgeons view magnetic resonance imaging (MRI) and computed tomography (CT) scans taken prior to an operation to establish where a tumor is located and to plan a surgical approach that will minimize damage to healthy tissues," says Dr. Steven Krosnick, an NIH expert in image-guided surgery. "But once the operation has begun, surgeons generally rely only on their eyes and sense of touch to distinguish tumor from healthy tissue."

Surgeons go through many years of training to understand the subtle cues that can distinguish tumor from normal surroundings. Sometimes the tumor is a slightly different color than healthy tissue, or it feels different. It might also bleed more readily or could contain calcium deposits. Even with these cues, however, surgeons do not always get it right.

"In a lot of cases, we leave tumor behind that could be safely removed if only we were able to better visualize it," says Dr. Daniel Orringer, a neurosurgeon at the University of Michigan.

In today's operating rooms, pathologists can often help surgeons determine if all of a tumor has been taken out. A pathologist may view the edges of the tissue under a microscope and look for cancer cells. If they are found, the surgeon will remove more tissue from the patient and send these again to the pathologist for review. This process can occur repeatedly while the patient remains on the operating table and continue until no cancer cells are detected.

"Each time a pathologist analyzes tissue during an operation, it can take up to 30 minutes because the tissue has to be frozen, thinly sliced, and stained so it can be viewed under the microscope," Krosnick says. "If multiple rounds of tissue are taken, it can greatly increase the length of the surgery."

In the days following an operation, the pathologist conducts a more thorough review of the tissue. If cancer cells are found at the margins, the patient may undergo a second surgery to remove cancer that was left behind.

Orringer is part of a research team that is testing a new technology that could help surgeons tell the difference between a tumor and healthy brain tissue during surgery. The team developed a special microscope with NIH support that shoots a pair of low-energy lasers at the tissue. That causes the chemical bonds in the tissue's molecules to vibrate. The vibrations are then analyzed by a computer and used to create detailed images of the tissue.

From a molecular point of view, the components of a tumor differ from those in healthy tissue. This specialized microscope can reveal differences between the tissues that cannot be seen with the naked eye.

"Our technology enables us to get a microscopic view of human tissues without taking them out of the body," Orringer says. "We can see cells, blood vessels, the connections between brain cells... all of the microscopic components that make up the brain."

Orringer and colleagues developed a computer program that can quickly analyze the images and assess whether or not cancer cells are present. This type of analysis could help surgeons decide whether all of a tumor has been cut out. To date, Orringer has used the specialized microscope to help remove cancer tissue in nearly 100 patients with brain tumors.

Other researchers are taking different approaches. For example, Dr. Quyen Nguyen—a head and neck surgeon at the University of California, San Diego—has developed a fluorescent molecule that is currently being tested in clinical trials. The patient receives an injection of the molecules before surgery. When exposed to certain types of light, these molecules cause cancer cells to glow, making them easier to spot and remove. The surgeon then uses a near-infrared camera to visualize the glowing tumor cells while operating.

Nguyen is also developing a fluorescent molecule to light up nerves. Accidental nerve injury during surgery can leave patients with loss of movement or feeling. In some cases, sexual function may be impaired.

"Nerves are really, really small, and they're often buried in soft tissue or encased within bone. When we have to do cancer surgery, they can be encased in the cancer itself," Nguyen says. The fluorescent molecule could help surgeons detect hard-to-spot nerves, so they can be protected. The nerve-tagging molecule is now being tested in animal studies.

Other NIH-funded researchers are focusing on ways to speed up cancer surgeries. Dr. Milind Rajadhyaksha, a researcher at Memorial Sloan Kettering Cancer Center, has developed a microscope technique to reduce the amount of time it takes to perform a common surgery for removing nonmelanoma skin cancers.

Each year about two million people in the United States undergo Mohs surgery, in which a doctor successively removes suspicious areas until the surrounding skin tissue is free of cancer. The procedure can take several hours, because each time more tissue is removed, it has to be prepared and reviewed under a microscope to determine if cancer cells remain. This step can take up to 30 minutes.

The technique developed by Rajadhyaksha shortens the time for assessing removed tissue to less than 5 minutes, which greatly reduces the overall length of the procedure. Tissue is mounted in a specialized microscope that uses a focused laser line to do multiple scans of the tissue. The resulting image "strips" are then combined, like a mosaic, into a complete microscopic image of the tissue.

About 1,000 specialized skin surgeries have already been performed guided by this technique. Rajadhyaksha is currently developing an approach that would allow doctors to use the technology directly on a patient's skin, before any tissue has been removed. This would allow doctors to identify the edges of tumors before the start of surgery and reduce the need for several presurgical "margin-mapping" biopsies.

There are many types of cancer surgeries, and researchers continue to work hard to develop better techniques.

Part 2 | **Preparing for Surgery**

Chapter 10 | What You Need to Know about Surgery

WHAT YOU SHOULD KNOW ABOUT YOUR OPERATION
What Kind of Anesthesia Will You Need?

Anesthesia is used so that surgery can be performed without unnecessary pain. Your surgeon can tell you whether the operation calls for local, regional, or general anesthesia and why this form of anesthesia is best for your procedure. Local anesthesia numbs only a part of your body and only for a short period of time. For example, when you go to the dentist, you may get a local anesthetic called "Novocain." It numbs the gum area around a tooth. Not all procedures done with local anesthesia are painless. Regional anesthesia numbs a larger portion of your body—for example, the lower part of your body—for a few hours. In most cases, you will be awake during the operation with regional anesthesia. General anesthesia numbs your entire body. You will be asleep during the whole operation if you have general anesthesia.

Anesthesia is quite safe for most patients. It is usually given by a specialized doctor (anesthesiologist) or nurse (nurse anesthetist). Both are highly skilled and have been trained to give anesthesia.

If you decide to have an operation, ask to meet with the person who will give you anesthesia. It is okay to ask what her or his qualifications are. Ask what the side effects and risks of having anesthesia are in your case. Be sure to tell her or him what

This chapter includes text excerpted from "Having Surgery? What You Need to Know," Agency for Healthcare Research and Quality (AHRQ), U.S. Department of Health and Human Services (HHS), October 1, 2005. Reviewed April 2020.

medical problems you have—including allergies and what med-icines you have been taking. These medicines may affect your response to the anesthesia. Be sure to include both prescription and over-the-counter (OTC) medicines, such as vitamins and supplements.

How Long Will It Take You to Recover?

Your surgeon can tell you how you might feel and what you will be able to do—or not do—the first few days, weeks, or months after surgery. Ask how long you will be in the hospital. Find out what kind of supplies, equipment, and help you will need when you go home. Knowing what to expect can help you get better faster.

Ask how long it will be before you can go back to work or start regular exercise again. You do not want to do anything that will slow your recovery. For example, lifting a 10-pound bag of potatoes may not seem to be "too much" a week after your operation, but it could be. You should follow your surgeon's advice to make sure you recover fully as soon as possible.

MAKING SURE YOUR SURGERY IS SAFE

Check with your insurance company to find out if you may choose a surgeon or hospital or if you must use ones selected by the insurer. Ask your doctor about which hospital has the best care and results for your condition if you have more than one hospital to choose from. Studies show that for some types of surgery, numbers count—using a surgeon or hospital that does more of a particular type of surgery can improve your chance of a good result.

Questions to Ask a Surgeon
WHAT ARE YOUR QUALIFICATIONS?

You will want to know that your surgeon is experienced and qual-ified to perform the operation. Many surgeons have taken special training and passed exams given by the national board of surgeons. Ask if your surgeon is "board certified" in surgery. Some surgeons also have the letters F.A.C.S. after their name. This means they are Fellows of the American College of Surgeons and have passed another review by surgeons of their surgical skills.

HOW MUCH EXPERIENCE DO YOU HAVE DOING THIS OPERATION?

One way to reduce the risks of surgery is to choose a surgeon who has been well trained to do the surgery and has plenty of experience doing it. You can ask your surgeon about her or his recent record of successes and complications with this surgery. If it is easier for you, you can discuss the surgeon's qualifications with your primary care doctor.

Chapter 11 | How to Get a Second Opinion

WHAT IS A SECOND OPINION?

A second opinion is when another doctor, in addition to your regular doctor gives her or his view about your health problem and how it should be treated. Getting a second opinion can help you make a more informed decision about your care. Medicare Part B (Medical Insurance) helps pay for a second opinion before surgery. When your doctor says you have a health problem that needs surgery, you have the right to:

- Know and understand your treatment choices
- Have another doctor look at those choices with you (second opinion)
- Participate in treatment decisions by making your wishes known

WHEN SHOULD YOU GET A SECOND OPINION?

If your doctor says you need surgery to diagnose or treat a health problem that is not an emergency, consider getting a second opinion. It is up to you to decide when and if you will have surgery. Medicare does not pay for surgeries or procedures that are not medically necessary, such as cosmetic surgery. This means that Medicare also would not pay for second opinions for surgeries or procedures that are not medically necessary.

This chapter includes text excerpted from "Getting a Second Opinion before Surgery," Centers for Medicare & Medicaid Services (CMS), September 2019.

Do not wait for a second opinion if you need emergency surgery. Some types of emergencies may require surgery right away, such as:
- Acute appendicitis
- Blood clots or aneurysms
- Accidental injuries

HOW DO YOU FIND A DOCTOR FOR A SECOND OPINION?
Make sure the doctor giving the second opinion accepts Medicare. To find a doctor for a second opinion:
- Visit Medicare.gov to find doctors who accept Medicare.
- Call 800-MEDICARE (800-633-4227). TTY users can call 877-486-2048. Ask for information about doctors who accept Medicare.
- Ask your doctor for the name of another doctor to see for a second opinion. Do not hesitate to ask—most doctors will encourage you to get a second opinion. You can also ask another doctor you trust to recommend a doctor for a second opinion.

WHAT SHOULD YOU DO BEFORE GETTING A SECOND OPINION?
Before you visit the second doctor:
- Ask the first doctor to send your medical records to the doctor giving the second opinion. That way, you may not have to repeat any tests you already had.
- Call the second doctor's office and make sure they have your records.
- Write down a list of questions to take with you to the appointment.
- Ask a family member or friend to go to the appointment with you.

During your visit with the second doctor:
- Tell the doctor what surgery your first doctor recommended.
- Tell the doctor what tests you already had.

- Ask the questions you have on your list and encourage your friend or loved one to ask any questions that she or he may have.

Important: The second doctor may ask you to have additional tests performed as a result of the visit. Medicare will help pay for these tests, just as it helps pay for other services that are medically necessary.

WHAT IF THE FIRST AND SECOND OPINIONS ARE DIFFERENT?

If the second doctor does not agree with the first, you may feel confused about what to do. In that case, you may want to:
- Talk more about your condition with your first doctor.
- Talk to a third doctor. Medicare helps pay for a third opinion if the first and second opinions are different.

Getting a second or third opinion does not mean you have to change doctors. You decide which doctor you want to do your surgery.

HOW MUCH DOES MEDICARE PAY FOR A SECOND OPINION?

Medicare Part B helps pay for a second (or third) opinion and related tests, just as it helps pay for other services that are medically necessary. If you have Part B and Original Medicare:
- Medicare pays 80 percent of the Medicare-approved amount.
- Your share is usually 20 percent of the Medicare-approved amount after you pay your yearly Part B deductible.

DO MEDICARE ADVANTAGE PLANS COVER SECOND OPINIONS?

If you are in a Medicare Advantage Plan, you have the right to get a second opinion. If the first two opinions are different, your plan will help pay for a third opinion. Even though you have the right to get a second opinion, keep these things in mind:
- Some plans will only help pay for a second opinion if you have a referral (a written okay) from your primary care doctor.

- Some plans will only help pay for a second opinion from a doctor who is in your plan's provider network.

Call Your Plan

Note: If you have Medicaid, it might also pay for you to get a second opinion before surgery. To find out, call your Medicaid office. You can get the phone number by:

- Visiting Medicare.gov/contacts
- Calling 800-MEDICARE (800-633-4227)
- TTY users can call 877-486-2048

Chapter 12 | **Choosing a Hospital**

STEPS TO CHOOSING A HOSPITAL

When you are sick, you may go to the closest hospital or the hospital where your doctor practices. But, which hospital is the best for your individual needs? Research shows that some hospitals do a better job taking care of patients with certain conditions than other hospitals. When you have a life-threatening emergency, always go to the nearest hospital.

However, if you are planning to have surgery, or if you have a condition, such as heart disease and know you may need hospital care in the future, use the steps mentioned below to learn about your hospital choices. Understanding your choices will help you have a more informed discussion with your doctor or other healthcare provider.

BEFORE YOU GET STARTED

Make the most of your appointments with your doctor or other healthcare providers to learn about your condition and healthcare needs:

- Before your appointment, make a list of things you want to talk to your doctor or healthcare provider about (such as recent symptoms, drug side effects, or other general health questions). Bring this list to your appointment.

This chapter includes text excerpted from "Guide to Choosing a Hospital," Centers for Medicare & Medicaid Services (CMS), December 2017.

- Bring any prescription drugs, over-the-counter (OTC) drugs, vitamins, and supplements to your appointment and review them with your doctor or healthcare provider.
- Take notes during your appointment. Then, take a moment to repeat back to the doctor or healthcare provider what they told you. Ask any questions you may have.
- Bring along a trusted family member or friend.
- Ask if there is any written information about your condition that you can take with you.
- Call the office if you have questions when you get home.

WHAT IS QUALITY HOSPITAL CARE?

Hospitals provide good quality care when they give you the care and treatments known to get the best results for your condition. Getting quality hospital care may help with your recovery and help you avoid other problems. Not all hospitals provide the same quality of care.

Most hospitals have programs to check and improve the quality of the care they provide. They may collect and monitor information from patient charts to see where they can improve patient care. They may survey patients about their hospital experience using the Hospital Consumer Assessment of Healthcare Providers and Systems (HCAHPS) survey. Many hospitals report the information they collect to their state and to Medicare.

Medicare, the states, and other hospital industry leaders review this information and help hospitals take steps to improve quality. Some of the information about hospital quality is available online.

HOW CAN YOU FIND INFORMATION ABOUT HOSPITAL QUALITY?

Visit Hospital Compare at Medicare.gov/hospitalcompare for information on hospital quality.

Hospital Compare gives you a "snapshot" of how well hospitals in your area, and around the nation, care for patients. Use this information when you talk to your doctor or other healthcare provider about which hospital is best for you.

HOW DOES HOSPITAL COMPARE WORK?

When you visit Hospital Compare, whether from your home computer, your tablet, or your smartphone, finding information about the quality of hospitals is just a couple of steps away:

- Click on "Find a hospital," and decide if you want to look for hospitals by the hospital name, city, state, or ZIP code.
- Select the hospitals you want to compare.

WHAT KIND OF INFORMATION IS ON HOSPITAL COMPARE?

You can compare hospitals based on these and more:

- What did other patients think about their hospital stay? Recently discharged patients responded to a national survey about their hospital experience. The survey asks questions, such as how well their hospital's doctors and nurses communicate with patients, and how well they manage their patients' pain.
- Did hospitals give timely and effective care? Find information, such as how often hospitals give recommended treatments for certain common conditions such as heart attack, heart failure, pneumonia, children's asthma, and surgery.
- Did patients get better? Learn how hospitals' rates of readmission, complications, and mortality (death) rates for certain conditions compared with the national rate.
- Is the hospital careful about giving people too many tests? Learn how each hospital uses outpatient medical imaging tests, such as computer tomography (CT) scans and magnetic resonance imaging (MRIs).

If you are in a Medicare Advantage Plan (such as HMO or PPO) or other Medicare health plan, Hospital Compare does not have information about whether your care will be covered in a certain hospital. Check with your plan.

The information on Hospital Compare is updated regularly. Check Hospital Compare often for the most up-to-date results and new information.

If you do not have a computer or Internet access, your local library, senior center, a family member, or friend may be able to help you. You can also call 800-MEDICARE (800-633-4227). TTY users can call 877-486-2048.

WHAT OTHER ORGANIZATIONS WORK TO IMPROVE HOSPITAL QUALITY?

Quality Improvement Organizations (QIOs) are organizations that employ a group of practicing doctors and other healthcare experts paid by the federal government to check and improve the care given to people with Medicare.

Some states and accrediting organizations also post information about the quality of their hospitals.

Chapter 13 | **Ambulatory Surgical Centers**

WHAT ARE AMBULATORY SURGICAL CENTERS?

Ambulatory surgical centers (ASCs), also known as "surgicenters," are healthcare facilities where surgical procedures that do not require hospital admission are carried out within the same day.

Until the introduction of ASCs, all surgeries in the United States were carried out in a hospital setting. Waiting periods for a surgery ranging from weeks to months were not uncommon and patients spent weeks recovering from their treatment. The ambulatory surgical centers were pioneered in the 1970s when two physicians opened a facility offering a low-cost and high-quality alternative to inpatient surgical services in hospitals. They presented ASCs as a better option for routine surgeries after being frustrated with scheduling issues, waiting periods, operating room nonavailability, and limited equipment at traditional hospitals.

Ambulatory surgical centers are not health clinics and do not provide diagnostic and primary healthcare services. They provide surgical intervention for patients whose physicians have recommended certain types of procedures for treatment.

HOW DO YOU CHOOSE QUALITY AMBULATORY CARE?

Your physician can help you determine if an ambulatory surgical center is the best option for your procedure and, if so, which facility is best. Also, take into account the following information to help you make the best choice:

"Ambulatory Centers," © 2017 Omnigraphics. Reviewed April 2020.

Questions Regarding Care

- Is this a state licensed facility? Is it accredited?
- Can your family members accompany and wait with you until you can go home?
- What are the risks and frequency of such surgeries at the facility?
- How is pain dealt with during surgery? Can you discuss this with the anesthesiologist?
- Ask for a copy or your legal rights and responsibilities and enquire if it will be explained to you in laymen terms.
- Will your treatment details remain confidential? What are the cases under which patient information is disclosed?
- Does this facility participate in your health insurance?

Questions Regarding Staff

- Are the doctors and nurses professionally qualified and do they have adequate experience?
- Are the healthcare staff trained in medical emergency procedures, such as cardiopulmonary resuscitation (CPR)?

Questions Regarding Emergency Care Postsurgery

- Is a 24-hour emergency telephone number available in case of an emergency? Will it be answered by a doctor or nurse in case you have questions?
- Does the facility have a disaster readiness plan? Can the facility handle a power failure or natural disaster?
- Does the facility have a transfer agreement with a local hospital?

WHAT ARE SOME COMMON SURGICAL PROCEDURES CARRIED OUT IN AMBULATORY SURGICAL CENTERS?

Common surgical specialties in an ambulatory setting include:
- Plastic surgery of the neck
- Cosmetic and facial surgeries such as chin reconstruction, augmentation and reduction of facial bones, and revision of the eyelids and sockets

- Endoscopic procedures of the nose, sinus, vascular, upper GI, small bowel, kidney, and ureter
- Laryngoscopy
- Colonoscopy
- Arthroscopy of the wrist, shoulder, hip, and knee
- Ophthalmological surgeries such as corneal transplantation, glaucoma surgery, cataract surgery, and ocular implantation

Frequently carried out surgical procedures include tonsillectomy, lens and cataract procedures, myringotomy, adenoidectomy, and semilunar knee cartilage removal.

WHAT ARE THE ADVANTAGES OF AMBULATORY SURGICAL CENTERS?

Depending on the procedure and the individual facility, an ambulatory surgical center can have the following benefits:

Cost. Outpatient surgical procedures at ASCs can cost one-half to one-third of what is charged at hospitals. Medicare beneficiaries may also pay lesser at ASCs compared to hospitals. Be aware that the cost varies based on the procedure and patients must consult with Medicare before preparing for their surgery.

Convenience. Generally, there is less paperwork and administrative concerns at ASCs. Also, doctors are in charge of setting standards for staffing, safety, operative procedures, and patient care rather than managerial staff as is the case in hospitals.

Efficiency. ASCs are generally more efficient at scheduling surgeries, getting equipment and materials ready for surgery. This is an advantage that surgeons benefit from. Surgeons can in fact take care of multiple patients at the same time that they take to treat one patient in a hospital environment.

WHAT ARE THE FEDERAL RULES GOVERNING AMBULATORY SURGICAL CENTERS?

Ambulatory surgical center facilities are governed by federal and state laws in the United States. The rules that apply to all other

healthcare facilities apply to ASCs as well. Adherence to standards of quality and safety in ASCs are governed by three processes. They are:
1. State licensure
2. Medicare certification
3. Voluntary accreditation

The rules for licensure of ASCs in each state varies. ASCs serving Medicare beneficiaries must be certified by the program. Medicare standards must be complied with initially and on an ongoing basis. ASCs also choose to be accredited with independent bodies such as the Joint Commission on Accreditation of Healthcare Organizations (JCAHO), the Accreditation Association for Ambulatory Health Care (AAAHC), the American Association for the Accreditation of Ambulatory Surgery Facilities (AAAASF), and the American Osteopathic Association (AOA). Accrediting agencies conduct onsite inspections and ASCs benchmark themselves to stay competent.

References

1. "Ambulatory Surgery Centers: A Positive Trend in Healthcare," American Society for Gastrointestinal Endoscopy (ASGE), n.d.
2. "Helping You Choose: Quality Ambulatory Care," The Joint Commission, October 2013.
3. "Ambulatory Surgery Centers," Advameg, Inc., n.d.
4. "What Are the 5 Most Common Ambulatory Surgeries?" Medical Transcription Billing, Corp, September 19, 2016.
5. "Using the Ambulatory Surgery Rate Codes in APGs," New York State Department of Health, April 2, 2009.

Chapter 14 | **How to Prepare for Surgery**

Patients and their family members or friends are important members of the care team. The care team also includes the doctors, nurses, and other healthcare professionals who help take care of you. Your role in the care team is to take the time to learn about your surgery—how to prepare, what is going to happen, and what to expect afterward. If you have questions, ask! Speaking up if you are concerned about anything is one of the things you can do to stay safe.

PREPARING FOR YOUR SURGERY

Before any surgical procedure, your doctor might ask you to take certain steps to get ready for surgery. Here are some tips to make sure you are prepared.

- **Medical instructions.** Talk with your doctor about your medications well before your surgery. Your doctor may want to stop or change some medications, such as blood thinners for a short time or may even want you to see another doctor before surgery. Your doctor's office will give you instructions to follow in the days before surgery. These instructions usually explain whether you need to stop medications or fill new prescriptions, when to stop eating and drinking before surgery, and other instructions. Be sure to follow all

This chapter includes text excerpted from "Getting Ready for Your Ambulatory Surgery," Agency for Healthcare Research and Quality (AHRQ), U.S. Department of Health and Human Services (HHS), August 2017.

directions carefully. If you are confused about anything, call your doctor's office and ask questions.

- **Medication and allergy list.** Prepare an up-to-date list of your current medications and any allergies and bring it with you on the day of surgery.
- **Preventing infection.** Your doctor may give you a prescription for an antibiotic to take before your surgery to help prevent infection. Be sure to fill any prescriptions before surgery and follow directions as prescribed. Do not wear deodorant, lotion, or perfume on the day of your surgery. Your doctor may also ask you to bathe with an antibacterial soap or solution.
- **Shaving.** Do not shave the area where you will have the surgery. If hair needs to be removed from the operating site, your care team will do this on the day of the surgery.
- **Tobacco and alcohol.** Do not use tobacco or drink alcohol for at least 24 hours before your surgery.
- **Fasting.** Ask your doctor how long you should go without eating or drinking before your surgery.
- **Personal items.** Be prepared to remove dentures, hearing aids, glasses, contact lenses, jewelry, and hair accessories. Leave them at home if you can. If you must wear them, bring a case to put them in while you have surgery (i.e., for glasses or contact lenses). Leave jewelry at home if you are concerned about losing it.
- **Support person.** Arrange to have someone, such as a family member or a trusted friend, go with you to the surgery center. This person will need to talk with the doctor after your surgery. Many medications used to keep you comfortable during surgery will affect your memory in the hours after surgery. Your support person can make sure you do not miss any important information, such as results and instructions.
- **Documents.** You may want to complete and sign an advance directive and healthcare proxy before surgery. These documents are available on the Internet and

from hospitals and many medical offices. If you prepare these, be sure to bring copies with you to the surgery center.

- **Personal information.** Make sure you bring your photo ID and health insurance information with you on the day of the surgery.

WHAT TO EXPECT ON THE DAY OF YOUR SURGERY

- **Admission.** When you arrive, you will check in with your photo ID and insurance information.
- **Preoperative (pre-op) area.** When it is your turn, you will move to a pre-op area. That is where a nurse will prepare you for surgery. The anesthesia provider, your doctor, and other members of your care team may talk with you during this time.
- **Staying safe.** Your care team will take steps to make sure your surgery is as safe as possible. For example, you might see a nurse using a surgical checklist or you may be asked more than once to verify what kind of surgery you are having and where on your body the surgery will be done. All members of your care team—including your support person or family members—should clean their hands. This can help keep you safe from surgical infections and other complications.

WHAT TO EXPECT AFTER THE SURGERY

- **Recovery.** After your procedure, you will probably be taken to a recovery area. That is where your care team can watch to make sure you are recovering well.
- **Talking with your surgeon or nurse.** Before you leave the recovery area, you and your support person should have the opportunity to ask questions. You may want to know about how the surgery went or who to call in case of questions. You should have a clear understanding of what you need to do in the recovery period and whether you will need help from others.

- **Discharge.** You will be discharged to go home after you
  have recovered from the anesthesia. Your vital signs
  should be stable, and any pain or nausea should be under
  control. You will likely be required to have someone drive
  you home. You will receive written instructions on what
  to do at home. These instructions may include things like
  a medication schedule, things to avoid (such as certain
  activities or foods), possible complications to look out for,
  when to follow-up with your doctor, and a number to call
  in case of problems.

Healthcare team members you may see in the surgery center could
include:
- **Attending physician or surgeon.** A medical doctor
  (MD) who leads the team. She or he has the final
  responsibility for your surgery. Other physicians, such
  as residents and fellows, may be involved in your care.
- **Physician's assistant (PA) or nurse practitioner
  (NP).** A licensed professional who helps the physician
  and can perform some of the duties of a physician,
  including surgery and pre- and post-procedure care.
- **Operating room nurse or circulating nurse.** A
  registered nurse who is in the surgery/procedure room
  to make sure that the procedure runs smoothly and
  safely.
- **Surgical technologists (scrub techs).** Personnel
  who set up the surgery/procedure room, prepare
  you for surgery, and assist the doctor by passing the
  instruments.
- **Anesthesiology team.** Personnel who are responsible
  for giving you the drugs that make you sleepy or
  sedated. The members of the anesthesia team vary and
  might include nurses, anesthesiologists, and certified
  registered nurse anesthetists (CRNAs).
- **Recovery room or postanesthesia care unit (PACU)
  nurse.** a nurse who monitors you immediately after
  surgery.

Chapter 15 | **Benefits of Prehabilitation in Surgery**

Major surgery usually causes a significant decline in functional capacity (ability to perform daily tasks) of the patient. Prehabilitation is the process of optimizing an individual's functional capacity to enable them to withstand a major surgery. It is a multimodal program that involves physical exercise along with nutritional and psychosocial interventions to enhance the body's fitness level in the preoperative period. It aims to increase preoperative functional reserve, resulting in better postoperative functional recovery and reduced complications.

The therapist performs a thorough preoperative assessment during the initial prehabilitation session. The pre- and post-operative functional and equipment needs required by the patient can be decided using this assessment. Depending on the patient's diagnosis and functional limitations, specific exercises, nutrition counseling, and strategies will be recommended to improve endurance and strength that can help lessen stress prior to the start of treatment.

COMPONENTS OF A PREHABILITATION PROGRAM

Several weeks may pass between the decision to proceed with a surgery and the surgery itself. This is considered the right time to positively influence a patient's health performance, which may, in turn, affect long-term survival. Recently, the advantages of a multimodal strategy are being realized through the following plan of actions:

- Medical optimization

"Benefits of Prehabilitation in Surgery," © 2020 Omnigraphics. Reviewed April 2020.

- Physical exercise
- Nutritional support
- Psychological support

These interventions are monitored by a multidisciplinary team of surgeons, physicians, anesthetists, physiotherapists, geriatricians, nutritionists, and psychologists. Functional capacity, nutritional status, and mood of the patient are assessed and tracked frequently throughout the program. These interventions should progress into the postoperative period as well.

TYPES OF PREHABILITATION

Depending on the type of surgery, prehabilitation can be classified into the following types:

Pelvic Floor Prehabilitation

Patients can benefit by performing exercises guided by a physical therapist in order to strengthen the pelvic floor muscles prior to pelvic surgeries such as prostatectomy, transurethral resection of the prostate (TURP), or bladder sling placement. The strengthening of the pelvic floor muscles using these exercises produces better outcomes after the surgery. The physical therapist helps establish a regular exercise routine before the surgery. They also provide advice on lifestyle modification, body mechanics training, and urge control techniques (to stop the bladder from contracting).

Cancer Prehabilitation

The primary aim of cancer prehabilitation is to decrease significant fatigue, pain, and disability caused by cancer treatment and to encourage cancer survivors to have the best quality of life (QOL) possible. The patients are provided with a comprehensive cancer prehabilitation and rehabilitation plan based on the type of cancer, and are supported by a team of certified clinicians and healthcare providers.

HEAD AND NECK CANCER PREHABILITATION

A change in the patient's ability to chew, swallow, or talk occurs as a result of treatment for head and neck cancers. Swallowing exercises are prescribed by a physical therapist prior to surgery and chemo-radiation. This enables the patient to eat properly after the surgery, which in turn prevents weight loss, improves overall energy and strength, and results in a faster recovery.

BREAST CANCER PREHABILITATION

A physical therapist can prescribe upper-body strengthening and range-of-motion exercises that may reduce the risk of post-operative pain and other complications, such as frozen shoulder. Prehabilitation can also emotionally support individuals dealing with a new diagnosis of breast cancer. The patients are also taught specific mind–body skills to decrease stress.

PREHABILITATION OUTCOMES

Safety. Physical exercises that are done as a part of prehabilitation are rarely known to cause complications, such as a stroke or myocardial infarction (MI), even among high-risk surgical patients. However, patients with a severe cardiorespiratory disease (such as unstable coronary artery disease or poorly controlled arrhythmias) are usually excluded, and they require tailored medical optimization before undertaking prehabilitation.

Cardiorespiratory fitness. Studies show that preoperative exercise training improves cardiorespiratory fitness. This helps achieve better postoperative outcomes and reduced surgical risks.

Resistance training. The resistance training in the preoperative period is feasible. Research shows an improvement in skeletal muscle strength, leading to improved postoperative physical function.

Respiratory muscle training. A program of preoperative inspiratory muscle training (IMT) reduces the risk of postoperative pulmonary complications, such as atelectasis (closure or collapse of lung) and pneumonia, along with a reduced length of hospital stay.

Smoking cessation. Patients who stop smoking at least four weeks before surgery are at a decreased risk of postoperative pulmonary complications. A cessation period of three to four weeks also decreases the risk of wound-healing complications.

Psychosocial preparation. Studies show that psychological prehabilitation does not affect usual surgical outcomes, including mortality and complication rates; however, it enhances the immunological function and an improvement in psychological outcomes and QOL.

Postoperative outcomes. Prehabilitation is known to minimize the rate of postoperative complications and the duration of hospital stay.

ADVANTAGES OF PREHABILITATION

Evidence-based research shows that prehabilitation:

- Helps a patient feel better and improves functional capacity before surgery
- Enables them to deal with the physical challenges faced following surgery
- Improves the patient's psychological outcomes
- Decreases hospital readmissions
- Reduces healthcare costs

References

1. "Understanding Prehabilitation," World Federation of Societies of Anesthesiologists (WFSA), December 27, 2018.
2. "Prehabilitation," Oxford University Press, August 16, 2017.
3. "What Is Prehabilitation," Cleveland Clinic Martin Health, June 19, 2017.
4. "Rehabilitation," OSF HealthCare, January 27, 2018.

Chapter 16 | Anesthesia

Chapter Contents

Section 16.1 | Anesthesia Basics

This section contains text excerpted from the following sources: Text beginning with the heading "What Is Anesthesia?" is excerpted from "Anesthesia," National Institute of General Medical Sciences (NIGMS), September 2017; Text beginning with the heading "Understanding How Anesthesia Helps" is excerpted from "Understanding Anesthesia," National Institute of General Medical Sciences (NIGMS), January 26, 2011. Reviewed April 2020.

WHAT IS ANESTHESIA?

Anesthesia is a medical treatment that prevents patients from feeling pain during surgery. It allows people to have procedures that lead to healthier and longer lives.

To produce anesthesia, doctors use drugs called "anesthetics." Scientists have developed a collection of anesthetic drugs with different effects. These drugs include general, regional, and local anesthetics. General anesthetics put patients to sleep during the procedure. Local and regional anesthetics just numb part of the body and allow patients to remain awake during the procedure.

Depending on the type of pain relief needed, doctors deliver anesthetics by injection, inhalation, topical lotion, spray, eye drops, or skin patch.

WHAT IS GENERAL ANESTHESIA?

General anesthesia affects the whole body, making patients unconscious and unable to move. Surgeons use it when they operate on internal organs and for other invasive or time-consuming procedures, such as back surgery. Without general anesthesia, many major, life-saving procedures would not be possible, including open-heart surgery, brain surgery, and organ transplants.

Doctors provide general anesthetics either directly into the bloodstream (intravenously) or as an inhaled gas. General anesthesia delivered intravenously will act quickly and disappear rapidly from the body. This allows patients to go home sooner after surgery. Inhaled anesthetics may take longer to wear off.

General anesthetics typically are very safe. But they can pose risks for some patients, such as the elderly or people with chronic illnesses, such as diabetes. Also, side effects may linger for several days in some patients, especially the elderly and children.

Serious side effects—such as dangerously low blood pressure—are much less common than they once were. Still, as with any medical procedure, some risks exist. To minimize these risks, specialized doctors called "anesthesiologists" carefully monitor unconscious patients and can adjust the amount of anesthetic they receive.

WHAT ARE LOCAL AND REGIONAL ANESTHESIA?
Doctors use local and regional anesthetics to block pain in a part of the body. With these anesthetics, patients stay conscious and comfortable. Usually, patients may go home soon after surgery.

Local anesthetics affect a small part of the body, such as a single tooth. They are often used in dentistry, for eye surgeries, such as cataract removal, and to remove small skin growths including warts and moles.

Regional anesthetics affect larger areas such as an arm, a leg, or everything below the waist. For example, this sort of anesthesia is used for hand and joint surgeries, to ease the pain of childbirth, or during a C-section delivery.

HOW DOES ANESTHESIA WORK?
Scientists are able to study how drugs affect specific molecules within cells. Most researchers agree that the drugs target proteins in the membranes around nerve cells. Because inhaled anesthetics have different effects than intravenous ones, scientists suspect that the two different types of drugs target different sets of proteins.

WHAT DO ANESTHESIOLOGISTS DO?
Anesthesiologists are doctors who carefully monitor patients throughout surgery and during recovery. They use highly advanced electronic devices that constantly display patients' blood pressure, blood oxygen levels, heart function, and breathing patterns. These devices have dramatically improved the safety of general anesthesia. They also make it possible to operate on many patients who used to be considered too sick to have surgery.

Anesthesiologists also provide pain relief for less invasive procedures such as those used to examine blood vessels and internal organs (endoscopy), and during labor and delivery.

As experts in pain management, anesthesiologists may advise patients and their doctors on how to manage pain.

HOW ARE ANESTHESIOLOGISTS TRAINED?

Like all medical doctors, anesthesiologists earn a college degree, often in a life sciences field, then a medical degree (M.D. or D.O.). After that, they complete a four-year residency program in anesthesiology. Many also train for an additional year or more in a specialty such as pain management, pediatric anesthesiology, or critical care medicine.

WHAT DOES THE FUTURE HOLD FOR ANESTHESIOLOGY?

Scientists are learning more about how anesthetics work at the most basic level. They are also studying the short- and long-term effects of these drugs on specific groups of people, such as the elderly and cancer survivors. These studies will reveal whether certain anesthetics are better than others for members of those groups.

Research on how a person's genetic makeup affects how she or he responds to anesthetics will allow doctors to further tailor drugs for each patient. In the future, scientists hope to design anesthetics that are safer, more effective, and more personalized.

Knowing how anesthetics affect pain and consciousness could also lead to new treatments for conditions that affect consciousness, such as epilepsy or coma. Studies of anesthesia may even help you better understand the nature of consciousness itself.

UNDERSTANDING HOW ANESTHESIA HELPS

Anesthesia helps many people during their lives, whether they need a local painkiller at the dentist, numbing eye drops for laser vision correction, or general anesthesia for major surgery. But, even though anesthetics have been used in many procedures for more than 150 years, doctors and scientists still do not know exactly how these medicines work in the body.

FINDING A SAFE WAY TO UNDERGO SURGERY

Before anesthesia, doctors and dentists operated on patients only in extreme circumstances and largely without the use of painkillers or sedatives.

Then, in 1846, dentist William T. G. Morton demonstrated the use of ether to put patients "to sleep" during surgery. The practice soon spread, but because doctors could not control the amount of ether inhaled, patients could wake up during surgery—or never wake again. Ether was also highly flammable.

The next few decades saw the introduction of less flammable anesthetic gases as well as the discovery of intravenous anesthetics with a controllable dosage. Still, well into the 1950s, dangerous side effects were common and included heart rhythm abnormalities, breathing problems, lowered blood pressure, nausea and vomiting.

Modern anesthetic techniques allow millions of Americans to safely undergo surgery with fewer and less serious side effects. New inhaled and intravenous general anesthetics act quickly and dissipate rapidly when stopped, while local and regional anesthetics that block specific nerves provide an alternative to general anesthesia.

Researchers funded by the National Institutes of Health (NIH) have helped identify and explore several components of general anesthesia—including sedation, unconsciousness, immobility, analgesia (lack of pain), and amnesia (lack of memory). And they have developed medicines that can provide one or more elements separately, allowing anesthesiologists to tailor painkiller regimens to individual procedures and patients.

AN ANESTHESIOLOGIST'S JOB IS NOT EASY

Since anesthesia can still cause complications and have body-wide effects, anesthesiologists carefully monitor patients throughout surgery using a variety of devices that display blood pressure, blood oxygen levels, heart function, and respiration. They adjust medications throughout the procedure to make sure each patient remains safe.

Anesthesiologists' jobs have expanded beyond the operating room as well, including caring for patients as they recover from surgery and providing anesthesia for nonsurgical procedures, such as colonoscopy and childbirth. They also advise other specialists on how to manage pain.

Section 16.2 | Regional Anesthesia for Postsurgical Pain

This section includes text excerpted from "Regional Anesthesia FAQs," U.S. Department of Veterans Affairs (VA), June 15, 2014. Reviewed April 2020.

WHAT IS REGIONAL ANESTHESIA?

"Regional anesthesia" is a targeted type of anesthesia. It involves injecting numbing medicine around nerves that provide sensation to specific regions or parts of your body (e.g., arm, leg, foot) and can be used instead of general anesthesia or in addition to general anesthesia as a way to control pain after surgery. Anesthesiologists can perform these procedures before surgery to prevent pain, or they can provide regional anesthesia as a "rescue" technique to relieve pain after surgery. Types of regional anesthesia procedures include spinal, epidural or peripheral nerve block. Depending on the type of numbing medicine (local anesthetic) used, a nerve block can last for a few hours or up to a whole day. For more painful surgeries, anesthesiologists can insert a tiny tube also known as a "catheter" that can continuously bathe the nerves in numbing medicine for an additional two to three days.

There are many advantages to regional anesthesia. Because you will have decreased sensation, you need to take less opioid (narcotic) pain medicines even though you will commonly have these medications prescribed to you. Patients who receive regional anesthesia also have less nausea, recover more quickly immediately after surgery, and sleep better overnight compared to patients who do not have regional anesthesia.

Even if you choose regional anesthesia instead of general anesthesia, you do not have to be "awake" during surgery. Anesthesiologists often combine regional anesthesia with either intravenous sedation or general anesthesia, both of which can allow you to "sleep" during surgery. You should discuss your preferences with your anesthesiologist prior to surgery.

There are always risks associated with performing any procedure. Fortunately, serious complications associated with regional anesthesia are exceedingly rare. Anesthesiology practices that specialize in regional anesthesia commonly have systems in place to prevent complications and treat them quickly if or when they occur.

WHAT CAN YOU EXPECT ON THE DAY OF SURGERY?

Before surgery (or on the day of surgery at the latest), you will meet with an anesthesiologist who will evaluate whether or not regional anesthesia is the right option for you. If you are eligible and desire regional anesthesia preoperatively, the anesthesiologist will perform your nerve block approximately 30 to 60 minutes before your surgery. Nerve blocks may be performed in a specialized area (block room) outside of the operating room. After your Intravenous therapy (IV) is inserted, your anesthesiologist may provide you with sedating medication during the performance of your nerve block. Before the procedure starts, your anesthesiologist will perform a "time-out" with you to confirm the correct site and side of your surgical procedure. It has become increasingly common for anesthesiologists to use ultrasound to identify your unique anatomy and safely inject numbing medication around the nerves. After the nerve block, your affected limb will "go to sleep" over the next 10 to 20 minutes.

WHAT ARE YOUR REGIONAL ANESTHESIA OPTIONS FOR HAND, WRIST, FOREARM, OR ELBOW SURGERY?

For hand, wrist, forearm, or elbow surgeries (e.g., carpal tunnel release, fracture repair, or tendon transfer) there are a few different locations in which to place the nerve block depending on the site of surgery and expected placement of the tourniquet (if utilized). Most commonly, the nerve block is performed above the collar bone (supraclavicular block) or below the collarbone (infraclavicular block). For extensive surgeries involving bones and/or joints, your anesthesiologist can place a catheter that will bathe the nerve in numbing medicine for an additional two to three days. An infraclavicular catheter may have advantages over the supraclavicular catheter in terms of pain control.

WHAT ARE YOUR REGIONAL ANESTHESIA OPTIONS FOR UPPER ARM OR SHOULDER SURGERY?

For surgeries involving the upper arm or shoulder, nerve blocks are most commonly performed in the neck (interscalene block). For extensive arthroscopic shoulder surgery and shoulder replacement, a catheter near the nerves that can deliver numbing medicine for two to three days is recommended. This type of pain relief helps you perform physical therapy and reduces your need for opioid (narcotic) pain medications.

WHAT ARE YOUR REGIONAL ANESTHESIA OPTIONS FOR KNEE SURGERY?

For surgeries involving the knee including total knee replacement, nerve blocks are routinely placed near the groin (femoral nerve block) or on the inside part of the thigh where the nerves to the front of the knee are located (adductor canal block). For patients having total knee replacement, your anesthesiologist may place a catheter to deliver numbing medicine near the nerves for two to three days. This type of pain relief will help you perform physical therapy, reduce your need for opioid (narcotic) pain medications, and decrease the time it takes for you to achieve discharge criteria. An adductor canal catheter may help patients walk further immediately after total knee replacement surgery compared to a femoral nerve catheter although both provide effective pain relief.

It is important to realize that any nerve block may also cause weak muscles. Therefore, after your nerve block, you must realize that you are at an increased risk of falling because your leg may not be strong enough to support your weight. Anesthesiology practices that provide regional anesthesia for pain relief after joint replacement are advised to have a comprehensive fall prevention program in place. However, in the immediate postoperative period it is important to always ask for assistance anytime you need to get out of bed. Do not attempt to walk by yourself.

WHAT ARE YOUR REGIONAL ANESTHESIA OPTIONS FOR HIP SURGERY?

For hip surgery, nerve blocks are performed above the groin crease near the nerves that affect the front and side of the hip (fascia iliaca block or femoral nerve block) or in the back (lumbar plexus block); both approaches provide similar pain relief. Alternatively, a spinal block with numbing and/or opioid pain medication may be placed.

It is important to realize that any nerve block may also cause weak muscles. Therefore, after your nerve block, you must realize that you are at increased risk of falling because your leg may not be strong enough to support your weight. Anesthesiology practices that provide regional anesthesia for pain relief after joint replacement are advised to have a comprehensive fall prevention program in place. However, in the immediate postoperative period it is important to always ask for assistance anytime you need to get out of bed. Do not attempt to walk by yourself.

WHAT ARE YOUR REGIONAL ANESTHESIA OPTIONS FOR FOOT OR ANKLE SURGERY?

For surgeries involving the foot or ankle, nerve blocks are most commonly performed in the area behind your knee (popliteal sciatic block) or at the level of the ankle (ankle block). For more invasive surgeries of this area (e.g., tendon/ligament repairs and fractures), your anesthesiologist may recommend a catheter near the nerves that can deliver numbing medicine into the area for two to three days. This type of pain relief helps you perform physical therapy and reduces your need for opioid (narcotic) pain medications.

WHAT ARE YOUR REGIONAL ANESTHESIA OPTIONS FOR FACIAL SURGERY?

For surgeries involving the face and neck, it may be possible to perform specific nerve blocks to minimize your postoperative pain. These may be performed by your anesthesiologist or surgeon. Common procedures that are suitable for these nerve blocks include skin cancer excision, endoscopic sinus surgery, septoplasty, and rhinoplasty. Your anesthesiologist will discuss these options with you on the day of surgery and determine if you are a good candidate for regional anesthesia.

WHAT ARE YOUR REGIONAL ANESTHESIA OPTIONS FOR CHEST OR ABDOMINAL SURGERY?

For major surgeries involving the chest or abdomen, your anesthesiologist may offer you an epidural or spinal block in addition to general anesthesia. Alternatively, special types of nerve block procedures, paravertebral blocks and transversus abdominis plane (TAP) blocks, have also been shown to provide effective pain relief after these surgeries. Your anesthesiologist will discuss these options with you on the day of surgery and determine if you are a good candidate for regional anesthesia.

HOW LONG WILL THE NUMBNESS FROM THE LOCAL ANESTHETIC MEDICATION LAST?

The intensity and duration of your block largely depends on the type of numbing medicine (local anesthetic) that was used, as well as whether you receive a single dose of medication or have a nerve block catheter in place. As a single dose, some local anesthetic medications provide a few hours of numbness while others can provide numbness that lasts up to a day.

WHAT SHOULD YOU KNOW ABOUT THE NERVE BLOCK CATHETER?

A nerve block catheter is a skinny tube placed near your nerves in order to continuously bathe your nerves with local anesthetic medication. The catheter is attached to a pump—the size of a small grapefruit or a similar type of device. This pump is filled with local anesthetic medication which is continuously delivered through the catheter to provide you with pain relief for two to three days. Once the medication runs out, the catheter should be removed. Removal is a simple procedure that you or a caretaker can do at home. Your anesthesiologist or another healthcare provider should follow-up with you daily and be available for any questions that you may have regarding the catheter and pump.

Catheters are more suitable for certain surgeries and nerve sites than others. Your anesthesiologist will help you determine whether or not this is a good option for you.

DOES IT HURT TO GET A NERVE BLOCK?

Getting a nerve block should be no more painful than getting an intravenous (IV). The practitioner will numb the skin before placing the nerve block and can also provide you with mild sedation prior to the procedure. Also, using ultrasound to locate the nerves during the procedure minimizes the amount of pain that you feel.

CAN YOU PUT THE NERVE BLOCK IN AFTER YOU ARE ASLEEP?

Although any of these procedures can be performed under general anesthesia, doing so prevents the patients from giving the feedback as the doctor works around your nerves. Placing the nerve block while you are "awake" (but, comfortably sedated) adds an additional measure of safety to the procedure.

IS IT SAFE TO GET A NERVE BLOCK?

There are always risks associated with performing any procedure. Fortunately, serious complications associated with regional anesthesia are exceedingly rare. Anesthesiology practices that specialize in regional anesthesia commonly have systems in place to prevent complications and treat them quickly if or when they occur. The practitioner performs this procedure in a sterile manner to minimize the risk of infection. The possibility of trauma to the nerves exists, but your anesthesiologist may take special precautions, including the use of ultrasound, to decrease this risk. Most commonly, patients report mild bruising or soreness from the site of injection.

Chapter 17 | Risks Associated with Surgery

Chapter Contents

Section 17.1 | Anesthesia Complications

This section includes text excerpted from "Cost Effectiveness Analysis of Anesthesia Providers," U.S. Department of Justice (DOJ), February 20, 2015. Reviewed April 2020.

Some adverse cases are highly publicized, anesthesia-related mortality rates have declined substantially during the past 2 decades to about 1 death for every 240,000 anesthetics. National estimates of anesthesia-related mortality in the United States for years 1999 to 2005 are 1.1 per million population per year and 8.2 per million hospital surgical discharges. National estimates of anesthesia complications for inpatients in 2005 found an incidence rate of 1.0 case per 1,000 admissions; of patients who developed complications, 0.9 percent died by discharge. The anesthetic agents and improved patient monitoring have contributed to these improved outcomes.

The Centers for Disease Control and Prevention (CDC) conducted a pilot study in 1980 and found the rate of adverse outcomes with anesthesia as a contributing factor was 6.25/10,000 procedures. The rate for adverse outcomes totally attributed to anesthesia was 1.25/10,000 procedures. The CDC concluded the low frequency of anesthesia-related adverse outcomes made the cost of a full-scale study prohibitive.

Research studies have found no significant differences in rates of anesthesia complications or mortality between certified registered nurse anesthetists (CRNA) and anesthesiologists or among delivery models for anesthesia that involve CRNAs, anesthesiologists, or both after controlling for other pertinent factors. There are limitations to the literature. Some researchers were not able to identify, precisely, the anesthesia delivery model. They might use the typical practice at a hospital rather than the anesthesia provider(s) for a specific procedure to identify delivery models. Sometimes the study identified those procedures which an anesthesiologist personally performed or directed, but may not distinguish whether medical direction was of CRNAs or anesthesiology residents. Given the low incidence of adverse anesthesia-related complications and anesthesia-related mortality rates in general, it is not surprising there are no studies that show a significant difference between CRNAs and anesthesiologists in patient outcomes.

157

Claims analysis for quality of care. In addition to reviewing the evidence from the literature, healthcare claims and discharge data were used to assess adverse anesthesia outcomes including death and anesthesia complications. Anesthesia complications were identified using the International Classification of Diseases, 9th Revision, Clinical Modification (ICD-9-CM) diagnosis codes.

The Ingenix national database contains integrated medical and financial claims data from commercial payers in 2008. A total of 52,636 claims that included anesthesia were reviewed. There were no complications arising from anesthesia in these claims. The National Survey of Ambulatory Surgery (NSAS) (2006) contains information about surgical and nonsurgical procedures performed on an ambulatory (outpatient) basis in hospitals or freestanding ambulatory surgery centers for 2006. There are 52,233 sampled visits, representing almost 35 million total visits in the United States. Only one visit resulted in a complication from anesthesia. For that visit, anesthesia was provided by an anesthesiologist and a CRNA. The Healthcare Cost and Utilization Project (HCUP) Nationwide Inpatient Sample (NIS) (2007) contains information for approximately 8 million hospital stays from about 1,000 hospitals sampled to represent a 20 percent stratified sample of United States community hospitals. The unit of observation is an inpatient stay record rather than one specific procedure. It does not include anesthesia provider information. The percentage of complications is very low at 0.12 percent for the sample and 0.11 percent for the national estimate.

Quality of care by anesthesia providers is excellent. The incidence of adverse anesthesia-related complications and anesthesia-related mortality rates is very low. Review of the literature revealed no studies that demonstrated a significant difference between CRNAs and anesthesiologists or differences between anesthesia delivery models in rates of anesthesia complications or mortality after controlling for hospital and patient factors.

Section 17.2 | **Wound Healing**

When you are discharged from the hospital after your surgery, your doctor will give you a set of instructions to follow to make sure your wound heals faster.

HOW TO KNOW THAT YOUR SURGICAL WOUND IS HEALING RIGHT

Make sure to keep an eye on your wound postsurgery. The wound may go through various phases and might not look normal while healing.

THE STAGES OF HEALING

Here are the three stages that your wound will go through before it starts healing:

Stage 1. Swelling is the first step to healing. The blood clots around the wound to prevent further flow of blood from the wound. White blood cells, which are known for controlling the infections, move into the wound and fight the bacteria. This phase lasts up to six days postsurgery, and you will find redness and pain around the area of the wound.

Stage 2. The rebuilding phase can last from four days to a month postsurgery. There is a possibility of the edges of the skin to pull together and start forming a scar in the place of the cut. You might also see some red bumps inside your wound. You will feel some sharp pain in your nerves that is caused due to your sensation returning back in your nerves. This feeling will slowly fade away over some time.

Stage 3. Remodeling is a phase that lasts between six months and two years; and during this stage, you will find some changes in your scar that looks thinner, flatter, and more like your usual skin color.

HOW TO KEEP YOUR WOUND CLEAN

There are some simple steps to follow to keep your would clean.

- Gently clean and dab the area around the wound with a soft cloth or gauze pad that is soaked in soapy water or sterile water and salt.
- Do not use skin cleansers, antibacterial soaps, or alcohol to clean the wound as they can damage the skin around the wound and delay the healing. You can wash your wound with a syringe. Fill the syringe with mild soap water or saltwater. This helps to drain away pus out of the wound and then pat it dry with clean gauze or a clean cloth.
- Keep your wound dry for the first 24 hours of your surgery; so skip a bath or shower after surgery. Check with your doctor about the complications of your wound before getting a shower or a bath.
- If your doctor has permitted to take a bath, then it is better to take a shower than a bath as soaking can soften your wound and cause it to open again.
- Do not pat the area with any other bath products before your wound heals.

WOUND INFECTIONS

Wound infections happen but are rare. You are likely to be prone to wound infections during the first month postsurgery.
There are different levels of wound infections and they can be classified as:
- **Superficial.** Only the skin area is infected.
- **Deep.** The infection goes deep down into the muscle and tissue.
- **Organ or space.** At this level of infection, it goes deep down to the organ or space you had surgery.

You will have the following symptoms if your wound is infected:
- Pain
- Fever
- Delay in healing
- Swelling near the wound
- Discharge of pus
- Skin redness

- Tenderness and warmth spreading around the wound

You are more prone to surgical infections if:
- You have diabetes
- You are obese or overweight
- You have a weak immune system
- You smoke
- You have a surgery that lasts for more than two hours

References

1. "How to Know Your Surgical Cut Is Healing Right," WebMD, November 8, 2018.
2. "How to Take Care of Your Wound after Surgery," WebMD, November 8, 2018.
3. "Surgical Wound Infection—Treatment," Utilization Review Accreditation Commission (URAC), March 4, 2020.

Section 17.3 | Thrombosis

This section includes text excerpted from "Your Guide to Preventing and Treating Blood Clots," Agency for Healthcare Research and Quality (AHRQ), U.S. Department of Health and Human Services (HHS), August 1, 2017.

Blood clots are a serious medical condition. It is important to know the signs and get treated right away. This section describes ways to prevent and treat blood clots, symptoms, and medication side effects as well as when to go to the emergency room.

Blood clots (also known as "deep vein thrombosis") most often occur in people who cannot move around well or who have had recent surgery or an injury.

CAUSES OF BLOOD CLOTS

Blood clots can form if you do not move around a lot. You may also get a blood clot if you:
- Have had recent surgery

- Are 65 years of age or older
- Take hormones, especially for birth control
- Have had cancer or are being treated for it
- Have broken a bone (hip, pelvis, or leg)
- Have a bad bump or bruise
- Are obese
- Are confined to bed or a chair much of the time
- Have had a stroke or are paralyzed
- Have a special port the doctor put in your body to give you medicine
- Have varicose or bad veins
- Have heart trouble
- Have had a blood clot before
- Have a family member who has had a blood clot
- Have taken a long trip (more than an hour) in a car, airplane, bus, or train

SYMPTOMS OF A BLOOD CLOT

You may have a blood clot if you see or feel:

- New swelling in your arm or leg
- Skin redness
- Soreness or pain in your arm or leg
- A warm spot on your leg

Blood clots can be dangerous. Blood clots that form in the veins in your legs, arms, and groin can break loose and move to other parts of your body, including your lungs. A blood clot in your lungs is known as "pulmonary embolism." If this happens, your life can be in danger.

A blood clot may have gone to your lungs if you suddenly have:

- A hard time breathing
- Chest pain
- A fast heartbeat
- Fainting spells
- A mild fever
- A cough, with or without blood

PREVENTING BLOOD CLOTS
You can help prevent blood clots if you:
- Wear loose-fitting clothes, socks, or stockings
- Raise your legs six inches above your heart from time to time
- Wear special stockings (known as "compression stockings") if your doctor prescribes them
- Do exercises your doctor gives you
- Change your position often, especially during a long trip
- Do not stand or sit for more than 1 hour at a time
- Eat less salt
- Try not to bump or hurt your legs and try not to cross them
- Do not use pillows under your knees
- Raise the bottom of your bed four to six inches with blocks or books
- Take all medicines the doctor prescribes you

TREATMENT OF BLOOD CLOTS
If you have been told you have a blood clot, your doctor may give you medicine to treat it. This type of medicine is known as a "blood thinner" also known as an "anticoagulant." In most cases, your doctor will tell you to follow this treatment plan:
- For the first week you will receive medicine called "heparin" that works quickly.
- This medicine is injected under the skin. You will learn how to give yourself these shots, or a family member or friend may do it for you.
- You will also start taking Coumadin—generic name: warfarin—pills by mouth. After about a week of taking both the shots and the pills, you will stop taking the shots. You will continue to take the Coumadin warfarin pills for about three to six months or longer.

SIDE EFFECTS OF BLOOD THINNERS
Blood thinners can cause side effects. Bleeding is the most common problem. Your doctor will watch you closely. If you notice

something wrong that you think may be caused by your medication, call your doctor.

Section 17.4 | Accidental Injury to Nearby Organs

Surgical patients face a risk of organ injury. This happens even when a surgical procedure is performed:
- For the right diagnosis
- In a perfect manner

Surgeries performed can either be minor or major and there bound to be complications. For some patients, the procedure leads to a more serious type of problem, such as the risk of organ injury.

INJURIES DURING ANESTHESIA
In major surgeries, the patient is subjected to general anesthesia, during which they experience unconsciousness and do not feel pain. Injuries during anesthesia are completely due to human error.

Some of the most common injuries caused are:

Dental Injury
Dental injuries occur when different kinds of dental equipment are used during surgery. Dental injuries are caused by the usage of the following equipment during surgery and they are:
- Laryngoscope
- Oropharyngeal airways
- Jaw clamping
- Oropharyngeal suction devices
- Dental props/mouth gags

Peripheral Nerve Injury

This type of injury occurs due to poor patient positioning while subjecting them to general anesthesia or to intra-neural injection during regional anesthesia.

Eye Injury

Corneal abrasion is the most common eye injury and it mostly heals without any long-term effects but occasionally leads to blurred areas in the field of view.

INJURIES CAUSED DUE TO LAPAROSCOPIC SURGERY

Laparoscopic surgeries have a number of advantages, however, undergoing these surgeries have its complications too. The complication rate is significantly influenced by the complexity of the surgery. Major complications include injuries to the vessels, bowel, and urinary tract.

VASCULAR INJURIES

The much-feared vascular complication of laparoscopic procedures is during the initiation of a pneumoperitoneum (the abnormal presence of air or other gas). The accident occurs when the veress needle (spring-loaded needle that is used to create pneumoperitoneum for laparoscopic surgery) is inserted before insufflation or when a trochar (a pen-shaped instrument with a sharp triangular point at one end) is inserted after insufflation (an act of blowing something such as gas, powder or vapor). Vascular injury from laparoscopy is the major cause of death with a mortality rate of around 15 percent.

BOWEL INJURIES

Bowel injury is a puncture to the bowel wall or tissue injury that results due to a delayed perforation from a laparoscopic procedure. Bowel injuries are the third cause of death from a laparoscopic surgery, and these injuries sometimes go unrecognized at the time of the procedure.

UROLOGICAL INJURIES

The urinary bladder is at most risk while performing laparoscopic gynecological surgery. This is because of its close proximity to the surgical area or due to the entry process while performing laparoscopic surgery.

AIR EMBOLISM

Air embolism occurs when air or gas enters into the vascular system. It is a rare but fatal complication that occurs during a variety of procedures and surgeries. This is more often associated with an iatrogenic complication (a complication that a person acquires after getting a medical treatment).

Air embolism is of two types and they are:

- **Venous air embolism.** This occurs when the air enters the venous structures and travels through the right heart to the pulmonary circulation.
- **Arterial air embolism.** This occurs when the air enters the artery and travels until the air is trapped at a point.

References

1. "Entry Complications in Laparoscopic Surgery," National Center for Biotechnology Information (NCBI), U.S. National Library of Medicine (NLM), 2009.
2. "Vascular Air Embolism," *International Journal of Critical Illness and Injury Science*, March 22, 2013.

Chapter 18 | Substance Use and Surgery

Section 18.1 | Alcohol Use and Heart Surgery

"Alcohol Use and Heart Surgery," © 2017 Omnigraphics. Reviewed April 2020.

It is important to disclose history of active alcohol use prior to heart surgery because it is associated with serious postsurgical complications. Alcohol use will likely impact planned recovery. It is crucial to let your surgeon know how many drinks you consume per day or per week. Excessive drinking is defined as having more than three drinks per day and is known to affect the outcome of surgery.

ALCOHOL USE AND SURGERY
What is a standard drink? It can be:
- 12 ounces of beer
- 5 ounces of wine
- 1.5 ounces of 80-proof liquor

When someone consumes more than three drinks a day, then it could lead to complications. This is true, especially for those who manifest alcohol withdrawal syndrome. Their central nervous system will "overreact" during withdrawal and will cause:
- Shakiness
- Sweating
- Hallucinations
- Other symptoms

If left untreated, it will result in life-threatening conditions such as:
- Tremors
- Seizures
- Delirium tremens
- Death

There is also a possibility of an alcoholic patient to be in the intensive care unit (ICU). They will take a longer time to recover from their surgery. Furthermore, heavy drinking also:
- Causes organ systems to malfunction
- Interferes with biochemical controls

This might lead to conditions harmful to survival after surgery.

WHAT ARE THE OUTCOMES OF ALCOHOL WITHDRAWAL TREATMENT BEFORE SURGERY?

Alcohol withdrawal treatment prior to surgery offers the following benefits:

- Strong doses of sedatives may not be needed
- Restraining devices may not be required
- Decrease in seizures and delirium tremens after surgery
- Ventilator support may not be needed for a long term
- Reduction in complications in organs and biochemical processes
- Reduction in falls and injuries
- Shorter stay after surgery for recovery

HOW TO UNDERSTAND THAT YOU COULD BE AT RISK FOR ALCOHOL WITHDRAWAL?

Once surgery is finalized as the course of treatment, you will be interviewed and asked to answer a questionnaire. Make sure you answer honestly all the questions in it. This could facilitate better treatment and increase your chances of full recovery. The information you provide is kept confidential and should not be a cause of concern.

WHEN CAN I DRINK ALCOHOL AFTER HEART SURGERY?

Consult with your doctor before you start drinking after surgery to be on the safer side. This way you can be assured that you will not be causing yourself any harm.

WILL ALCOHOL INTERACT WITH PRESCRIBED MEDICATION?

Alcohol interacts with medication, potentially changing its effects depending on the type of medication you have been prescribed. Mixing alcohol with certain medications is possibly lethal, particularly painkillers and sleep medication. Excessive alcohol also affects coagulation of blood. And you should be careful if you have been prescribed anticoagulants, such as Warfarin.

IS IT SAFE TO DRINK AFTER FULL RECOVERY?

It is fine to drink within recommended limits after recovery from heart surgery. However, check with your doctor to make sure it is indeed safe for you to drink. If you have been diagnosed with certain types of cardiomyopathy you will be advised to avoid drinking completely.

Some drinks known as "caffeinated alcoholic drinks" contain caffeine and overwork the heart. They are not advisable if you've been diagnosed with tachycardias and arrhythmias.

DOES DRINKING IN MODERATION HAVE ITS BENEFITS?

Excessive drinkers statistically carry more risk of cardiovascular complications compared to teetotalers. On the other hand, some studies have indicated that moderate drinkers are at 25 percent lesser risk of complications postsurgery compared to patients who do not drink at all.

Men are advised not to have more than two drinks a day and women should restrict themselves to one a day.

References

1. "Alcohol and Heart Surgery," Cleveland Clinic, n.d.
2. "Advisory: Alcohol Screening and Management Protocols," Commonwealth of Massachusetts, Board of Registration in Medicine (BORIM), July 2013.
3. "Heart Conditions and Alcohol," British Heart Foundation (BHF), n.d.
4. "Alcohol and Heart Health," American Heart Association (AHA), January 12, 2015.

Section 18.2 | **Smoking and Surgery**

"Smoking and Surgery," © 2020 Omnigraphics. Reviewed April 2020.

It is evident that smoking causes serious health problems, and the habit of smoking before surgery will affect your quality of recovery and outcome after surgery. Healthcare providers and doctors strongly recommend their patients to quit smoking before two months of surgery. The earlier you quit, the healthier you will be to undergo a surgery. The levels of the chemicals, such as nicotine and carbon monoxide drop, and thereby it improves blood flow and reduces the likelihood of problems.

IMPORTANCE OF QUITTING SMOKING BEFORE SURGERY

When a person smokes, their heart and lungs do not function the way they should and it, in turn, increases their risk of having pneumonia and breathing problems during and after surgery. Smoking decreases the flow of blood that affects the healing. The wounds are less likely to heal and more likely to get infected as smoking affects the immune system and increases the chance of infection after surgery.

There are some specific complications that are more likely to occur in smokers than in nonsmokers. For instance:

- In an orthopedic surgery, the bones can take longer to heal
- In a plastic surgery, there is a higher chance of scarring
- In a breast reconstruction surgery, they are more likely to lose implants
- In a spinal fusion surgery, there is a higher chance of infection and bone fracture

Secondhand smoke can also cause harm during surgery. Children are the most affected due to secondhand smoking.

COMMON RISK FACTORS

Continuing to smoke right up until the day of surgery can bring a lot of risk factors.

- Smoking can starve the heart and lungs of oxygen.
- It can form blood clots in the veins.
- There is a higher risk of lung complications, such as pneumonia and lung collapse.
- The healing of bones, skin, and the wound will be delayed.
- There will be a change in the breakdown of certain drugs in your blood.

References

1. "Why You Should Quit Smoking before Having Surgery," Truth Initiative, March 6, 2017.
2. "Smoking: Surgery Risks and Anesthesia Complications," American Society of Anesthesiologists (ASA), January 26, 2018.
3. "Smoking and Surgery," Queensland Government, May 3, 2015.

Chapter 19 | **Blood Typing and Blood Transfusion**

BASICS OF BLOOD TRANSFUSION

A blood transfusion is a common, safe medical procedure in which healthy blood is given to you through an intravenous (IV) line that has been inserted in one of your blood vessels.

Your blood carries oxygen and nutrients to all parts of your body. Blood transfusions replace blood that is lost through surgery or injury or provide it if your body is not making blood properly. You may need a blood transfusion if you have anemia, sickle cell disease, a bleeding disorder such as hemophilia, or cancer. For people in critical condition, blood transfusions can be lifesaving.

Four types of blood products may be given through blood transfusions: whole blood, red blood cells, platelets, and plasma. Most of the blood used for transfusions comes from whole blood donations given by volunteer blood donors. A person can also have her or his own blood collected and stored a few weeks before surgery in case it is needed.

After a doctor determines that you need a blood transfusion, she or he will test your blood to make sure that the blood you are given matches your blood type. A small needle is used to insert an IV line in one of your blood vessels. Through this line, you

This chapter contains text excerpted from the following sources: Text under the heading "Basics of Blood Transfusion" is excerpted from "Blood Transfusion," National Heart, Lung, and Blood Institute (NHLBI), December 10, 2019; Text beginning with the heading "Key Facts" is excerpted from "Blood Safety Basics," Centers for Disease Control and Prevention (CDC), February 4, 2019; Text under the heading "Understanding Blood Type and Transfusion" is © 2016 Omnigraphics. Reviewed April 2020.

receive healthy blood. Blood transfusions usually take one to four hours to complete. You will be monitored during and after the procedure.

Blood transfusions are usually very safe, because donated blood is carefully tested, handled, and stored. However, there is a small chance that your body may have a mild to severe reaction to the donor blood. Other complications may include fever, heart or lung complications, alloimmunization, and rare but serious reactions in which donated white blood cells attack your body's healthy tissues. Some people have health problems from getting too much iron from frequent transfusions. There is also a very small chance of getting an infectious disease, such as hepatitis B or C or human immunodeficiency virus (HIV) through a blood transfusion. For HIV, that risk is less than one in 1 million. Scientific research and careful medical controls make the supply of donated blood very safe. Blood transfusions are among the most common medical procedures in the nation.

KEY FACTS

- Each day life-saving blood transfusions are needed in hospitals and emergency treatment facilities across the United States.
- There are more than 13.2 million blood donors in the United States, resulting in a total of 17.2 million transfused blood product units per year.
- Most patients do not experience any side effects from blood transfusions. On rare occasions, blood transfusions can cause adverse reactions in the patients receiving blood.
- Although the United States blood supply is safer than ever before, some bacteria, viruses, prions, and parasites can be transmitted by blood transfusions.
- Each donor is screened for risk of transmissible disease by questionnaire, and each unit of blood donated in the United States is routinely screened for various infectious disease pathogens using the U.S. Food and Drug Association (FDA) approved assays.

SCREENING DONATED BLOOD

Blood donors are asked a set of standard questions prior to donating blood to assist in determining if they are in good health and free of any diseases that could be transmitted by blood transfusion. If the donor's answers indicate they are not well or are at risk for having a disease transmissible by blood transfusion, they are not allowed to donate blood.

If the donor is eligible to donate, the donated blood is tested for blood type (ABO group) and Rh type (positive or negative). This is to make sure that patients receive blood that matches their blood type. Before transfusion, the donor and blood unit are also tested for certain proteins (antibodies) that may cause adverse reactions in a person receiving a blood transfusion.

All blood for transfusion is tested for evidence of certain infectious disease pathogens, such as hepatitis B and C viruses and HIV. The tests used to screen donated blood are listed below.

UNDERSTANDING BLOOD TYPE AND TRANSFUSIONS
Blood Typing

Blood typing is a classification system used to sort human blood according to the kinds of antigens (blood proteins) found on red blood cells. There are four primary types of blood: A, B, AB, and O. Each blood type is further classified by an Rh positive or negative designation. Rh refers to "Rhesus factor" and indicates the presence (positive) or absence (negative) of a specific protein found on the surface of red blood cells. Blood type is an inherited trait.

Blood typing is important because not all blood types are compatible with each other. Giving the wrong blood type to a person through a blood transfusion can result in serious complications and even death. Blood typing is especially important for pregnant women. If the expectant mother is Rh-negative and the expectant father is Rh-positive, the mother will need to receive treatment to help protect the fetus from complications that could arise from a mix of incompatible blood types.

Table 19.1. Tests Used to Screen Donated Blood

Infectious Disease Pathogen	Laboratory Tests Used	Frequency of Tests
Hepatitis B virus (HBV)	Hepatitis B surface antigen (HBsAg) detection Hepatitis B core antibody (anti-HBc) detection Nucleic acid amplification testing (NAT) for HBV	Every donation
Hepatitis C virus (HCV)	Hepatitis C virus antibody (anti-HCV) detection Nucleic acid amplification testing (NAT) for HCV	Every donation
Human Immunodeficiency virus Types 1 and 2 (HIV)	HIV-1 and HIV-2 antibody (anti-HIV-1 and anti-HIV-2) detection Nucleic acid amplification testing (NAT) for HIV-1	Every donation
Human T-Lymphotropic Virus Types I and II (HTLV)	HTLV-I and HTLV-II antibody (anti-HTLV-I and anti-HTLV-II) detection	Every donation
Treponema pallidum (syphilis)	Anti-treponemal antibody detection	Every donation
West Nile virus (WNV)	Nucleic acid amplification testing (NAT) for WNV	Every donation
Zika Virus (ZIKV)	Nucleic acid amplification testing (NAT) for ZikV.	Every donation
Bacterial Contamination	Bacterial culture	Every platelet donation
Babesia	Nucleic acid amplification test (NAT) and antibody for *B. microti*	Performed on donations in Babesia-endemic regions
Trypanosoma cruzi (Chagas disease)	*T. cruzi* antibody detection	All first-time donors tested

Table 19.1. Continued

Infectious Disease Pathogen	Laboratory Tests Used	Frequency of Tests
Cytomegalovirus (CMV)	CMV antibody detection	Performed on some donations for special needs recipients

Testing Blood Type

Blood type tests are performed for a variety of reasons. Some of the most common include:

- Classification of donated blood
- Preparation for a blood transfusion or any surgery
- Preparation for organ transplant
- When a woman is pregnant or plans to become pregnant
- Identification of individuals (for example, determining blood relations)

The two most common blood typing tests are the ABO and the Rh tests.

The ABO test examines red blood cells in order to classify the blood as A, B, AB, or O. Blood that is type A contains the A antigen, and type B contains the B antigen. These two blood types are incompatible. Each contains antibodies that will attack and destroy the cells of the other. Type AB blood contains both A and B antigens, meaning that it is compatible with both A and B blood types. People with type AB blood can receive blood from anyone of any blood type, making type AB the "universal recipient." Type O blood contains no antigens, and can be given to anyone of any blood type. For this reason, type O blood is known as the "universal donor."

To test for blood type, a small amount of blood is mixed with serum containing blood antibodies and observed to see if the sample blood cells agglutinate (stick together). Blood cells that stick together when mixed with Anti-A serum is classified as type A. Type B blood cells stick together when mixed with Anti-B serum. Type AB blood cells stick together when mixed with both Anti-A and Anti-B serums. Blood cells that do not stick together when mixed with Anti-A or Anti-B serums is classified as type O.

A second blood type test is performed to verify the results of the first test. In the second test, known as "back-typing," a small amount of the blood being tested is mixed with a small amount of blood that has already been classified as type A or type B and observed for agglutination (sticking together). If the sample blood cells stick together when mixed with type B blood, the sample is identified as type A. Conversely, if the sample blood cells stick together when mixed with type A blood, the sample is identified as type B. If the sample blood cells stick together when mixed with either type A or type B blood, the sample is identified as type AB. If the sample blood cells do not stick together when mixed with type A or type B blood, the sample is identified as type O.

The Rh test is performed by mixing a small blood sample with a serum that contains anti-Rh serum. If the sample blood cells stick together when mixed with anti-Rh serum, the blood is Rh-positive. If the sample blood cells do not stick together when mixed with anti-Rh serum, the blood is Rh-negative. People with Rh-negative blood can only receive Rh-negative blood; people with Rh-positive blood can receive either Rh-positive or Rh-negative blood.

The results of both kinds of blood type testing are used for complete identification of blood type. For example, type A blood that is Rh-positive is A-positive, type B blood that is Rh-negative is B-negative, and so on.

Blood Type Compatibility

- A person with A-negative blood can receive types A-negative and O-negative blood.
- A person with A-positive blood can receive types A-negative, A-positive, O-negative, and O-positive blood.
- A person with B-negative blood can receive types B-negative and O-negative blood.

- A person with B-positive blood can receive types B-negative, B-positive, O-negative, and O-positive blood.
- A person with AB-negative blood can receive types AB-negative and O-negative blood.
- A person with AB-positive blood can receive any type of blood.
- A person with O-negative blood can only receive type O-negative blood.
- A person with O-positive blood can receive O-negative or O-positive blood.

References

1. Gersten, Todd. "Blood Typing," MedlinePlus, National Institutes of Health (NIH), February 24, 2014.
2. "Blood Type Test," WebMD, September 9, 2014.

Chapter 20 | Reducing Anxiety before Surgery

It is natural to feel anxious before surgery no matter how major or minor the procedure is. Even though most of the surgeries occur with relatively few complications, patients tend to feel anxious beforehand. Sometimes, the fear becomes significant, with the patient experiencing physical symptoms including chest pain, racing heart, and nausea.

The source of this anxiety could be an unknown fear, a previous bad experience with surgery, or fear about the outcome of surgery. It is important not to become overwhelmed by anxiety before surgery. While a magic cure for anxiety does not exist, but things, such as relaxation techniques and support from family, friends, and hospital staff go a long way in reducing presurgery stress.

WHAT ARE THE EFFECTS OF ANXIETY BEFORE SURGERY?

For many patients, it is hard not to have anxious feeling about the inherent risks of surgery. Anxiety leads to stress and other related symptoms such as a fast pulse, racing heart, nervous stomach, sleeplessness, and shortness of breath. These symptoms might make it difficult for the patient to properly prepare for surgery or to remember postsurgery instructions.

WHAT CAN BE DONE TO RELIEVE ANXIETY BEFORE SURGERY?

Anxiety is a normal human response. The body is conditioned to protect itself by going into a defensive stance or escaping from danger. This is known as the "fight-or-flight response" and it is responsible for causing the physiological responses in the body when you are anxious. Unfortunately, they are not of much use when no inherent danger exists. Most people learn to adapt to frightening situations over time, but surgery can often be a new and anxiety-inducing event.

Taking the following steps may help ease your anxiety.

Share Your Fears

Talking about your fears is the first step in controlling it. Sharing your thoughts lifts the burden from your mind and results in relief. Also, seek information and determine if there is any basis to your fears or if they are simply unfounded. Talk to the hospital clinical counselor or physician assistant or nurse about your fears. They will be able to understand your anxiety and help alleviate it.

Understand the Surgical Procedure

Fear of the unknown is a primary cause of anxiety and the best way to handle it is to understand what you are getting into. Talk to the surgeon and get to know the surgical procedure and what to expect when it is over. If you are searching the Internet for information, be sure you are sourcing it from credible websites. It is the unanswered questions that cause anxiety. Understanding what you will undergo will calm your nerves. Though it may be clear that surgery is essential for you, it is easy to be confused by medical jargon. Make sure you understand why you need surgery and do not be afraid to get a second opinion.

Learn about Anesthesia

Educate yourself about anesthesia. You may not get a chance to meet the anesthesiologist the day before surgery. So, make an appointment with her or him beforehand. Understand what choices will be available to you. Research the kind of anesthesia you will be given using authoritative websites. You may not have much choice in anesthesia because, after an evaluation of all factors involved, the specific kind of anesthesia to be used is decided only shortly before surgery.

Keep Yourself Busy

Prepare yourself to avoid stress. Take care of chores at home before surgery. Clean your house or if possible make a thorough clean up. Take care of your work and apply for leave if needed. If you have kids, make arrangements for their care while you are in recovery. Tell your partner about things to take care at home, such as cooking meals, so that your absence will not be felt.

Distract Yourself

It is easy to dwell on negative thoughts and brood over them. Don't let your imagination get the better of you. Use common distraction techniques such as reading a book, watching a TV show or movie, or listening to your favorite music. This should keep your mind relaxed and delay your thoughts about surgery until much later.

Use Relaxation Techniques

If you are prone to anxiety, then find out about specific techniques to reduce it. Breathing exercises, meditation, and mindfulness help reduce anxiety, stress, and lowers blood pressure. Such techniques have been scientifically proven to reduce stress and anxiety.

Allow Hospital Staff to Help You

Doctors and nurses at the hospital are well aware of patients' potential anxiety. Most staff try to make wait times minimal and your stay as pleasant as possible. Hospitals have counselors and volunteers on call to offer support and assistance. Make use of their services. Personal coping strategies serve the purpose best, but they tend to be different for each individual.

Do Not Smoke before Surgery

Smoking before surgery is linked to complications and is best avoided even though you think it will help relax you. Smoking adversely affects healing of wounds and you should begin nicotine replacement therapy a few months before surgery if possible in order to reduce risk of complications.

Use of Sedatives

If you are admitted to the hospital the night before surgery you might be given a sedative, usually a benzodiazepine, to make you sleep better and to control anxiety. Sedatives make you drowsy and can cause nausea but they also make you relax and reduce anxiety. You may also be given a sedative an hour or two before anesthesia is administered.

HELPING YOUR CHILD WHO IS ANXIOUS ABOUT SURGERY

It is very important to address concerns about surgery in children because this usually translates to better outcomes after surgery. Children tend to emulate the attitude of parents when it comes to surgery, be it good or bad. If a parent is fearful or anxious, chances are the child becoming fearful too. Children should be told about the surgery in advance and allowed to ask questions. Any anxiety or fearfulness about surgery should be put to rest. It is best not to surprise a child because it could result in a lasting fear of healthcare. Also, it is better to sound positive and upbeat about surgery with your child. She or he should know what the advantages are that will come after surgery.

The approach adopted with children varies with age. Very young children need to be informed just a few days before surgery. Slightly older children may already know what surgery entails and should be given enough opportunities to voice their doubts and fears with doctors and parents. Older children may know the surgical procedure in detail from books, TV, or the Internet. They should meet the surgeon with their parent for a 'reality check' so they understand what the procedure actually entails. Most hospitals offer a presurgery tour and information presentations to relieve anxiety before surgery.

References

1. "What Can Help Relieve Anxiety before Surgery?" PubMed Health, IQWiG (Institute for Quality and Efficiency in Health Care), May 21, 2014.
2. "5 Ways to Calm Your Nerves before Surgery," The Healthcare Management Trust, July 26, 2016.
3. TahoeDoc. "How to Calm Yourself Down before a Day Surgery Procedure," HealDove, April 28, 2017.
4. Whitlock, Jennifer., RN, MSN, FNP-C. "Understanding and Dealing with a Fear of Surgery," VeryWell, April 21, 2016.

Chapter 21 | **Understanding Informed Consent**

INFORMED CONSENT PROCESS

For patients who have decision-making capacity, the informed consent process involves the following outlined procedures. The same process applies to surrogates who make decisions for patients who lack decision-making capacity.

Informing the Patient

During the informed consent process, the practitioner must:
- Provide information that a patient, in similar circumstances, would reasonably want to know.
  - For treatments and procedures that are low risk and are within broadly-accepted standards of medical practice, it is sufficient to obtain oral consent for the entire treatment or procedure without explicitly discussing each of its component elements; for example, a practitioner may obtain consent for a panel of routine blood tests without explicitly discussing that the panel includes tests for sodium, potassium, and chloride.
  - Information about certain tests must be considered "information that a patient in similar circumstances would reasonably want to know" because these tests are particularly sensitive and

This chapter includes text excerpted from "Informed Consent for Clinical Treatments and Procedures," U.S. Department of Veterans Affairs (VA), August 14, 2009. Reviewed April 2020.

may have consequences that the patient might reasonably want to avoid. These tests include, but are not limited to, specific tests to identify illicit drug use, alcohol intoxication, Methicillin-Resistant Staphylococcus aureus (MRSA), and inheritable genetic abnormalities. For these tests, practitioners must obtain specific consent and follow the informed consent process as outlined in the remainder of this paragraph. Signature consent is not required; oral consent is sufficient and must be documented in the patient's electronic health record.

- Describe the recommended treatment or procedure in language that is understandable to the patient. **NOTE:** An interpreter must be provided, if necessary, to achieve this purpose.
- Give a clear and concise explanation of the patient's condition(s) or diagnosis(es) that relates to the recommended treatment or procedure.
- Describe the name, nature, and details of the recommended treatment or procedure, and the indications for that course of action, including the likelihood of success of the recommended treatment or procedure for that particular patient.
- Describe the expected benefits and known risks associated with the recommended treatment or procedure, including problems that might occur during recuperation. For example, discuss the risks of teratogenicity to the fetus when prescribing medications to women of childbearing age. Risks of minor seriousness do not have to be described, unless they commonly occur. Risks that are extremely unlikely do not have to be described, unless the patient requests that information, or unless such risks may result in death or permanent disability.
- Describe reasonable alternative treatments and procedures. The practitioner must:

- Explain why the recommended treatment is thought to be more beneficial to the patient than the alternatives.
- Describe any expected benefits and known risks associated with the alternative treatments and procedures.
- Discuss reasonable alternatives including:
  - The option of no treatment or procedure and the expected benefits and known risks of that option; and
  - Potential emergency responses to known complications of the treatment or procedure that the patient may wish to forgo (e.g., blood transfusion for bleeding during an operation, hysterectomy for complications of an obstetrical procedure, open-heart surgery for complications of an angioplasty).
- Identify by name and profession the practitioner who has primary responsibility for the relevant aspect of the patient's care. Also, identify by name and profession any other individuals responsible for authorizing or performing the treatment or procedure under consideration.
- Advise the patient if another practitioner will need to be substituted for any of those named. If the need for a substitution is known prior to initiating a treatment or procedure that requires signature consent, the patient must be informed of the change and this discussion and the patient's assent must be documented in the patient's electronic health record.
- Advise the patient if the recommended treatment is novel or unorthodox (e.g., nontraditional medicine, alternative medicine for which evidence of efficacy is lacking, and innovative surgical procedures that are not widely used).
- Advise the patient, when relevant, of the patient's responsibilities when undertaking the treatment or

procedure (e.g., taking medications at home, changing own bandages).

- Obtain specific consent for any aspect of the recommended treatment or procedure that involves research.
- Ensure that the patient indicates understanding of the information provided. For example, the practitioner may ask the patient to describe the recommended treatment or procedure in the patient's own words.
- Encourage the patient to ask questions.
- Document all actions, as appropriate.

PROMOTING VOLUNTARY DECISION-MAKING

- The practitioner must promote the patient's voluntary decision-making during the informed consent process. The practitioner must not unduly pressure or coerce the patient into consenting to a particular treatment or procedure, but must instead convey that the patient is free to choose among any recommended treatments and procedures, including no treatment, or to revoke a prior consent without prejudice to the patient's access to future healthcare or other benefits.
- The practitioner is prohibited from attempting to persuade a patient to consent to a particular treatment or procedure by denying, or threatening to deny, the patient access to another procedure or treatment. However, in cases where in the medical judgment of the practitioner a particular treatment or procedure cannot be safely provided or performed without another treatment or procedure also being provided or performed, access to the first treatment or procedure may be made contingent on the patient's consent to the second treatment or procedure.
- Patients must not, as part of the routine practice of obtaining informed consent, be asked to sign consent forms "on the gurney" or after they have been sedated in preparation for a procedure. Exceptions may occur when there is an urgent clinical need.

DOCUMENTING THE INFORMED CONSENT PROCESS

Prior to undertaking any treatment or procedure, the practitioner must obtain informed consent and document the informed consent process in the patient's electronic health record. For certain treatments or procedures, the practitioner must also obtain the patient's signature consent.

- **Treatments and procedures that require only oral informed consent**
  - Treatments and procedures that are low risk and within broadly-accepted standards of medical practice (e.g., administration of most drugs, vaccines, or for the performance of minor procedures, such as routine x-rays) require oral informed consent, but do not require signature consent. Both oral informed consent and signature consent must be documented in the patient's electronic health record. In accordance with policy on documentation of patient records, documentation must be sufficient to serve as a basis to plan patient care, support diagnoses, and warrant treatment. In most cases, a brief statement such as "patient consented to treatment plan" is sufficient for these purposes.
  - For tests that provide information that is particularly sensitive or may have significant consequences for the patient, the patient's oral consent to each test must be explicitly documented. **NOTE:** If specific consent is not obtained or documented, and the patient subsequently objects to the test, the patient must be notified of the patient's right to request that information pertaining to the test be expunged from the patient's electronic health record.
- **Treatments and procedures that require signature consent** Prior to undertaking certain treatments and procedures, the practitioner must document the informed consent process in detail and obtain the patient's signature on an authorized consent form.

193

- The patient's signature consent must be obtained for treatments and procedures that:
  - Can be reasonably expected to produce significant pain or discomfort to the patient
  - Can be reasonably expected to produce pain or discomfort to the patient that is substantial enough to require sedation, anesthesia, or narcotic analgesia
  - Can be reasonably considered to have a significant risk of complication or morbidity
  - Require injections of any substance into a joint space or body cavity (excluding the intravascular space)

NOTE: When sedation or anesthesia is administered in conjunction with a treatment or procedure, a single consent form that includes general information on anesthesia, along with information on the primary procedure or treatment, is sufficient.

- Documentation of the informed consent process for treatments and procedures that require signature consent must include all of the following elements:
  - The practitioner's assessment of whether the patient has decision-making capacity.
  - The name(s) of all the practitioner(s) immediately responsible for the performance of the procedure, and if applicable, the supervision of the treatment or procedure, such as the resident physician and the attending physician.
  - A brief description of the recommended treatment or procedure.
  - A statement that relevant aspects of the treatment or procedure, including indications, benefits, risks, and alternatives including no treatment, have been discussed with the patient in language that the patient can understand; and that the patient indicated comprehension of the discussion.
  - A statement that the patient had an opportunity to ask questions.

- A statement that the practitioner refrained from using coercion.
- The date and time the discussion took place and whether the patient consented to the treatment or procedure.
- The written or valid electronic signature of the patient or the patient's authorized surrogate.
- The written or valid electronic signature of the practitioner writing the note (including the practitioner's legibly written name).
- The signatures need not be witnessed, except when the patient's or surrogate's signature is indicated on the authorized consent form by an "X," in which case two adult witnesses (not including the practitioner) are required to sign the form. The signatures of these witnesses on the form attests only to the fact that the witnesses saw the patient or surrogate and the practitioner sign the form. **NOTE:** If an individual cannot physically document consent, a member of the treatment team may sign on the patient's behalf and document the circumstances of the signature in a progress note. The signing health professional's signature must be witnessed by two adults.
- A properly-executed authorized consent form is valid for a period of 60 calendar days from the date signed. If during this 60-day period there is a significant change in the patient's condition that would reasonably be expected to alter the diagnosis or therapeutic decision, the consent is automatically rescinded and the informed consent process must be repeated for subsequent treatment.
  - Rescission of consent must be documented in the patient's electronic health record.
  - The practitioner who obtained consent or the practitioner responsible for the treatment or procedure for which consent was obtained must certify or verify the patient's rescission.

- When the patient chooses an alternative treatment, including no treatment, or revokes consent. The patient may choose among recommended or alternative treatments and procedures that are consistent with accepted professional standards, including no treatment. Or the patient may revoke a prior consent, even if that decision may increase the risk of serious illness or death, without prejudice to the patient's access to future healthcare or other benefits.
  - If the patient chooses an alternative treatment or procedure, including no treatment, that increases the risk of illness or death, or revokes a prior consent, the progress note must document the patient's reason(s), if known, and the expected outcome.
  - Whenever a patient revokes a prior consent, the responsible practitioner must:
    - Write an addendum to the progress note associated with the prior consent. The addendum must state that the patient revoked the informed consent, document the date of the revocation, as well as the signing date(s) of any form(s) invalidated by this decision. The note must describe the substance of the discussion with the patient, and the reasons for the revocation.
    - Request that the responsible party (typically, the Chief, Health Information Management Service) re-title the progress note associated with the revoked informed consent such that the first word of the note title is "Rescinded" followed by the local note title terminology. For example, change the note title "Informed Consent—General Surgery" to "Rescinded Informed Consent—General Surgery."

Chapter 22 | Ensuring Patient Safety

Chapter Contents

Section 22.1 | Tips to Prevent Medical Errors

This section includes text excerpted from "20 Tips To Help Prevent Medical Errors: Patient Fact Sheet," Agency for Healthcare Research and Quality (AHRQ), U.S. Department of Health and Human Services (HHS), August 2018.

Medical errors can occur anywhere in the healthcare system: in hospitals, clinics, surgery centers, doctors' offices, nursing homes, pharmacies, and patients' homes. Errors can involve medicines, surgery, diagnosis, equipment, or lab reports.

One in seven Medicare patients in hospitals experience a medical error. They can happen during even the most routine tasks, such as when a hospital patient on a salt-free diet is given a high-salt meal.

Most errors result from problems created by today's complex healthcare system. But errors also happen when doctors and patients have problems communicating. These tips tell what you can do to get safer care.

WHAT YOU CAN DO TO STAY SAFE
Hospital Stays

- If you are in a hospital, consider asking all healthcare workers who will touch you whether they have washed their hands.

  Handwashing can prevent the spread of infections in hospitals.
  - When you are being discharged from the hospital, ask your doctor to explain the treatment plan you will follow at home.

This includes learning about your new medicines, making sure you know when to schedule follow-up appointments, and finding out when you can get back to your regular activities.

It is important to know whether or not you should keep taking the medicines you were taking before your hospital stay. Getting clear instructions may help prevent an unexpected return trip to the hospital.

Surgery

- If you are having surgery, make sure that you, your doctor, and your surgeon all agree on exactly what will be done.
- Having surgery at the wrong site (for example, operating on the left knee instead of the right) is rare. But even once is too often. The good news is that wrong-site surgery is 100 percent preventable. Surgeons are expected to sign their initials directly on the site to be operated on before the surgery.
- If you have a choice, choose a hospital where many patients have had the procedure or surgery you need.
- Research shows that patients tend to have better results when they are treated in hospitals that have a great deal of experience with their condition.

Other Steps

- **Speak up if you have questions or concerns**
  You have a right to question anyone who is involved with your care
- **Make sure that someone, such as your primary care doctor, coordinates your care**
  This is especially important if you have many health problems or are in the hospital
- **Make sure that all your doctors have your important health information**
  Do not assume that everyone has all the information they need
- **Ask a family member or friend to go to appointments with you**
  Even if you do not need help now, you might need it later
- **Know that "more" is not always better**
  It is a good idea to find out why a test or treatment is needed and how it can help you. You could be better off without it.

- **If you have a test, do not assume that no news is good news**
  Ask how and when you will get the results
- **Learn about your condition and treatments by asking your doctor and nurse and by using other reliable sources**
  For example, treatment options based on the latest scientific evidence are available from the Effective healthcare Website. Ask your doctor if your treatment is based on the latest evidence.

Section 22.2 | Strategies to Reduce Medication Errors

This section includes text excerpted from "Working to Reduce Medication Errors," U.S. Food and Drug Administration (FDA), August 23, 2019.

A medication error is defined as "any preventable event that may cause or lead to inappropriate medication use or patient harm while the medication is in the control of the healthcare professional, patient, or consumer," according to the National Coordinating Council for Medication Error Reporting and Prevention (NCC MERP).

Medication errors can occur throughout the medication-use system such as, when prescribing a drug, upon entering information into a computer system, when the drug is being prepared or dispensed, or when the drug is given to or taken by a patient.

The U.S. Food and Drug Administration (FDA) receives more than 100,000 U.S. reports each year associated with a suspected medication error. FDA reviews the reports and classifies them to determine the cause and type of error. The reports come from drug manufacturers, and healthcare professionals and consumers through MedWatch—the Agency's safety information and adverse event reporting program. Serious harmful results of a medication error may include:

- Death
- Life-threatening situation
- Hospitalization
- Disability
- Birth defect

LOOKING FOR WAYS TO REDUCE MEDICATION ERRORS

The FDA looks for ways to prevent medication errors. Before drugs are approved for marketing, FDA reviews the drug name, labeling, packaging, and product design to identify and revise information that may contribute to medication errors. For example, FDA reviews:

- Proposed proprietary (brand) names to minimize confusion among drug names. With the help of simulated prescriptions and computerized models, FDA determines the acceptability of proposed proprietary names to minimize medication errors associated with product name confusion.
- Container labels to help healthcare providers and consumers select the right drug product. If a drug is made in multiple strengths—e.g., 5 mg, 10 mg, and 25 mg—the labels of those three containers should be easy to differentiate. The label design may use different colors or identify the strength in large bold numbers and letters.
- Prescribing and patient information to ensure the directions for prescribing, preparing, and use are clear and easy to read.

After drugs are approved for marketing in the United States, FDA monitors and evaluates medication error reports. FDA may require a manufacturer to revise the labels, labeling, packaging, product design, or proprietary name to prevent medication errors. FDA may also issue communications alerting the public about a medication error safety issue, by way of Drug Safety Communications, Drug Safety Alerts, Medication Guides and Drug Safety Podcasts.

The FDA collaborates with external stakeholders, regulators, patient safety organizations, such as the Institute for Safe Medication Practices (ISMP), standard-setting organizations, such as the U.S. Pharmacopeia, and researchers to understand the causes of medication errors, the effectiveness of interventions to prevent them, and to address broader safety issues that may contribute to medication errors.

GETTING THE RIGHT DRUG TO THE RIGHT PATIENT

The FDA also put into place rules requiring barcodes on certain drug and biological product labels. Barcodes allow healthcare professionals to use barcode scanning equipment to verify that the right drug—in the right dose and right route of administration—is being given to the right patient at the right time. This system is intended to help reduce the number of medication errors that occur in hospitals and other healthcare settings.

The FDA has published several guidances to help manufacturers design their drug labels, labeling, packaging, and select drug names in a way to minimize or eliminate hazards that can contribute to medication errors. For example, in 2016, the FDA issued a final guidance titled, Safety Considerations for Product Design to Minimize Medication Errors. To avoid errors and encourage safe use of drugs, the guidance recommendations include:

- Tablets and other oral dosage forms should have distinct and legible imprint codes so healthcare providers and consumers can verify the drug product and strength.
- Oral syringes and other dosing devices copackaged with a liquid oral dosage form should be appropriate for the doses to be measured. Dosing errors have been reported when an oral syringe is labeled in milligrams but the dose is prescribed in milliliters.
- The package design should protect the consumer against incorrect use. Medications applied to the skin (topical) should not be packaged in containers that look like the containers usually associated with eye, ear, nasal, or oral products. Similar looking containers have

resulted in people putting a topical product in the eye, ear, nose, and mouth.

OVER-THE-COUNTER AND PRESCRIPTION DRUG LABELING

According to a Harris Interactive Market Research Poll conducted for the National Council on Patient Information and Education and released in January 2002, consumers tend to overlook important label information on over-the-counter (OTC) drugs. In response to that report, the FDA now requires a standardized "Drug Facts" label on more than 100,000 OTC drug products. Modeled after the Nutrition Facts label on foods, Drug Facts helps consumers compare and select OTC medicines, and follow instructions. The label clearly lists active ingredients, inactive ingredients, uses, warnings, dosage, directions, and other information, such as how to store the medicine.

In 2006, the FDA revised its rules for the content and format of prescribing information for prescription drug and biological products. The new look helps healthcare professionals find the information they need more easily and quickly. The FDA also makes updated prescribing information available on the Web at Drugs@FDA.

CONSUMERS PLAY AN IMPORTANT ROLE

Consumers can also play an important role in reducing medication errors. Here are some drug safety tips:

- Know the various risks and causes for medication errors.
- Find out what drug you are taking and what it is for. Rather than simply letting the doctor write you a prescription and send you on your way, be sure to ask the name of the drug and the purpose of the drug.
- Find out how to take the drug and make sure you understand the directions. Ask if the medicine needs to be kept in the refrigerator.
- Check the container's label every time you take a drug. This is especially important if you are taking several

drugs because it will lower your risk of accidentally taking the wrong medicine.

- Keep drugs stored in their original containers. Many pills look alike, so keeping them in their original containers will help know the name of the drug and how to take them. If you are having trouble keeping multiple medications straight, ask your doctor or pharmacist about helpful aids.
- Keep an updated list of all medications taken for health reasons, including OTC drugs, supplements, medicinal herbs, and other substances. Give a copy of this list to your healthcare provider.
- Be aware of the risk of drug/drug or drug/food interactions.
- If in doubt or you have questions about your medication, ask your pharmacist or other healthcare provider.
- Report suspected medication errors to MedWatch.

Section 22.3 | Preventing Healthcare-Associated Infections

This section includes text excerpted from "Getting Medical Care? How to Avoid Getting an Infection," Centers for Disease Control and Prevention (CDC), March 2, 2020.

GETTING MEDICAL CARE? HOW TO AVOID GETTING AN INFECTION
Learn 10 Things You Can Do to Avoid Getting an Infection

People receiving medical care sometimes develop infections so serious they may lead to sepsis or death. It can happen in any medical facility such as a hospital, outpatient clinic, dialysis center, or long-term care facility.

These are called "healthcare-associated infections"—and are often associated with devices used in medical procedures, such as catheters or ventilators.

Healthcare-associated infections can be caused by bacteria that are resistant to antibiotics, making them difficult to treat. Although national progress is being made to prevent these infections, there is more to do, especially in fighting antibiotic-resistant bacteria. As a patient, you can help prevent the spread of infections and improve antibiotic use.

HERE ARE 10 THINGS YOU CAN DO TO PROTECT YOURSELF AND YOUR LOVED ONES

1. **Speak up.** Talk to your doctor about any questions or worries. Ask what they are doing to protect you.
2. **Keep hands clean.** Make sure everyone, including friends and family, clean their hands before touching you. If you do not see your healthcare providers clean their hands, ask them to do so.
3. **Ask each day if your central line catheter or urinary catheter is necessary.** Leaving a catheter in place too long increases the chances you will get an infection. Let your doctor or nurse know immediately if the area around the central line becomes sore or red, or if the bandage falls off or looks wet or dirty.
4. **Prepare for surgery.** Let your doctor know about any medical problems you have. Ask your doctor how she or he prevents surgical site infections.
5. **Ask your healthcare provider,** "Will there be a new needle, new syringe, and a new vial for this procedure or injection?" Insist that your healthcare providers never reuse a needle or syringe on more than one patient.
6. **Get Smart about antibiotics.** Antibiotics only treat bacterial infections–they do not work for viruses like the ones that cause colds and flu. Ask your healthcare provider if there are steps you can take to feel better without using antibiotics. If you are prescribed an antibiotic, make sure to take the prescribed antibiotic exactly as your healthcare provider tells you and do not skip doses.
7. **Watch out for deadly diarrhea (aka Clostridium difficile).** Tell your doctor if you have 3 or more diarrhea

episodes in 24 hours, especially if you have been taking an antibiotic.

8. **Know the signs and symptoms of infection.** Some skin infections, such as Methicillin-resistant *Staphylococcus aureus* (MRSA), appear as redness, pain, or drainage at an IV catheter site or surgery site and come with a fever. Infections can also lead to sepsis, a complication caused by the body's overwhelming and life-threatening response to an infection.

9. **Get Vaccinated.** Getting yourself, family, friends, and caregivers vaccinated against the flu and other infections prevents spread of disease.

10. **Cover your mouth and nose.** When you sneeze or cough, germs can travel three feet or more. Use a tissue to avoid spreading germs with your hands.

Healthcare-associated infections are not only a problem for healthcare facilities—they represent a public-health issue. Many people and organizations are working together to attack these largely preventable infections. The Centers for Disease Control and Prevention (CDC) is committed to preventing healthcare-associated infections and making healthcare safer for everyone.

Chapter 23 | What Medicare Covers If You Are Having Surgery

If you are enrolled in Original Medicare, it is not always easy to find out if Medicare will cover a service or supply that you need. Generally, Medicare covers services (such as lab tests, surgeries, and doctor visits) and supplies (such as wheelchairs and walkers) that Medicare considers "medically necessary" to treat a disease or condition.

What Medicare covers may be based on several factors, like:
- Federal laws describing Medicare benefits, or state laws that tell what services a particular type of practitioner is licensed to provide
- National coverage decisions made by Medicare about whether a particular item or service is covered nationally under Medicare's rules
- Local coverage decisions made by local companies in each state that process claims for Medicare. These companies decide whether an item or service is medically necessary and should be covered in that area under Medicare's rules.

There may be other coverage rules and policies that also apply. Some services may only be covered when you get them in certain settings, or covered for patients with certain conditions. For

This chapter includes text excerpted from "Learning What Medicare Covers and How Much You Pay," Centers for Medicare & Medicaid Services (CMS), July 2019.

example, some surgeries, like organ transplants, can only be done in certain approved hospitals. If you are in a Medicare Advantage Plan or other Medicare health plan, you may have different rules, but your plan must give you at least the same coverage as Original Medicare.

WHERE CAN YOU LEARN MORE ABOUT WHAT MEDICARE COVERS?

- Talk to your doctor or other healthcare provider about why you need the service or supply and ask whether she or he thinks Medicare will cover it. Your doctor or provider knows more than anyone about your individual medical needs.
- Check your "Medicare & You" handbook mailed to you each fall. Your handbook has this information:
  - A general list of services covered by Medicare Part A (Hospital Insurance) such as inpatient hospital stays, home health services, hospice care, and care in a skilled nursing facility
  - A general list of services covered by Medicare Part B (Medical Insurance) such as preventive services, lab tests, x-rays, doctor services, and more
  - Information on getting Medicare benefits through private health plans (Part C) and Medicare prescription drug coverage (Part D)
  - General information on coinsurance and copayment amounts
  - Yearly deductibles for Part A and Part B services, and other costs under Part C and Part D
  To view or download this booklet, visit Medicare.gov/publications. You can also call 800-MEDICARE (800-633-4227). TTY users can call 877-486-2048.
- Call 800-MEDICARE to see if they have information on any related local or national coverage policies.

If there is a service or supply that Medicare usually covers that your doctor, healthcare provider, or supplier thinks Medicare would not cover in your specific case, she or he must give you a Medicare notice, like an "Advance Beneficiary Notice of Noncoverage," and ask you to sign it. Read this notice carefully to understand your options and payment responsibilities. You will be asked if you want to get the items or services listed on the notice and you will have to pay for them if Medicare does not.

Note: The type of notice you get depends on the healthcare setting and services you are getting.

IF YOU ARE HAVING SURGERY, HOW DO YOU FIND OUT HOW MUCH YOU WILL HAVE TO PAY?

For surgeries or procedures, it may be difficult to know the exact costs in advance because no one knows exactly the amount or type of services you will need. For example, if you experience complications during surgery, your costs could be higher.

If you are having surgery or a procedure, there are some things you can do in advance to determine approximately what your share of the cost may be:

- Ask the doctor or healthcare provider if they can tell you how much the surgery or procedure will cost and how much you will have to pay. Learn how Medicare covers inpatient versus outpatient hospital services. Visit Medicare.gov or call 800-MEDICARE (800-633-4227). TTY users can call 877-486-2048.
- Look at your last "Medicare Summary Notice" to see if you met the deductible for Part A (Hospital Insurance) if you expect to be admitted to the hospital, or the deductible for Part B (Medical Insurance) for a doctor's visit and other outpatient care. You will need to pay the deductible amounts before Medicare will start to pay. After Medicare starts to pay, you may have copayments for the care you get.
- Check with any other insurance you may have such as Medicare Supplement Insurance (Medigap), Medicaid, or an employer retiree insurance plan, to see what they will pay. If you belong to a Medicare health plan, contact the plan for more information.

- Call the hospital or facility and ask them to tell you the copayment for the specific surgery or procedure the doctor is planning. It is important to remember that if you need other unexpected services, your costs may be higher.
- Ask your doctor, surgeon, or other healthcare provider, or their staff what kind of care or services you may need after your surgery or procedure and how much you will have to pay.

HOW CAN YOU KEEP YOUR COSTS DOWN?

- Make sure that your Medicare card is valid and that you have paid your Medicare Part B premium.
- Ask your doctor, other healthcare provider, or supplier if they accept assignment. Assignment means your doctor, provider, or supplier has signed an agreement with Medicare (or is required by law) to accept the Medicare-approved amount as full payment for covered services. This can help keep your costs down.
- If you have limited income and resources, you might qualify for Extra Help to pay for some of your healthcare and prescription drug costs.

Chapter 24 | Advance Care Planning

Advance care planning is not just about old age. At any age, a medical crisis could leave you too ill to make your own healthcare decisions. Even if you are not sick now, planning for healthcare in the future is an important step toward making sure you get the medical care you would want, if you are unable to speak for yourself and doctors and family members are making the decisions for you. Many Americans face questions about medical treatment but may not be capable of making those decisions, for example, in an emergency or at the end of life. This chapter explain the types of decisions that may need to be made in such cases and questions you can think about now so you are prepared later. It can helps you think about who you would want to make decisions for you if you cannot make them yourself. It will also discusses ways you can share your wishes with others. Knowing who you want to make decisions on your behalf and how you would decide might take some of the burden off family and friends.

WHAT IS ADVANCE CARE PLANNING?

Advance care planning involves learning about the types of decisions that might need to be made, considering those decisions ahead of time, and then letting others know—both your family and your healthcare providers—about your preferences. These preferences are often put into an advance directive, a legal document that goes into effect only if you are incapacitated and unable to speak

This chapter includes text excerpted from "Advance Care Planning: Healthcare Directives," National Institute on Aging (NIA), National Institutes of Health (NIH), January 15, 2018.

for yourself. This could be the result of disease or severe injury—no matter how old you are. It helps others know what type of medical care you want.

An advance directive also allows you to express your values and desires related to end-of-life care. You might think of it as a living document—one that you can adjust as your situation changes because of new information or a change in your health.

ADVANCE CARE PLANNING DECISIONS

Sometimes advance care planning decisions must be made about the use of emergency treatments to keep you alive. Doctors can use several artificial or mechanical ways to try to do this. Decisions that might come up at this time relate to:

- Cardiopulmonary resuscitation (CPR)
- Ventilator use
- Artificial nutrition (tube feeding) and artificial hydration (IV, or intravenous, fluids)
- Comfort care

What is CPR? Cardiopulmonary resuscitation might restore your heartbeat if your heart stops or is in a life-threatening abnormal rhythm. It involves repeatedly pushing on the chest with force, while putting air into the lungs. This force has to be quite strong, and sometimes ribs are broken or a lung collapses. Electric shocks, known as "defibrillation," and medicines might also be used as part of the process. The heart of a young, otherwise healthy person might resume beating normally after CPR. Often, CPR does not succeed in older adults who have multiple chronic illnesses or who are already frail.

Using a ventilator as emergency treatment. Ventilators are machines that help you breathe. A tube connected to the ventilator is put through the throat into the trachea (windpipe) so the machine can force air into the lungs. Putting the tube down the throat is called "intubation." Because the tube is uncomfortable, medicines are often used to keep you sedated while on a ventilator. If you are expected to remain on a ventilator for a long time, a doctor may perform a tracheotomy or "trach" (rhymes with "make").

During this bedside surgery, the tube is inserted directly into the trachea through a hole in the neck. For long-term help with breathing, a trach is more comfortable, and sedation is not needed. People using such a breathing tube are not able to speak without special help because exhaled air does not go past their vocal cords.

Using artificial nutrition and hydration near the end of life. If you are not able to eat, you may be fed through a feeding tube that is threaded through the nose down to your stomach. If tube feeding is still needed for an extended period, a feeding tube may be surgically inserted directly into your stomach. Hand-feeding (sometimes called "assisted oral feeding") is an alternative to tube feeding. This approach may have fewer risks, especially for people with dementia.

If you are not able to drink, you may be provided with intravenous (IV) fluids. These are delivered through a thin plastic tube inserted into a vein.

Artificial nutrition and hydration can be helpful if you are recovering from an illness. However, studies have shown that artificial nutrition toward the end of life does not meaningfully prolong life. Artificial nutrition and hydration may also be harmful if the dying body cannot use the nutrition properly.

What is comfort care at the end of life? Comfort care is anything that can be done to soothe you and relieve suffering while staying in line with your wishes. Comfort care includes managing shortness of breath; limiting medical testing; providing spiritual and emotional counseling; and giving medication for pain, anxiety, nausea, or constipation.

GETTING STARTED WITH ADVANCE CARE PLANNING

Start with advance care planning by thinking about what kind of treatment you do or do not want in a medical emergency. It might help to talk with your doctor about how your current health conditions might influence your health in the future. For example, what decisions would you or your family face if your high blood pressure leads to a stroke. You can ask your doctor to help you understand and think through your choices before you put them in writing. Discussing advance care planning decisions with your doctor is free through Medicare during your annual wellness visit. Private health insurance may also cover these discussions.

If you do not have any medical issues now, your family medical history might be a clue to help you think about the future. Talk with your doctor about decisions that might come up if you develop health problems similar to those of other family members.

In considering treatment decisions, your personal values are key. Is your main desire to have the most days of life? Or, would your focus be on quality of life, as you see it? What if an illness leaves you paralyzed or in a permanent coma and you need to be on a ventilator? Would you want that?

What makes life meaningful to you? If your heart stops or you have trouble breathing, would you want to undergo life-saving measures if it meant that, in the future, you could be well enough to spend time with your family? Would you be content if the emergency leaves you simply able to spend your days listening to books on tape or gazing out the window?

But, there are many other scenarios that would help you decide:

- If a stroke leaves you unable to move and then your heart stops, would you want CPR? What if you were also mentally impaired by a stroke—does your decision change?
- What if you are in pain at the end of life? Do you want medication to treat the pain, even if it will make you more drowsy and lethargic?
- What if you are permanently unconscious and then develop pneumonia? Would you want antibiotics and to be placed on a ventilator?

For some people, staying alive as long as medically possible, or long enough to see an important event like a grandchild's wedding, is the most important thing. An advance directive can help to make that possible. Others have a clear idea about when they would no longer want to prolong their life. An advance directive can help with that, too.

Your decisions about how to handle any of these situations could be different at age 40 than at age 85. Or, they could be different if you have an incurable condition as opposed to being generally healthy. An advance directive allows you to provide instructions for these types of situations and then to change the instructions as you get older or if your viewpoint changes.

MAKING YOUR ADVANCE CARE WISHES KNOWN

There are two main elements in an advance directive—a living will and a durable power of attorney for healthcare. There are also other documents that can supplement your advance directive. You can choose which documents to create, depending on how you want decisions to be made. These documents include:

- Living will
- Durable power of attorney for healthcare
- Other advance care planning documents

Living will. A living will is a written document that helps you tell doctors how you want to be treated if you are dying or permanently unconscious and cannot make your own decisions about emergency treatment. In a living will, you can say which of the procedures you would want, which ones you would not want, and under which conditions each of your choices applies.

Durable power of attorney for healthcare. A durable power of attorney for healthcare is a legal document naming a healthcare proxy, someone to make medical decisions for you at times when you are unable to do so. Your proxy, also known as a "representative," "surrogate," or "agent," should be familiar with your values and wishes. This means that she or he will be able to decide as you would when treatment decisions need to be made. A proxy can be chosen in addition to or instead of a living will. Having a healthcare proxy helps you plan for situations that cannot be foreseen, like a serious auto accident.

Some people are reluctant to put specific health decisions in writing. For them, naming a healthcare agent might be a good approach, especially if there is someone they feel comfortable talking with about their values and preferences. A named proxy can evaluate each situation or treatment option independently.

Other advance care planning documents. You might also want to prepare documents to express your wishes about a single medical issue or something not already covered in your advance directive. A living will usually covers only the specific life-sustaining treatments discussed earlier. You might want to give your healthcare proxy specific instructions about other issues, such as blood transfusion or kidney dialysis. This is especially important if your doctor suggests that, given your health condition, such treatments might be needed in the future.

Medical issues that might arise at the end of life include:
- DNR orders
- Organ and tissue donation
- POLST and MOLST forms

A **DNR (do not resuscitate) order** tells medical staff in a hospital or nursing facility that you do not want them to try to return your heart to a normal rhythm if it stops or is beating unsustainably using CPR or other life-support measures. Sometimes this document is referred to as a "DNAR (do not attempt resuscitation)" or an "AND (allow natural death)" order. Even though a living will might say CPR is not wanted, it is helpful to have a DNR order as part of your medical file if you go to a hospital. Posting a DNR next to your bed might avoid confusion in an emergency situation. Without a DNR order, medical staff will make every effort to restore your breathing and the normal rhythm of your heart.

A similar document, called a **"DNI (do not intubate) order,"** tells medical staff in a hospital or nursing facility that you do not want to be put on a breathing machine.

A **nonhospital DNR order** will alert emergency medical personnel to your wishes regarding measures to restore your heartbeat or breathing if you are not in the hospital.

Organ and tissue donation allow organs or body parts from a generally healthy person who has died to be transplanted into people who need them. Commonly, the heart, lungs, pancreas, kidneys, corneas, liver, and skin are donated. There is no age limit for organ and tissue donation. You can carry a donation card in your wallet. Some states allow you to add this decision to your driver's license. Some people also include organ donation in their advance care planning documents.

At the time of death, family members may be asked about organ donation. If those close to you, especially your proxy, know how you feel about organ donation, they will be ready to respond. There is no cost to the donor's family for this gift of life. If the person has requested a DNR order but wants to donate organs, she or he might have to indicate that the desire to donate supersedes the DNR. That is because it might be necessary to use machines to keep the heart beating until the medical staff is ready to remove the donated organs.

POLST and MOLST forms provide guidance about your medical care preferences in the form of a doctor's orders. Typically you create a POLST (Physician Orders for Life-Sustaining Treatment) or MOLST (Medical Orders for Life-Sustaining Treatment) when you are near the end of life or critically ill and know the specific decisions that might need to be made on your behalf. These forms serve as a medical order in addition to your advance directive. They make it possible for you to provide guidance that healthcare professionals can act on immediately in an emergency.

A number of states use POLST and MOLST forms, which are filled out by your doctor or sometimes by a nurse practitioner or physician's assistant. The doctor fills out a POLST or MOLST after discussing your wishes with you and your family. Once signed by your doctor, this form has the same authority as any other medical order. Check with your state department of health to find out if these forms are available where you live.

HOW TO CHOOSE YOUR HEALTHCARE PROXY

If you decide to choose a proxy, think about people you know who share your views and values about life and medical decisions. Your proxy might be a family member, a friend, your lawyer, or someone in your social or spiritual community. It is a good idea to also name an alternate proxy. It is especially important to have a detailed living will if you choose not to name a proxy.

You can decide how much authority your proxy has over your medical care—whether she or he is entitled to make a wide range of decisions or only a few specific ones. Try not to include guidelines that make it impossible for the proxy to fulfill her or his duties. For example, it is probably not unusual for someone to say in conversation, "I don't want to go to a nursing home," but think carefully about whether you want a restriction like that in your advance directive. Sometimes, for financial or medical reasons, that may be the best choice for you.

Of course, check with those you choose as your healthcare proxy and alternate before you name them officially. Make sure they are comfortable with this responsibility.

MAKING YOUR HEALTHCARE DIRECTIVES OFFICIAL

Once you have talked with your doctor and have an idea of the types of decisions that could come up in the future and whom you would like as a proxy, if you want one at all, the next step is to fill out the legal forms detailing your wishes. A lawyer can help but is not required. If you decide to use a lawyer, do not depend on her or him to help you understand different medical treatments. Start the planning process by talking with your doctor.

Many states have their own advance directive forms. Your local Area Agency on Aging can help you locate the right forms. You can find your area agency phone number by calling the Eldercare Locator toll-free at 800-677-1116 or by visiting eldercare.acl.gov.

Some states require your advance directive to be witnessed; a few require your signature to be notarized. A notary is a person licensed by the state to witness signatures. You might find a notary at your bank, post office, or local library, or call your insurance agent. Some notaries charge a fee.

Some states have registries that can store your advance directive for quick access by healthcare providers, your proxy, and anyone else to whom you have given permission. Private firms also will store your advance directive. There may be a fee for storing your form in a registry. If you store your advance directive in a registry and later make changes, you must replace the original with the updated version in the registry.

Some people spend a lot of time in more than one state—for example, visiting children and grandchildren. If that is your situation, consider preparing an advance directive using forms for each state—and keep a copy in each place, too.

WHAT TO DO AFTER YOU SET UP YOUR ADVANCE DIRECTIVE

Give copies of your advance directive to your healthcare proxy and alternate proxy. Give your doctor a copy for your medical records. Tell close family members and friends where you keep a copy. If you have to go to the hospital, give staff there a copy to include in your records. Because you might change your advance directive in the future, it is a good idea to keep track of who receives a copy. Review your advance care planning decisions from time to time— for example, every 10 years, if not more often. You might want to revise your preferences for care if your situation or your health changes. Or, you might want to make adjustments if you receive a serious diagnosis; if you get married, separated, or divorced; if your spouse dies; or if something happens to your proxy or alternate. If your preferences change, you will want to make sure your doctor, proxy, and family know about them.

BE PREPARED

What happens if you have no advance directive or have made no plans and you become unable to speak for yourself? In such cases, the state where you live will assign someone to make medical decisions on your behalf. This will probably be your spouse, your parents if they are available, or your children if they are adults. If you have no family members, the state will choose someone to represent your best interests.

Always remember. An advance directive is only used if you are in danger of dying and need certain emergency or special measures to keep you alive, but you are not able to make those decisions on your own. An advance directive allows you to make your wishes about medical treatment known.

It is difficult to predict the future with certainty. You may never face a medical situation where you are unable to speak for yourself and make your wishes known. But having an advance directive may give you and those close to you some peace of mind.

Chapter 25 | **Medical Tourism**

GOING ABROAD FOR MEDICAL CARE

"Medical tourism" refers to traveling to another country for medical care. It is estimated that thousands of United States residents travel abroad for medical care each year. Many factors influence the decision to seek medical care overseas. Some people travel for care because treatment is cheaper in another country. Others may be immigrants to the United States who prefer to return to their home country for healthcare. Still, others may travel to receive a procedure or therapy not available in the United States. The most common procedures that people undergo on medical tourism trips include cosmetic surgery, dentistry, and heart surgery.

RISKS OF MEDICAL TOURISM

The specific risks of medical tourism depend on the area being visited and the procedures performed, but some general issues have been identified:

- Communication may be a challenge. Receiving care at a facility where you do not speak the language fluently might increase the chance that misunderstandings will arise about your care.
- Medication may be counterfeit or of poor quality in some countries.

This chapter includes text excerpted from "Medical Tourism: Getting Medical Care in Another Country," Centers for Disease Control and Prevention (CDC), October 23, 2017.

- Antibiotic resistance is a global problem, and resistant bacteria may be more common in other countries than in the United States.
- Flying after surgery can increase the risk for blood clots.

WHAT YOU CAN DO

- If you are planning to travel to another country for medical care, see a travel medicine provider at least four to six weeks before the trip to discuss general information for healthy travel and to learn about specific risks related to the procedure and to travel before and after the procedure.
- Make sure that any current medical conditions you have are well controlled, and that your regular healthcare provider knows about your plans for travel and medical care overseas.
- Check the qualifications of the healthcare providers who will be doing the procedure and the credentials of the facility where the procedure will be done. Remember that foreign standards for healthcare providers and facilities may be different from those of the United States. Accrediting groups, including Joint Commission International (JCI), DNV International Accreditation for Hospitals, and the International Society for Quality in Healthcare (ISQua), have lists of standards that facilities need to meet to be accredited.
- Make sure you have a written agreement with the healthcare facility or the group arranging the trip, defining what treatments, supplies, and care are covered by the costs of the trip.
- If you go to a country where you do not speak the local language, determine ahead of time how you will communicate with your doctor and other people who are caring for you.
- Take with you copies of your medical records that include the lab and other studies done related to the condition for

which you are obtaining care and any allergies you may have.

- Bring copies of all your prescriptions and a list of all the medicines you take, including their brand names, generic names, manufacturers, and dosages.
- Arrange for follow-up care with your local healthcare provider before you leave.
- Before planning vacation activities such as sunbathing, drinking alcohol, swimming, or taking long tours, find out if those activities are permitted after surgery.
- Get copies of all your medical records before you return home.

Part 3 | Common Types of Surgery and Surgical Procedures

Chapter 26 | **Head and Neck Surgery**

Chapter Contents

Section 26.1 | Treating Head and Neck Cancers

This section includes text excerpted from "Head and Neck Cancers," National Cancer Institute (NCI), March 29, 2017.

WHAT ARE CANCERS OF THE HEAD AND NECK?

Cancers that are known collectively as head and neck cancers usually begin in the squamous cells that line the moist, mucosal surfaces inside the head and neck (for example, inside the mouth, the nose, and the throat). These squamous cell cancers are often referred to as "squamous cell carcinomas" of the head and neck. Head and neck cancers can also begin in the salivary glands, but salivary gland cancers are relatively uncommon. Salivary glands contain many different types of cells that can become cancerous, so there are many different types of salivary gland cancer.

WHAT ARE THE SIDE EFFECTS OF SURGERY?

Surgery for head and neck cancers often changes the patient's ability to chew, swallow, or talk. The patient may look different after surgery, and the face and neck may be swollen. The swelling usually goes away within a few weeks. However, if lymph nodes are removed, the flow of lymph in the area where they were removed may be slower and lymph could collect in the tissues, causing additional swelling; this swelling may last for a long time.

After a laryngectomy (surgery to remove the larynx) or other surgery in the neck, parts of the neck and throat may feel numb because nerves have been cut. If lymph nodes in the neck were removed, the shoulder and neck may become weak and stiff.

OTHER FORMS OF HEAD AND NECK CANCER SURGERIES

Depending on the location of the cancer and the type of treatment, rehabilitation may include physical therapy, dietary counseling, speech therapy, and/or learning how to care for a stoma. A "stoma" is an opening into the windpipe through which a patient breathes after a laryngectomy—surgery to remove the larynx.

Sometimes, especially with cancer of the oral cavity, a patient may need reconstructive and plastic surgery to rebuild bones or tissues. However, reconstructive surgery may not always be possible because of damage to the remaining tissue from the original surgery or from radiation therapy. If reconstructive surgery is not possible, a prosthodontist may be able to make a prosthesis (an artificial dental and/or facial part) to restore satisfactory swallowing, speech, and appearance. Patients will receive special training on how to use the device.

Eating may be difficult after treatment for head and neck cancer. Some patients receive nutrients directly into a vein after surgery or need a feeding tube until they can eat on their own. A feeding tube is a flexible plastic tube that is passed into the stomach through the nose or an incision in the abdomen. A nurse or speech-language pathologist can help patients learn how to swallow again after surgery.

Section 26.2 | Brain Tumor Surgery

This section contains text excerpted from the following sources: Text beginning with the heading "Neurosurgery" is excerpted from "Brain and Spinal Cord Tumors: Hope Through Research," National Institute of Neurological Disorders and Stroke (NINDS), December 31, 2019; Text under the heading "Types of Tumor and It is Standard Treatment" is excerpted from "Standard Treatment and Surgery Codes," Surveillance, Epidemiology, and End Results Program (SEER), National Cancer Institute (NCI), October 30, 2003. Reviewed April 2020.

NEUROSURGERY

Surgery is usually the first step in treating an accessible tumor—one that can be removed without unacceptable risk of neurological damage. Surgery is aimed at removing all or as much tumor as possible (called "resecting" or "excising") and can often slow worsening of neurological function.

An inaccessible or inoperable tumor is one that cannot be removed surgically because of the risk of severe nervous system damage during the operation. These tumors are frequently located deep within the brain or near vital structures, such as the brain stem.

A biopsy is sometimes performed to help doctors determine how to treat a tumor. A brain biopsy involves surgically removing a small part of the skull to sample the tumor tissue. Biopsies can sometimes be performed by a needle inserted through a small hole. A small piece of tissue remains in the hollow needle when it is removed from the body. A pathologist will stain and examine the tissue for certain changes that signal cancer and grade it to reflect the degree of malignancy.

If the sample is cancerous, the surgeons will remove as much of the tumor as possible. For some primary brain tumors it is not possible to surgically remove all malignant cells. Malignant brain tumors commonly recur from cells that have spread from the original tumor mass into the surrounding brain tissue. In contrast, many benign tumors and secondary metastatic tumors can be completely removed surgically.

In some cases, a surgeon may need to insert a shunt into the skull to drain any dangerous buildup of cerebrospinal fluid (CSF) caused by the tumor. A shunt is a flexible plastic tube that is used to divert the flow of CSF from the central nervous system to another part of the body, where it can be absorbed as part of the normal circulatory process.

Fortunately, research has led to advances in neurosurgery that make it possible for doctors to completely remove many tumors that were previously thought to be inoperable. These new techniques and tools let neurosurgeons operate within the tight, vulnerable confines of the central nervous system (CNS). Some tools used in the operating room include a surgical microscope, the endoscope (a small viewing tube attached to a video camera), and miniature precision instruments that allow surgery to be performed through a small incision in the brain or spine.

Intraoperative MRI uses a special type of MRI to provide a real-time evaluation of the surgery. Constantly updated images that are provided during surgery let doctors see how much tumor material has been removed. Intraoperative MRI can also help doctors choose the best surgical approaches and monitor any complications during surgery.

Navigation equipment used in computer-guided, or stereo-tactic, neurosurgery gives doctors a precise, three-dimensional map of an individual's spine or brain as the operation progresses. A computer uses preoperative diagnostic images of the individual to reduce the risk of damage to surrounding tissue.

Intraoperative nerve monitoring tests, such as evoked potentials use real-time recordings of nerve cell activity to determine the role of specific nerves and monitor brain activity as the surgery progresses. Small electrodes are used to stimulate a nerve and measure its electrical response (or evoked potential). Some surgeries may be done while the individual is awake under monitored anesthesia care, rather than under general anesthesia. This allows doctors to monitor the individual's speech and motor functions as a tumor is being removed.

A possible side effect of surgery is swelling around the site of the tumor, and can be treated with steroids. Bleeding into the tumor site or infection are other serious risks of brain surgery.

In the case of metastatic tumors, doctors usually treat the original cancer. However, if there are only one or two metastases to the brain or if a metastatic tumor causes serious disability or pain, doctors may recommend surgery—even if the original cancer has not been controlled.

Surgery may be the beginning and end of your treatment if the biopsy shows a benign tumor. If the tumor is malignant, doctors often recommend additional treatment, including radiation and chemotherapy, or one of several experimental treatments.

TYPES OF TUMOR AND ITS STANDARD TREATMENT
Table 26.1. Standard Treatment and Surgery Codes

Tumor	Treatment
Astrocytoma, noninfil.	S(+R)
Astrocytoma, anaplastic	S+R
Astrocytoma, high grade	S+R(+C)
Glioblastoma multiforme	S+R+C
Brain stem glioma	R
Ependymoma, w-d	S(+R)
Ependymoma, anaplastic	S+R
Oligodendroglioma	S(+R)
Oligodendroglioma, anaplastic	S+R(+C)
Mixed glioma	S+R(+C)
Medulloblastoma	S(+R)
Pineal parenchymal tumor	S+R(+C)
CNS germ cell tumor	S(+R)
Craniopharyngioma	S(+R)
Meningioma, w-d	S(+R)
Meningioma, malignant	S+R

R = Radiation therapy
S = Surgery
C = Chemotherapy
( ) = Optional treatments

Section 26.3 | **Middle Ear Infections**

This section contains text excerpted from the following sources: Text Under the heading "Myringotomy" is excerpted from "Myringotomy," U.S. Department of Veterans Affairs (VA), July 2005. Reviewed April 2020; Text under the heading "Background and Objectives" is excerpted from "Tympanostomy Tubes in Children With Otitis Media," Effective Healthcare Program, Agency for Healthcare Research and Quality (AHRQ), May 2017; Text under the heading "Ear Tubes under Local Anesthesia to Treat Ear Infection" is excerpted from "FDA Approves System for the Delivery of Ear Tubes under Local Anesthesia to Treat Ear Infection," U.S. Food and Drug Administration (FDA), November 25, 2019.

OTITIS MEDIA

Otitis media is often preceded by a viral upper respiratory tract infection that causes eustachian tube obstruction, negative middle ear pressure, and accumulation of fluid in the normally air-filled space of the middle ear. Acute otitis media (AOM) is defined as the presence of fluid in the middle ear with signs and symptoms of an acute infection, such as fever and ear pain. Otitis media with effusion (OME) is defined as the presence of fluid in the middle ear behind an intact tympanic membrane without signs and symptoms of an acute infection. OME is defined as chronic OME, if effusion persists for three months or longer. Acute otitis media and chronic OME have shared causes. Children with chronic OME are prone to recurrent AOM episodes, and after an AOM episode all children have OME for some time. Chronic OME can result in hearing deficits, which puts a child at risk for speech and language delays, behavioral changes, and poor academic achievement. Recurrent AOM has been shown to impact quality of life (QOL) for patients and their caregivers. Certain children, including those with Down syndrome and cleft palate, have a very high risk for middle ear disease. The American Academy of Otolaryngology—Head and Neck Surgery (AAO-HNS).

Clinical practice guideline (CPG) identifies a subpopulation of children who may be at increased risk for speech, language, or learning problems from otitis media because of baseline sensory, physical, cognitive, or behavioral factors.

Myringotomy with tympanostomy tube (TT) placement is the most common ambulatory surgery performed on children in the United States, with 667,000 TT placed in children under the age of 15 in 2006. The proceedings of the National Summit on Overuse, convened in 2012, based on sample of continually enrolled children into a treatment pathways database and a Medicaid database, reported that 2.5 percent of all U.S. children 2 years old and older had TT inserted in 2010.

The effectiveness of TT for chronic OME and recurrent AOM is likely influenced by many factors that affect the prognosis for middle ear disease in children, including current age, age at first diagnosis, frequency of respiratory tract infections, and day care exposure.

The AAO-HNS CPG recommends that clinicians offer TT to children with recurrent AOM who have middle ear effusion at the time of assessment for tube candidacy, and that clinicians do not perform TT insertion when middle ear effusion is not present.

TT placement may result in acute otorrhea in some patients and conversely watchful waiting may result in continued episodes of recurrent AOM, which may include tympanic membrane perforation and otorrhea.

In children with TTs, episodes of otorrhea that reflect acute bacterial infection may be otherwise asymptomatic and less troublesome than AOM episodes in children with intact eardrums. However, otorrhea may be associated with a foul odor, fever, or pain, and it may negatively affect quality of life. Treatment is aimed at eradicating bacterial infection and reducing the duration and severity of symptoms.

MYRINGOTOMY

A myringotomy is a tiny opening made in the eardrum so fluid can drain from the middle ear.

Why Is It Done?

The eustachian tube is the narrow passage between the middle ear and the space behind the nose. Repeated infections can block the eustachian tube. Prolonged blockage may cause some discomfort, decreased hearing, and fluid formation in the middle ear space.

How Is It Done?

The doctor makes a very small opening in your eardrum and suctions (vacuums) out the fluid. This relieves pressure and lets air flow through the middle ear. A small tube may be placed in this opening to help drainage and air flow.

Care after Tube Placement

If you are given a prescription for ear drops, use them as prescribed. Follow these steps to put the drops in your ear:

- Lie down on your side.
- Gently pull the ear up, back, and out to straighten the ear canal.
- Use the dropper to put the prescribed number of drops into your ear.
- Remain on your side for about five minutes to let the drops work their way into the ear canal.

The tube falls out as the eardrum heals, this is normal.

EAR TUBES UNDER LOCAL ANESTHESIA TO TREAT EAR INFECTION

The U.S. Food and Drug Administration (FDA) has approved a new system for the delivery of tympanostomy tubes, commonly referred to as "ear tubes," that can be inserted into the eardrum to treat recurrent ear infections (i.e., otitis media). The Tubes Under Local Anesthesia (Tula) System is the first ear tube delivery system that can be performed in young children using local anesthesia in a physician's office setting. The Tula System consists of the anesthetic Tymbion, Tusker Medical tympanostomy tubes, and several devices needed for the delivery of the ear tubes and the anesthetic into the ear drum.

"Today's approval offers patients an option for the treatment of recurrent ear infections that does not require general anesthesia. As millions of children suffer from ear infections every year, it is important to have safe and effective treatments available to this susceptible patient population," said Jeff Shuren, M.D., director of the FDA's Center for Devices and Radiological Health (CDRH). "This approval has the potential to expand patient access to a treatment that can be administered in a physician's office with local anesthesia and minimal discomfort."

Ear infections are common in children, with the National Institute of Deafness and other Communication Disorders (NIDCD) estimating that 5 in 6 children will have at least one ear infection before their third birthday. While healthcare professionals frequently prescribe antibiotics as a treatment, if antibiotics fail to treat an ear infection, or if infections continue to occur, a doctor may recommend a surgical procedure to place a small tube in the eardrum. In young children, the delivery of an ear tube has traditionally been performed in a hospital setting or surgery center and required the patient to receive general anesthesia.

The Tula System enables the delivery of an ear tube to patients under local anesthesia in a physician's office setting, therefore, avoiding the administration of general anesthesia. The Tula System uses a small electrical current to deliver a local anesthetic into the ear drum prior to tube insertion. It is approved for use in both adults and children as young as six months of age.

The FDA evaluated data provided by the sponsor from 222 pediatric patients to assess the effectiveness of the Tula System for the delivery of ear tubes. The procedural success rate was 86 percent and 89 percent in children younger than age 5 and between ages 5 to 12 years old, respectively. The most common adverse event observed was inadequate anesthesia during the procedure. The Tula System should not be used in patients younger than six months of age or patients who have allergies to some local anesthetics. This product is not intended for patients who may have preexisting issues with their eardrum, such as a perforated eardrum.

Section 26.4 | Cochlear Implant Surgery

This section contains text excerpted from the following sources: Text beginning the heading "What is a cochlear implant?" is excerpted from "Cochlear Implants," National Institute on Deafness and Other Communication Disorders (NIDCD), March 6, 2017; Text beginning with the heading "What happens before surgery?" is excerpted from "Before, during, and after Implant Surgery," U.S. Food and Drug Administration (FDA), December 29, 2017. Text beginning with the heading "What are the Benefits of Cochlear Implants?" is excerpted from "Benefits and Risks of Cochlear Implants," U.S. Food and Drug Administration (FDA), August 28, 2018.

WHAT IS A COCHLEAR IMPLANT?

A cochlear implant is a small, complex electronic device that can help to provide a sense of sound to a person who is profoundly deaf or severely hard-of-hearing. The implant consists of an external portion that sits behind the ear and a second portion that is surgically placed under the skin. An implant has the following parts:

- A microphone, which picks up sound from the environment
- A speech processor, which selects and arranges sounds picked up by the microphone
- A transmitter and receiver/stimulator, which receive signals from the speech processor and convert them into electric impulses
- An electrode array, which is a group of electrodes that collects the impulses from the stimulator and sends them to different regions of the auditory nerve

An implant does not restore normal hearing. Instead, it can give a deaf person a useful representation of sounds in the environment and help her or him to understand speech.

HOW DOES A COCHLEAR IMPLANT WORK?

A cochlear implant is very different from a hearing aid. Hearing aids amplify sounds so they may be detected by damaged ears. Cochlear implants bypass damaged portions of the ear and directly stimulate the auditory nerve. Signals generated by the implant are sent by way of the auditory nerve to the brain, which recognizes the signals as sound. Hearing through a cochlear implant is different

Ear with cochlear implant

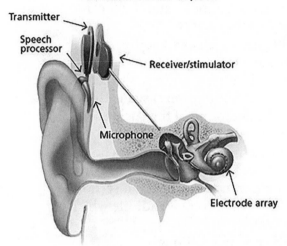

Transmitter

Speech
processor

Receiver/stimulator

Microphone

Electrode array

Figure 26.1. Ear with Cochlear Implant

from normal hearing and takes time to learn or relearn. However, it allows many people to recognize warning signals, understand other sounds in the environment, and understand speech in person or over the telephone.

WHO GETS COCHLEAR IMPLANTS

Children and adults who are deaf or severely hard-of-hearing can be fitted with cochlear implants. As of December 2012, approximately 324,200 registered devices have been implanted worldwide. In the United States, roughly 58,000 devices have been implanted in adults and 38,000 of them in children. (Estimates provided by the U.S. Food and Drug Administration (FDA), as reported by cochlear implant manufacturers.)

WHAT HAPPENS BEFORE SURGERY

Primary care doctors usually refer patients to ear, nose, and throat doctors (ENT doctors or otolaryngologists) to test them to see if they are candidates for cochlear implants.

Tests often done are:
- Examination of external, middle, and inner ear for signs of infection or abnormality
- Various tests of hearing, such as an audiogram
- A trial of hearing aid use to assess its potential benefit
- Exams to evaluate middle and inner ear structures
  - **CT (computerized tomography) scan.** This type of x-ray helps the doctor see if the cochlea has a normal shape. This scan is especially important if the patient has a history of meningitis because it helps see if there is new bone growth in the cochlea that could interfere with the insertion of the implant. This scan also may indicate which ear should be implanted.
  - **MRI (magnetic resonance imaging) scan**
- Psychological examination to see if the patient can cope with the implant
- Physical exam to prepare for general anesthesia

WHAT HAPPENS DURING SURGERY

The doctor or other hospital staff may:
- Insert some intravenous (IV) lines
- Shave or clean the scalp around the site of the implant
- Attach cables, monitors and patches to the patient's skin to monitor vital signs
- Put a mask on the patient's face to provide oxygen and anesthetic gas
- Administer drugs through the IV and the face mask to cause sleep and general anesthesia
- Awaken the patient in the operating room and take her or him to a recovery room until all the anesthesia is gone

WHAT HAPPENS AFTER SURGERY

Immediately after waking, a patient may feel:
- Pressure or discomfort over her (or his) implanted ear

- Dizziness
- Sick to the stomach (have nausea)
- Disoriented or confused for a while
- A sore throat for a while from the breathing tube used during general anesthesia

Then, a patient can expect to:
- Keep the bandages on for a while
- Have the bandages be stained with some blood or fluid
- Go home in about a day after surgery
- Have stitches for a while
- Get instructions about caring for the stitches, washing the head, showering, and general care and diet
- Have an appointment in about a week to remove the stitches and have the implant site examined
- Have the implant "turned on" (activated) about 3 to 6 weeks later

CAN A PATIENT HEAR IMMEDIATELY AFTER THE OPERATION?
No. Without the external transmitter part of the implant a patient cannot hear. The clinic will give the patient the external components about a month after the implant surgery in the first programming session.

WHY IS IT NECESSARY TO WAIT THREE TO SIX WEEKS AFTER THE OPERATION BEFORE RECEIVING THE EXTERNAL TRANSMITTER AND SOUND PROCESSOR?
The waiting period provides time for the operative incision to heal completely. This usually takes three to six weeks. After the swelling is gone, your clinician can do the first fitting and programming.

WHAT HAPPENS DURING THE INITIAL PROGRAMMING SESSION
An audiologist adjusts the sound processor to fit the implanted patient, tests the patient to ensure that the adjustments are correct, determines what sounds the patient hears, and gives information on the proper care and use of the device.

IS IT BENEFICIAL IF A FAMILY MEMBER PARTICIPATES IN THE TRAINING PROGRAM?

Yes. A family member should be included in the training program whenever possible to provide assistance. The family member should know how to manage the operations of the sound processor.

DO PATIENTS HAVE MORE THAN ONE IMPLANT?

Usually, patients have only one ear implanted, though a few patients have implants in both ears.

HOW CAN YOU HELP MY CHILD RECEIVE THE MOST BENEFIT FROM THEIR COCHLEAR IMPLANT?

- Try to make hearing and listening as interesting and fun as possible.
- Encourage your child to make noises.
- Talk about things you do as you do them.
- Show your child that she or he can consciously use and evaluate the sounds she or he receives from her or his cochlear implant.
- Realize that the more committed you, your child's teachers, and your health professionals are to helping your child, the more successful she or he will be.

WHAT CAN YOU EXPECT A COCHLEAR IMPLANT TO ACHIEVE IN MY CHILD?

As a group, children are more adaptable and better able to learn than adults. Thus, they can benefit more from a cochlear implant. Significant hearing loss slows a child's ability to learn to talk and affects overall language development. The vocal quality and intelligibility of speech from children using cochlear implants seems to be better than from children who only have acoustic hearing aids.

HOW IMPORTANT IS THE ACTIVE COOPERATION OF THE PATIENT?

Extremely important. The patient's willingness to experience new acoustic sounds and cooperate in an auditory training program are critical to the degree of success with the implant. The duration and complexity of the training varies from patient to patient.

WHAT ARE THE RISKS OF COCHLEAR IMPLANTS?
General Anesthesia Risks
- General anesthesia is drug-induced sleep. The drugs, such as anesthetic gases and injected drugs, may affect people differently. For most people, the risk of general anesthesia is very low. However, for some people with certain medical conditions, it is more risky.

Risks from the Surgical Implant Procedure
- **Injury to the facial nerve.** This nerve goes through the middle ear to give movement to the muscles of the face. It lies close to where the surgeon needs to place the implant, and thus it can be injured during the surgery. An injury can cause a temporary or permanent weakening or full paralysis on the same side of the face as the implant.
- **Meningitis.** This is an infection of the lining of the surface of the brain. People who have abnormally formed inner ear structures appear to be at greater risk of this rare, but serious complication.
- **Cerebrospinal fluid leakage.** The brain is surrounded by fluid that may leak from a hole created in the inner ear or elsewhere from a hole in the covering of the brain as a result of the surgical procedure.
- **Perilymph fluid leak.** The inner ear or cochlea contains fluid. This fluid can leak through the hole that was created to place the implant.
- **Infection** of the skin wound
- **Blood or fluid collection** at the site of surgery
- **Attacks of dizziness or vertigo**
- **Tinnitus,** which is a ringing or buzzing sound in the ear
- **Taste disturbances.** The nerve that gives taste sensation to the tongue also goes through the middle ear and might be injured during the surgery.

- **Numbness** around the ear
- **Reparative granuloma.** This is the result of localized inflammation that can occur if the body rejects the implant.

There may be other unforeseen complications that could occur with long-term implantation that cannot be predicted.

OTHER RISKS ASSOCIATED WITH THE USE OF COCHLEAR IMPLANTS
People with a Cochlear Implant

- **May hear sounds differently.** Sound impressions from an implant differ from normal hearing, according to people who could hear before they became deaf. At first, users describe the sound as "mechanical," "technical," or "synthetic." This perception changes over time, and most users do not notice this artificial sound quality after a few weeks of cochlear implant use.
- **May lose residual hearing.** The implant may destroy any remaining hearing in the implanted ear.
- **May have unknown and uncertain effects.** The cochlear implant stimulates the nerves directly with electrical currents. Although this stimulation appears to be safe, the long-term effect of these electrical currents on the nerves is unknown.
- **May not hear as well as others** who have had successful outcomes with their implants
- **May not be able to understand language well.** There is no test a person can take before surgery that will predict how well she or he will understand language after surgery.
- **May have to have it removed** temporarily or permanently if an infection develops after the implant surgery. However, this is a rare complication.
- **May have their implant fail.** In this situation, a person with an implant would need to have additional surgery to resolve this problem and would be exposed to the risks of surgery again.

- **May not be able to upgrade** their implant when new external components become available. Implanted parts are usually compatible with improved external parts. That way, as advances in technology develop, one can upgrade her or his implant by changing only its external parts. In some cases, though, this would not work and the implant will need changing.
- **May not be able to have some medical examinations and treatments.** These treatments include:
  - **MRI imaging.** MRI is becoming a more routine diagnostic method for early detection of medical problems. Even being close to an MRI imaging unit will be dangerous because it may dislodge the implant or demagnetize its internal magnet. The FDA has approved some implants, however, for some types of MRI studies done under controlled conditions.
  - Neurostimulation
  - Electrical surgery
  - Electroconvulsive therapy
  - Ionic radiation therapy
- **Will depend on batteries** for hearing. For some devices new or recharged batteries are needed every day.
- **May damage their implant.** Contact sports, automobile accidents, slips and falls, or other impacts near the ear can damage the implant. This may mean needing a new implant and more surgery. It is unknown whether a new implant would work as well as the old one.
- **May find them expensive.** Replacing damaged or lost parts may be expensive.
- **Will have to use it for the rest of life.** During a person's lifetime, the manufacturer of the cochlear implant could go out of business. Whether a person will be able to get replacement parts or other customer service in the future is uncertain.
- **May have lifestyle changes because** their implant will interact with the electronic environment. An implant may:
  - Set off theft detection systems
  - Set off metal detectors or other security systems

- Be affected by cellular phone users or other radio transmitters
- Have to be turned off during takeoffs and landings in aircraft
- Interact in unpredictable ways with other computer systems
- **Will have to be careful of static electricity.** Static electricity may temporarily or permanently damage a cochlear implant. It may be a good practice to remove the processor and headset before contact with static generating materials such as children's plastic play equipment, TV screens, computer monitors, or synthetic fabric. For more details regarding how to deal with static electricity, contact the manufacturer or implant center.
- **Have less ability to hear** both soft sounds and loud sounds without changing the sensitivity of the implant. The sensitivity of normal hearing is adjusted continuously by the brain, but the design of cochlear implants requires that a person manually change sensitivity setting of the device as the sound environment changes.
- **May develop irritation** where the external part rubs on the skin and have to remove it for a while
- **Cannot let the external parts get wet.** Damage from water may be expensive to repair and the person may be without hearing until the implant is repaired. Thus, the person will need to remove the external parts of the device when bathing, showering, swimming, or participating in water sports.
- **May hear strange sounds** caused by its interaction with magnetic fields, like those near airport passenger screening machines

Section 26.5 | Endoscopic Sinus Surgery

This section includes text excerpted from "Endoscopic Sinus Surgery," U.S. Department of Veterans Affairs (VA), July 2013. Reviewed April 2020.

SINUSES

Your sinuses are air-filled spaces in the bones of the face and head. The sinuses drain mucous through small openings that are linked to the inside of the nose. They play a big role in how humans breathe and make mucous. Mucous does not drain well when you have swelling of the lining of the nose and sinuses. An acute or chronic infection can result. When medical therapies and sinus rinses do not clear up the swelling, surgery may be needed to open up the sinuses and allow them to drain. Some people grow polyps (small growth sticking out from the mucous lining). Surgery may be needed to remove the polyps.

ENDOSCOPIC SINUS SURGERY

During an endoscopic sinus surgery, you will be given medicine to keep you asleep and free from pain. There will be no incisions (cuts) made on the outside of your nose. All surgery is done through your nostrils, using scopes. Your doctor can see the images on a monitor. The opening to each sinus that is blocked will be opened. Any polyps are removed. This is a detailed surgery and must be done carefully. The surgery may take three to four hours. If the divider between the two sides of your nose (the nasal septum) is too crooked it may have to be straightened. This will allow drainage of all the sinuses. This is called "septoplasty," and will add an extra hour to the procedure.

At the end of the surgery, your sinuses will still be oozing a little blood. Nasal packings or foam are placed in your nostrils to stop the bleeding. If you have nasal packing (like a nasal tampon) surgeon will see you back in a few days to take it out. You need to stop taking aspirin, ibuprofen (Advil or Motrin), naproxen (Alleve) and similar medicines at least one week before surgery. These medicines can cause bleeding.

Sinus surgery is usually safe. There is a one percent risk of a major complication. Problems that may happen due to sinus surgery can be: blindness, double vision, injury to brain tissue, and leakage of fluid from around the brain. More common minor problems are scarring, need for more surgery, decreased sense of smell, and nosebleeds.

You can go home the same day of surgery. You will need someone to drive you home.

AFTER YOUR SURGERY INSTRUCTIONS
Nosebleed Safety Measures

You may have a slow trickle of blood down your throat or out of the front of your nose for a few days. You need to see your surgeon right away if you are having a lot of bleeding or it seems too much to you. If you are having bothersome oozing, it can help to spray oxymetazoline (Afrin) 2 sprays in each nostril. You can use the spray up to 4 times a day during the first week. Only use the spray for 1 week. Oxymetazoline constricts blood vessels and can decrease bleeding. However, if used longer than a week it can hurt the lining of your nose and cause nasal congestion that is only relieved by more oxymetazoline. To decrease the risk of nosebleeds after surgery:

- Sneeze with your mouth open.
- Do not blow your nose for at least 1 week after surgery. You may gently wipe the front of your nose, or gently use a Sinus Rinse bottle to cleanse the inside of your nose.
- Keep your head elevated to lessen swelling. This is especially important at night. You could raise the head of your bed, sleep with 2 to 3 pillows, or sleep in a recliner. Avoid bending over.
- If you take medicines to control your blood pressure, make sure to take them as ordered. High blood pressure will make nosebleeds more likely.
- Do not lift anything more than 10 pounds. Do not strain yourself in any way with vigorous activity, sex, or exercise for 2 weeks after surgery.

- You need to stop taking aspirin, ibuprofen (Advil or Motrin), naproxen (Alleve) and similar medicines at least one week after surgery. These medicines can increase the risk of nosebleeds.

Nasal/Sinus Rinses

After surgery you need to keep your nasal cavities moist, to help blood clots dissolve and loosen crusting. Your surgeon may ask you to use nasal saline (salt water). You should use it as often during the day as you remember, or at least 4 to 5 times per day.

Your surgeon may ask you to do saline sinus rinses after surgery. You can use an over-the-counter (OTC) system such as NeilMed® Sinus Rinse. Start rinses gently the evening after surgery. If the nose seems to be blocked, stop rinsing and gently try again the next day. This will really help dissolve clots and help nasal breathing and healing.

Activity

You need to avoid activity that raises your blood pressure for two weeks. Things that can raise your blood pressure are heavy lifting, hard exercise, and sex. This could cause a nosebleed.

Diet

You may eat your regular diet after surgery, as long as your stomach is not upset from the anesthesia. If it is, wait until you feel better before you start eating solid foods.

Pain

Pain is usually mild to moderate the first 24 to 48 hours. Then it will decrease. You may not need a strong narcotic pain medicines. The sooner you reduce your narcotic pain medicines use, the faster you will heal. As your pain lessens, try using extra-strength acetaminophen (Tylenol) instead of your narcotic medicines. It is best to reduce your pain to a level you can manage, rather than to get rid of the pain completely. Please start at a lower dose of narcotic pain medicines, and increase the dose only if the pain remains uncontrolled. Decrease the dose if the side effects are too severe.

Do not drive, operate dangerous machinery, or do anything dangerous if you are taking narcotic pain medication (such as oxycodone, hydrocodone, morphine, etc.) This medication affects your reflexes and responses, just like alcohol.

CALL YOUR SURGEON: IF YOU HAVE

- **Any concerns**. The U.S. Department of Veterans Affairs (VA) offers advice that you call your surgeon rather than worry at home, or get into trouble.
- Fever over 101.5°F
- Any changes in your vision
- Headaches
- Leakage of clear fluid from your nose
- Excessive bleeding
- Pain that continues to increase instead of decrease
- Problem urinating
- If you have chest pain or difficulty breathing, do not call—go to the nearest emergency room right away.

POSTOPERATIVE APPOINTMENT

You will need to have your nasal cavities and sinuses checked and possibly cleaned out at your postoperative visit. Usually surgeons need to see you in clinic about 7 to 10 days after surgery.

Section 26.6 | **Tonsillectomy and Adenoidectomy**

This section includes text excerpted from "Tonsillectomy and Adenoidectomy," U.S. Department of Veterans Affairs (VA), July 2013. Reviewed April 2020.

TONSILS

A tonsillectomy is surgery to remove your tonsils. The tonsils are 2 large lumps of tissue in the back of your throat. Tonsils are part of the immune system. Your body can do fine without them. Your tonsils may need to be taken out if you have frequent tonsil infections, if the tonsils are too large, or if there is concern for cancer.

You will be asleep under general anesthesia while your tonsils are being taken out. She or he places tools inside your mouth to keep it open and to keep your tongue out of the way. Your doctor uses tools to take your tonsils out. The doctor uses tools to stop the bleeding in the areas where tissue was removed. Rarely, a tooth can be chipped or dislodged even though tooth protectors are used during surgery. You may have tongue numbness or taste change after surgery which sometimes can takes weeks to improve. The biggest risk from tonsillectomy is bleeding. Up to 10 percent of adults will need to come back and be treated for bleeding after tonsillectomy. Very rarely, a patient can have severe bleeding after surgery that leads to death.

The surgery usually lasts an hour or less. Having tonsils removed as an adult is more painful than it is for a child. You may have a very severe sore throat for two weeks or more after surgery.

You will usually go home the same day of surgery. You will need someone to drive you home.

If your tonsillectomy was done because of concerns about tonsil cancer, your surgeon or a resident surgeon will call you with the result of the biopsy as soon as it is available.

If you have not heard the results within that time, please call the ear-nose-throat (ENT) clinic to request the results.

ADENOIDS

Adenoids are small lumps of tissue on the top of your throat. Many people no longer have adenoids by the time they are adults.

Adenoids are removed in a similar way to tonsils. The pain after this surgery is usually less than after tonsillectomy. You may have ear pain after adenoidectomy.

ACTIVITY

No straining, heavy lifting, or vigorous exercise for two weeks after surgery.

DIET

You should follow a soft diet for two weeks. This means nothing sharp, for example, no Doritos, popcorn, nuts, etc. Any liquid or soft food is fine.

PAIN

Throat pain may be moderate to severe.

Do not drive, operate dangerous machinery, or do anything dangerous if you are a taking narcotic pain medicines (examples are oxycodone, hydrocodone, morphine, etc.) These drugs affect your reflexes and responses, just like alcohol.

HEALING PROCESS

It is normal to have bad breath as your throat heals after surgery. This may last several weeks. It is also normal to have a grey/white coating where your tonsils were as you heal. This will clear up within a few weeks.

CALL YOUR SURGEON: IF YOU HAVE

- **Any concerns**. The U.S. Department of Veterans Affairs (VA) offers advice that you call your doctor rather than worry at home, or get into trouble.
- Persistent fever over 101.5°F
- Unable to eat or drink
- Difficulty urinating
- Neck stiffness

- If you have chest pain or difficulty breathing, do not call—you will need to go to the nearest emergency room immediately.

Bleeding

The time that you are most at risk for bleeding is within 24 hours after surgery, and again 5 to 7 days after surgery. At 5 to 7 days after surgery, scabs in your throat can peel off and cause serious bleeding. If you have a tiny amount of blood in your saliva, you can stay at home and keep an eye on it. Go back to a liquid diet for the remainder of the day. If you have bright red blood from your mouth or throat, you will need to be seen by your surgeon. If it is severe, go to the nearest emergency room.

Section 26.7 | Thyroid Surgery

This section includes text excerpted from "Thyroidectomy," U.S. Department of Veterans Affairs (VA), July 2013. Reviewed April 2020.

THYROID GLAND

Your thyroid gland is in the front lower part of your neck. It makes hormones that help make your body work right. Your thyroid gland has two sections. Each section has parathyroid glands.

THYROIDECTOMY

Thyroid nodules (round hard lump of cells) are common. If a nodule has cancer in it, then the half of the thyroid gland with the nodule must be taken out. The surgery is needed to find out if it is cancerous. If you have cancer, your thyroid gland, as well as tissue and lymph nodes around the gland may be taken out. Some people have a big thyroid that causes problems swallowing or breathing. This is called a "goiter" and is not cancer. If you have a goiter you may need surgery to take it out.

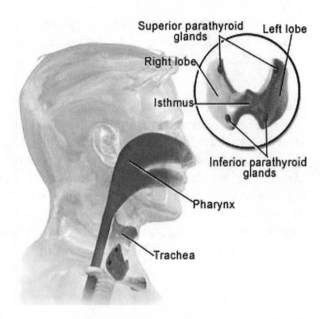

Figure 26.2. Thyroid and Parathyroid Glands

Your surgeon makes an incision (cut) in the lower area of your neck. The exact size of the cut varies, so you may ask your surgeon to show you. The surgeon then carefully cuts out the thyroid lobe(s.) Your surgeon will find your vocal cord nerve and work around it. There are tiny glands called "parathyroid glands" that are carefully cut away from the gland and left in the neck. If your whole thyroid needs to be taken out, the same process is carried out on the other side.

Your vocal cord is usually not harmed by the surgery. Your voice may be hoarse or weak after surgery. Only 10 to 30 percent will be hoarse after surgery. Less than 5 percent will always be hoarse after the surgery. The surgeon will check your vocal cords at your postoperative visit so try not to worry about it until then.

Your parathyroid glands may not work as well as they should after surgery. This can cause your calcium blood levels to drop too low. This can be life-threatening. This may be a problem for a short time, or it may be long lasting. Up to 30 percent of patients will have problems with their parathyroid glands. It is rare to have long lasting problems with your parathyroid.

If you have just one half of your thyroid removed (thyroid lobectomy, or hemithyroidectomy) then you may go home the same day of surgery. You will need someone to drive you home. You will stay in the hospital at least 1 night if you had to have your whole thyroid taken out (total thyroidectomy). Your blood calcium levels will be checked every 6 hours. If they are stable, you can go home the next day. If they are too low, the surgeon will have to give you calcium and vitamin D supplements until your levels become stable. This may take 2 to 3 days, rarely more.

If you have had your whole thyroid taken out, you will have to take a thyroid hormone pill every day for the rest of your life. The exact dose of the medicine may need to be adjusted over time. The surgeon will ask your primary care doctor or endocrinologist (a doctor who treats diseases that affect your glands) to check blood tests 6 weeks after starting your thyroid hormone. Your dose of the thyroid hormone medicine will be adjusted as needed. Sometimes, your endocrinologist does not want you to start taking this hormone pill until the tests come back showing you do not have cancer. In that case, your surgeon will let you know.

POST OPERATIVE INSTRUCTIONS
Incision

Please keep the incision dry for 3 days, and then you may shower and pat the incision dry. You may use Q-tips or gauze dipped in a ½ hydrogen peroxide and ½ water mixture to remove any dried blood over the incision. After washing, apply a thin film of an antibacterial ointment, such as Polysporin. Apply the ointment 2 times a day. However, if your surgeon used skin glue you may shower right away, and you do not need to use antibiotic ointment. The skin glue will slowly peel off after 1 to 2 weeks. If it has not at all come off by your postoperative appointment, the surgeon will remove it at that time.

Please avoid any activity that pulls across the incision, such as shaving, for at least 2 weeks. The rest of the face may be shaved. The staples and/or stitches will be taken out 1 to 2 weeks after surgery at your postoperative appointment in the ear-nose-throat (ENT) clinic.

Drain

Some patients go home with a thin drain tube and an egg shaped collecting bulb called a "JP drain." The tube should be gently stripped every 4 hours. A nurse will teach you how to do this before you leave the hospital. When the JP drain looks half full or at least 2 times a day, please empty the bulb into a small plastic measuring cup. Then write down the amount in the cup. Pour the fluid in the sink or toilet. When the amount of fluid emptied from the drain is 30 ml (or 2 tablespoons) or less in a 24-hour period, the drain is ready to be taken out. If the drain is in place for 1 week it needs to be taken out no matter how much fluid got drained. Call the ENT clinic to have the drain taken out. If it is a weekend or holiday, call the ENT resident doctor on call to have the drain taken out.

The fluid from the JP drain should be red, pink, or straw colored (yellow.) If it is milky or looks like pus, you need to be seen by your surgeon right away.

Head of Bed

Please raise the head of your bed 30 to 45 degrees or sleep in a recliner for the first 3 to 4 days to decrease swelling. The skin above the incision may look swollen after lying down for a few hours.

Activity

No straining, heavy lifting, or vigorous exercise for 2 weeks after surgery.

Diet

You may eat your regular diet after surgery.

Pain

Your pain can be mild to moderate the first 24 to 48 hours. The pain usually lessens after that. Many patients complain more about a sore throat from the breathing tube used during surgery then about pain from the surgery itself. Your pain will get better in 1 to 2 days and is best treated with throat lozenges.

You may not need strong narcotic pain medication. The sooner you reduce your narcotic pain medication use, the faster you will heal. As your pain lessens, try using extra-strength acetaminophen (Tylenol) instead of your narcotic med. It is best to reduce your pain to a level you can manage, rather than to get rid of the pain completely. Please start at a lower dose of narcotic pain med, and increase the dose only if the pain remains uncontrolled. Decrease the dose if the side effects are too severe.

Do not drive, operate dangerous machinery, or do anything dangerous if you are taking narcotic pain medication (such as oxy-codone, hydrocodone, morphine, etc.) This medication affects your reflexes and responses, just like alcohol.

CALL YOUR SURGEON: IF YOU HAVE

- **Any concerns**. The U.S. Department of Veterans Affairs (VA) offers advice that you call your surgeon rather than worry at home, or get into trouble.
- Any numbness or tingling around your mouth, in your fingers or toes, or anywhere. This may be a sign of low blood calcium levels. If you have muscle cramping and/ or curling of your fingers or toes, this could be even more seriously low blood calcium levels. This can be a life-threatening problem. You must go have your blood calcium levels drawn immediately. You should not drive if you are having these symptoms. You need to have someone drive you to the nearest emergency room (ER), if possible. If you live too far away, go to a nearby ER. Have the ER staff call your surgeon after drawing your blood calcium and giving you extra calcium if needed. Bring these postoperative instructions with you to show to them. If your blood calcium gets too low, you could have seizures or your heart could stop, so you must take this seriously.
- Fever over 101.5°F

- Foul smelling discharge from your incision
- Large amount of bleeding
- More than expected swelling of your neck
- Increased warmth or redness around the incision
- Problems urinating
- Pain that continues to increase instead of decrease
- Choking or coughing with food or liquid

POSTOPERATIVE APPOINTMENT

If you have stitches, you will need to have them taken out at your postoperative visit 7 to 10 days after surgery. If you have skin glue, you need to be seen about 2 to 3 weeks after surgery.

Chapter 27 | Eye Surgery

Chapter Contents

Section 27.1 | Cataract Surgery

This section contains text excerpted from the following sources: Text beginning with the heading "What Are Cataracts?" is excerpted from "Cataracts," National Eye Institute (NEI), August 3, 2019; Text beginning with the heading "Who Needs Cataract Surgery?" is excerpted from "Cataract Surgery," National Eye Institute (NEI), May 29, 2019.

WHAT ARE CATARACTS?

A cataract is a cloudy area in the lens of your eye. Cataracts are very common as you get older. In fact, more than half of all Americans aged 80 or older either have cataracts or have had surgery to get rid of cataracts.

At first, you may not notice that you have a cataract. But, over time, cataracts can make your vision blurry, hazy, or less colorful. You may have trouble reading or doing other everyday activities.

The good news is that surgery can get rid of cataracts. Cataract surgery is safe and corrects vision problems caused by cataracts.

WHAT ARE TYPES OF CATARACTS?

Most cataracts are age-related—they happen because of normal changes in your eyes as you get older. But, you can get cataracts for other reasons—for example, after an eye injury or after surgery for another eye problem (like glaucoma).

No matter what type of cataract you have, the treatment is always surgery.

WHAT ARE THE SYMPTOMS OF CATARACTS?

You might not have any symptoms at first when cataracts are mild. But, as cataracts grow, they can cause changes in your vision. For example, you may notice that:

- Your vision is cloudy or blurry.
- Colors look faded.
- You cannot see well at night.
- Lamps, sunlight, or headlights seem too bright.
- You see a halo around lights.
- You see double (this sometimes goes away as the cataract gets bigger).

- You have to change the prescription for your glasses often.
- These symptoms can be a sign of other eye problems, too. Be sure to talk to your eye doctor if you have any of these problems.

Over time, cataracts can lead to vision loss.

WHO NEEDS CATARACT SURGERY?

Your doctor will probably suggest cataract surgery if you have vision loss that gets in the way of everyday activities such as reading, driving, or watching TV.

Sometimes, your doctor might recommend cataract surgery even if your cataracts are not the main cause of your vision problems. For example, cataracts might need to be removed so that your doctor can see the back of your eye. If you have another eye condition, like diabetic retinopathy or age-related macular degeneration (AMD), your doctor will need to see the back of your eye to help you manage it.

Cataracts are not a medical emergency, and you do not need to rush to have surgery to remove them. Ask your doctor about the risks and benefits of cataract surgery to decide if it is right for you.

HOW DO YOU PREPARE FOR CATARACT SURGERY?

At your doctor's office before the day of the surgery, your doctor will do some tests to measure the size and shape of your eye. You may need to use some special eye drops before the surgery, and your doctor may tell you not to eat anything the night before your surgery.

You would not be able to drive yourself home after the surgery, and you will need a friend or family member to make sure you get home safely—so be sure to bring someone with you.

If you have cataracts in both eyes, you will need to have surgery on each eye at a separate time, usually about four weeks apart.

WHAT HAPPENS DURING CATARACT SURGERY

During surgery, the doctor will remove the cloudy lens from your eye and replace it with an artificial lens (called an "intraocular lens"). The surgery lasts about one hour and is almost painless.

Usually, you will be awake during cataract surgery. You might notice lights or motion, but you would not be able to see what your doctor is doing.

When you get this surgery, your doctor will:

- Put numbing drops into your eye to keep you from feeling anything
- Use tiny tools to cut into your eye, break up the lens, and take it out
- Place the new artificial lens in your eye

Right after surgery, you will need to rest in a recovery area outside the operating room for a little while. Before you go home, the medical team will check to make sure you do not have any problems with your eye.

WHAT HAPPENS AFTER CATARACT SURGERY

Your doctor will explain how to protect your eye after cataract surgery. They will give you eye drops to help your eye heal and you may need to wear a special eye shield or glasses. You may need to avoid some activities for a few weeks, like touching your eye, bending over, or lifting heavy things.

Your eye may feel a bit itchy or uncomfortable and sensitive to light and touch. After 1 or 2 days, your eye should feel better.

Call your doctor right away if you notice any of these problems after surgery:

- Vision loss
- Bad pain that would not go away even if you take medicine for it
- Very red eyes
- Flashes of light or a lot of floaters (specks) in your vision

- Most people are completely healed eight weeks after their surgery. Your doctor will schedule checkups to make sure your eye is healing correctly.

WILL YOUR VISION BE NORMAL AFTER CATARACT SURGERY?

About 9 in 10 people who get cataract surgery see better afterward, but your vision might be blurry at first while your eye recovers.

Some people notice that colors seem brighter after cataract surgery. This is because the artificial lens is clear, while your natural lens had a yellow or brown tint from the cataract.

Once your eye is completely healed, you might need a new prescription for glasses or contact lenses to see clearly.

WHAT ARE THE RISKS OF CATARACT SURGERY?

Cataract surgery is one of the most common, safe, and effective types of surgery done in the United States. But, like any surgery, there are risks, including:

- Swelling, bleeding, or infections
- Vision loss or double vision
- Unusual changes in eye pressure
- Retinal detachment
- Secondary cataract (posterior capsule opacity)

Your doctor can treat these problems if they are caught early. Be sure to go to all of your checkups, and call your doctor if you notice anything wrong with your eyes or your vision.

WHAT IS SECONDARY CATARACT?

After cataract surgery, some people may develop a condition known as "secondary cataract," or "posterior capsule opacification." Secondary cataracts are not actually cataracts, because they are caused by cloudiness on the outside of your lens, not the inside—but, they make your vision cloudy. Secondary cataracts can appear weeks, months, or even years after cataract surgery—but, they are easy to fix with a laser treatment in the doctor's office.

Section 27.2 | **Glaucoma Surgery**

This section includes text excerpted from "Glaucoma Surgery," National Eye Institute (NEI), June 26, 2019.

Glaucoma is a group of eye diseases that can cause vision loss and blindness by damaging the nerve in the back of your eye called the "optic nerve."

If glaucoma medicines and laser treatment have not helped to treat your glaucoma, your doctor may recommend surgery. Surgery cannot cure glaucoma or undo vision loss, but it can help protect your vision and stop it from getting worse.

There are a few different types of surgery for glaucoma that can help lower the pressure in your eye:

- Trabeculectomy
- Glaucoma implant surgery
- Minimally invasive glaucoma surgery (MIGS)

If you need glaucoma surgery in both eyes, your doctor will only do surgery on one eye at a time.

WHAT IS TRABECULECTOMY?

This type of surgery is usually used to treat open-angle glaucoma. It is done in a hospital and usually takes less than an hour.

The surgeon will create a tiny opening in the top of your eye, under your eyelid where no one will see it. This opening allows extra fluid in your eye to drain away, lowering pressure in your eye.

Usually, you will be awake during this surgery—but, you will get numbing medicine and medicine to help you relax. You can usually go home the same day, but you will need someone to drive you home.

WHAT IS GLAUCOMA IMPLANT SURGERY?

This type of surgery is used to treat several types of glaucoma, including congenital glaucoma, neovascular glaucoma, and glaucoma caused by an injury. It is done in a hospital and usually takes 1 to 2 hours.

In this operation, the surgeon implants a tiny tube, or shunt, onto the white of your eye. The tube helps extra fluid drain out of your eye, lowering your eye pressure.

Usually, you will be awake during this surgery—but, you will get numbing medicine and medicine to help you relax. You can usually go home the same day, but you will need someone to drive you home.

WHAT IS MINIMALLY INVASIVE GLAUCOMA SURGERY?

If you have mild glaucoma, your doctor may recommend a new approach known as "minimally invasive glaucoma surgery (MIGS)." This also lowers eye pressure, but it is safer and helps you recover faster.

There are different types of MIGS, so ask your eye doctor about whether MIGS may be an option for you.

WHAT HAPPENS AFTER SURGERY?

Your doctor will prescribe eye drops to help prevent swelling and infections, and you will need to use them for several weeks. These eye drops are different from other glaucoma eye drops you may already use.

While you recover, you may need to avoid some activities for 2 to 4 weeks, like lifting anything heavy. You will also need check-ups with your doctor to make sure your eye is healing well.

WILL YOU NEED SURGERY AGAIN?

For some people, the benefits of surgery last a long time. For others, the opening in the eye begins to close up and they need surgery again. You will need regular check-ups with your doctor to test your eye pressure. That way, your doctor will be able to act fast if you need more treatment.

Research shows that trabeculectomy lowers eye pressure in 6 to 8 in 10 people who have it. It may work best in people who have not had eye surgery—such as surgery for glaucoma, retina surgery, eye muscle surgery, or some types of cataract surgery—or eye trauma.

WHAT ARE THE SIDE EFFECTS OF SURGERY FOR GLAUCOMA?

Glaucoma surgery can have side effects, just like any operation. For example, your eye may be swollen and sore for a while.

Other possible risks include:

- Cataract
- Problems with the cornea (the clear surface layer of your eye)
- Eye pressure that is too low
- Vision loss

Section 27.3 | Macular Degeneration Surgery

This section includes text excerpted from "Macular Hole," National Eye Institute (NEI), July 8, 2019.

WHAT IS A MACULAR HOLE?

A macular hole is a small break in the macula, located in the center of the eye's light-sensitive tissue called "retina." The macula provides the sharp, central vision we need for reading, driving, and seeing fine detail.

A macular hole can cause blurred and distorted central vision. Macular holes are related to aging and usually occur in people over age 60.

Is a Macular Hole the Same as Age-Related Macular Degeneration?

No. Macular holes and age-related macular degeneration are two separate and distinct conditions, although the symptoms for each are similar. Both conditions are common in people 60 and over. An eye care professional will know the difference.

ARE THERE DIFFERENT TYPES OF A MACULAR HOLE?

Yes. There are three stages to a macular hole:

- Foveal detachments (Stage I). Without treatment, about half of Stage I macular holes will progress

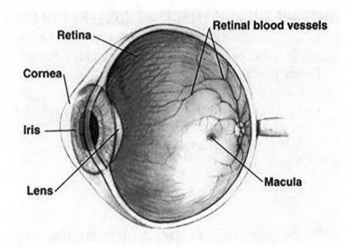

Figure 27.1. Macular Hole

- Partial-thickness holes (Stage II). Without treatment, about 70 percent of Stage II macular holes will progress
- Full-thickness holes (Stage III)

The size of the hole and its location on the retina determine how much it will affect a person's vision. When a Stage III macular hole develops, most central and detailed vision can be lost. If left untreated, a macular hole can lead to a detached retina, a sight-threatening condition that should receive immediate medical attention.

WHAT ARE THE SYMPTOMS OF A MACULAR HOLE?
Macular holes often begin gradually. In the early stage of a macular hole, people may notice a slight distortion or blurriness in their straight-ahead vision. Straight lines or objects can begin to look bent or wavy. Reading and performing other routine tasks with the affected eye become difficult.

WHAT CAUSES A MACULAR HOLE?
Most of the eye's interior is filled with vitreous, a gel-like substance that fills about 80 percent of the eye and helps it maintain a round shape.

The vitreous contains millions of fine fibers that are attached to the surface of the retina. As we age, the vitreous slowly shrinks and pulls away from the retinal surface. Natural fluids fill the area where the vitreous has contracted. This is normal. In most cases, there are no adverse effects. Some patients may experience a small increase in floaters, which are little "cobwebs" or specks that seem to float about in your field of vision.

However, if the vitreous is firmly attached to the retina when it pulls away, it can tear the retina and create a macular hole. Also, once the vitreous has pulled away from the surface of the retina, some of the fibers can remain on the retinal surface and can contract. This increases tension on the retina and can lead to a macular hole. In either case, the fluid that has replaced the shrunken vitreous can then seep through the hole onto the macula, blurring and distorting central vision.

Macular holes can also occur in other eye disorders, such as high myopia (nearsightedness), injury to the eye, retinal detachment, and, rarely, macular pucker.

Is Your Other Eye at Risk?

If a macular hole exists in one eye, there is a 10 to 15 percent chance that a macular hole will develop in your other eye over your lifetime. Your doctor can discuss this with you.

WHAT IS THE TREATMENT FOR A MACULAR HOLE?

Although some macular holes can seal themselves and require no treatment, surgery is necessary in many cases to help improve vision. In this surgical procedure—known as "vitrectomy"—the vitreous gel is removed to prevent it from pulling on the retina and replaced with a bubble containing a mixture of air and gas. The bubble acts as an internal, temporary bandage that holds the edge of the macular hole in place as it heals. Surgery is performed under local anesthesia and often on an out-patient basis.

Following surgery, patients must remain in a face-down position, normally for a day or two, but sometimes for as long as two-to-three weeks. This position allows the bubble to press against the macula and be gradually reabsorbed by the eye, sealing the hole.

As the bubble is reabsorbed, the vitreous cavity refills with natural eye fluids.

Maintaining a face-down position is crucial to the success of the surgery. Because this position can be difficult for many people, it is important to discuss this with your doctor before surgery.

What Are the Risks of Surgery?

The most common risk following macular hole surgery is an increase in the rate of cataract development. In most patients, a cataract can progress rapidly, and often becomes severe enough to require removal. Other less common complications include infection and retinal detachment either during surgery or afterward, both of which can be immediately treated.

For a few months after surgery, patients are not permitted to travel by air. Changes in air pressure may cause the bubble in the eye to expand, increasing pressure inside the eye.

How Successful Is This Surgery?

Vision improvement varies from patient to patient. People that have had a macular hole for less than six months have a better chance of recovering vision than those who have had one for a longer period. Discuss vision recovery with your doctor before your surgery. Vision recovery can continue for as long as three months after surgery.

What If You Cannot Remain in a Face-Down Position after the Surgery?

If you cannot remain in a face-down position for the required period after surgery, vision recovery may not be successful. People who are unable to remain in a face-down position for this length of time may not be good candidates for a vitrectomy. However, there are a number of devices that can make the "face-down" recovery period easier on you. There are also some approaches that can decrease the amount of "face-down" time. Discuss these with your doctor.

Section 27.4 | Laser Eye Surgery (LASIK) for Refractive Disorders

This section contains text excerpted from the following sources: Text beginning with the heading "The Eye and Vision Errors" is excerpted from "What Is Lasik?" U.S. Food and Drug Administration (FDA), July 11, 2018; Text beginning with the heading "Compilation of Patient Information " is excerpted from "What Should I Expect before, during, and after Surgery?" U.S. Food and Drug Administration (FDA), July 11, 2018; Text beginning with the heading; "Know What Makes You a Poor Candidate" is excerpted from "LASIK Surgery Checklist," U.S. Food and Drug Administration (FDA), July 11, 2018.

THE EYE AND VISION ERRORS

The parts of the eye. Indicated are the conjunctiva, sclera, choroid, optic nerve, retina, chamber angle, lens, cilary body, vitreous humor, aqueous humor, iris, pupil, cornea.

The cornea is a part of the eye that helps focus light to create an image on the retina. It works in much the same way that the lens of a camera focuses light to create an image on film. The bending and focusing of light is also known as "refraction." Usually, the shape of the cornea and the eye are not perfect and the image on the retina is out-of-focus (blurred) or distorted. These imperfections in the focusing power of the eye are known as "refractive errors." There are three primary types of refractive errors: myopia, hyperopia and astigmatism. Persons with myopia, or nearsightedness, have more difficulty seeing distant objects as clearly as near objects. Persons with hyperopia, or farsightedness, have more difficulty seeing near objects as clearly as distant objects. Astigmatism is a distortion of the image on the retina caused by irregularities in the cornea or lens of the eye. Combinations of myopia and astigmatism or hyperopia and astigmatism are common. Glasses or contact lenses are designed to compensate for the eye's imperfections. Surgical procedures aimed at improving the focusing power of the eye are called "refractive surgery." In LASIK surgery, precise and controlled removal of corneal tissue by a special laser reshapes the cornea changing its focusing power.

OTHER TYPES OF REFRACTIVE SURGERY

Radial keratotomy (RK) and photorefractive keratectomy (PRK) are other refractive surgeries used to reshape the cornea. In RK,

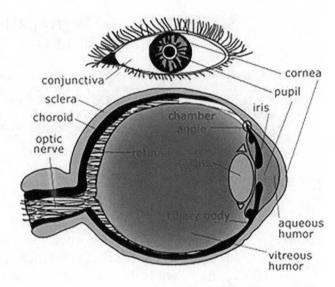

conjunctiva
sclera
choroid
optic nerve
chamber angle
retina
lens
ciliary body
cornea
pupil
iris
aqueous humor
vitreous humor

Figure 27.2. Anatomy of Eye

a very sharp knife is used to cut slits in the cornea changing its shape. PRK was the first surgical procedure developed to reshape the cornea, by sculpting, using a laser. Later, LASIK was developed. The same type of laser is used for LASIK and PRK. Often the exact same laser is used for the two types of surgery. The major difference between the two surgeries is the way that the stroma, the middle layer of the cornea, is exposed before it is vaporized with the laser. In PRK, the top layer of the cornea, called the "epithelium," is scraped away to expose the stromal layer underneath. In LASIK, a flap is cut in the stromal layer and the flap is folded back.

Another type of refractive surgery is thermokeratoplasty in which heat is used to reshape the cornea. The source of the heat can be a laser, but it is a different kind of laser than is used for LASIK and PRK. Other refractive devices include corneal ring segments that are inserted into the stroma and special contact lenses that temporarily reshape the cornea (orthokeratology).

COMPILATION OF PATIENT INFORMATION

What to expect before, during, and after surgery will vary from doctor to doctor and patient to patient. This section is a compilation of patient information developed by manufacturers and healthcare professionals, but cannot replace the dialogue you should have with your doctor. Read this information carefully and with the checklist, discuss your expectations with your doctor.

Before Surgery

If you decide to go ahead with LASIK surgery, you will need an initial or baseline evaluation by your eye doctor to determine if you are a good candidate. This is what you need to know to prepare for the exam and what you should expect:

If you wear contact lenses, it is a good idea to stop wearing them before your baseline evaluation and switch to wearing your glasses full-time. Contact lenses change the shape of your cornea for up to several weeks after you have stopped using them depending on the type of contact lenses you wear. Not leaving your contact lenses out long enough for your cornea to assume its natural shape before surgery can have negative consequences. These consequences include inaccurate measurements and a poor surgical plan, resulting in poor vision after surgery. These measurements, which determine how much corneal tissue to remove, may need to be repeated at least a week after your initial evaluation and before surgery to make sure they have not changed, especially if you wear RGP or hard lenses. If you wear:

- Soft contact lenses, you should stop wearing them for 2 weeks before your initial evaluation.
- Toric soft lenses or rigid gas permeable (RGP) lenses, you should stop wearing them for at least 3 weeks before your initial evaluation.
- Hard lenses, you should stop wearing them for at least 4 weeks before your initial evaluation.
- Before your initial exam, stop wearing contact lenses. 4 weeks before initial exam, hard (PMMA) lenses. 3 weeks before, rigid gas permeable (RGP) lenses. 2 weeks before, soft lenses.

You should tell your doctor:
- About your past and present medical and eye conditions

- About all the medications you are taking, including over-the-counter medications and any medications you may be allergic to

Your doctor should perform a thorough eye exam and discuss:
- Whether you are a good candidate
- What the risks, benefits, and alternatives of the surgery are
- What you should expect before, during, and after surgery
- What your responsibilities will be before, during, and after surgery

You should have the opportunity to ask your doctor questions during this discussion. Give yourself plenty of time to think about the risk/benefit discussion, to review any informational literature provided by your doctor, and to have any additional questions answered by your doctor before deciding to go through with surgery and before signing the informed consent form.

You should not feel pressured by your doctor, family, friends, or anyone else to make a decision about having surgery. Carefully consider the pros and cons.

The day before surgery, you should stop using:
- Creams
- Lotion
- Makeup
- Perfumes

These products as well as debris along the eyelashes may increase the risk of infection during and after surgery. Your doctor may ask you to scrub your eyelashes for a period of time before surgery to get rid of residues and debris along the lashes.

Also, before surgery, arrange for transportation to and from your surgery and your first follow-up visit. On the day of surgery, your doctor may give you some medicine to make you relax. Because this medicine impairs your ability to drive and because your vision may be blurry, even if you do not drive make sure someone can bring you home after surgery.

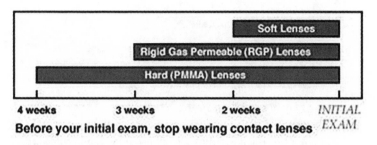

Figure 27.3. Contact Lens—Baseline Evaluation Chart

DURING SURGERY

The surgery should take less than 30 minutes. You will lie on your back in a reclining chair in an exam room containing the laser system. The laser system includes a large machine with a microscope attached to it and a computer screen.

A numbing drop will be placed in your eye, the area around your eye will be cleaned, and an instrument known as a "lid speculum" will be used to hold your eyelids open.

Your doctor may use a mechanical microkeratome (a blade device) to cut a flap in the cornea.

If a mechanical microkeratome is used, a ring will be placed on your eye and very high pressures will be applied to create suction to the cornea. Your vision will dim while the suction ring is on and you may feel the pressure and experience some discomfort during this part of the procedure. The microkeratome, a cutting instrument, is attached to the suction ring. Your doctor will use the blade of the microkeratome to cut a flap in your cornea. Microkeratome blades are meant to be used only once and then thrown out. The microkeratome and the suction ring are then removed.

Your doctor may use a laser keratome (a laser device), instead of a mechanical microkeratome, to cut a flap on the cornea.

If a laser keratome is used, the cornea is flattened with a clear plastic plate. Your vision will dim and you may feel the pressure and experience some discomfort during this part of the procedure. Laser energy is focused inside the cornea tissue, creating thousands

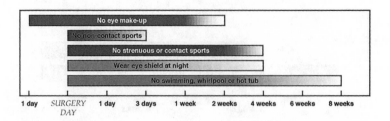

Figure 27.4. Good Practices to Follow before and after Surgery

of small bubbles of gas and water that expand and connect to separate the tissue underneath the cornea surface, creating a flap. The plate is then removed.

You will be able to see, but you will experience fluctuating degrees of blurred vision during the rest of the procedure. The doctor will then lift the flap and fold it back on its hinge, and dry the exposed tissue.

The laser will be positioned over your eye and you will be asked to stare at a light. This is not the laser used to remove tissue from the cornea. This light is to help you keep your eye fixed on one spot once the laser comes on.

When your eye is in the correct position, your doctor will start the laser. At this point in the surgery, you may become aware of new sounds and smells. The pulse of the laser makes a ticking sound. As the laser removes corneal tissue, some people have reported a smell similar to burning hair. A computer controls the amount of laser energy delivered to your eye. Before the start of surgery, your doctor will have programmed the computer to vaporize a particular amount of tissue based on the measurements taken at your initial evaluation. After the pulses of laser energy vaporize the corneal tissue, the flap is put back into position.

A shield should be placed over your eye at the end of the procedure as protection, since no stitches are used to hold the flap in place. It is important for you to wear this shield to prevent you from rubbing your eye and putting pressure on your eye while you sleep, and to protect your eye from accidentally being hit or poked until the flap has healed.

AFTER SURGERY

Immediately after the procedure, your eye may burn, itch, or feel like there is something in it. You may experience some discomfort, or in some cases, mild pain and your doctor may suggest you take a mild pain reliever. Both your eyes may tear or water. Your vision will probably be hazy or blurry. You will instinctively want to rub your eye, but do not! Rubbing your eye could dislodge the flap, requiring further treatment. In addition, you may experience sensitivity to light, glare, starbursts or halos around lights, or the whites of your eye may look red or bloodshot. These symptoms should improve considerably within the first few days after surgery. You should plan on taking a few days off from work until these symptoms subside. You should contact your doctor immediately and not wait for your scheduled visit, if you experience severe pain, or if your vision or other symptoms get worse instead of better.

You should see your doctor within the first 24 to 48 hours after surgery and at regular intervals after that for at least the first six months. At the first postoperative visit, your doctor will remove the eye shield, test your vision, and examine your eye. Your doctor may give you one or more types of eye drops to take at home to help prevent infection and/or inflammation. You may also be advised to use artificial tears to help lubricate the eye. Do not resume wearing a contact lens in the operated eye, even if your vision is blurry.

You should wait one to three days following surgery before beginning any noncontact sports, depending on the amount of activity required, how you feel, and your doctor's instructions.

To help prevent infection, you may need to wait for up to two weeks after surgery or until your doctor advises you otherwise before using lotions, creams, or make-up around the eye. Your doctor may advise you to continue scrubbing your eyelashes for a period of time after surgery. You should also avoid swimming and using hot tubs or whirlpools for 1 to 2 months.

Strenuous contact sports such as boxing, football, karate, etc., should not be attempted for at least four weeks after surgery. It is important to protect your eyes from anything that might get in them and from being hit or bumped.

During the first few months after surgery, your vision may fluctuate.
- It may take up to three to six months for your vision to stabilize after surgery.
- Glare, haloes, difficulty driving at night, and other visual symptoms may also persist during this stabilization period. If further correction or enhancement is necessary, you should wait until your eye measurements are consistent for two consecutive visits at least three months apart before re-operation.
- It is important to realize that although distance vision may improve after re-operation, it is unlikely that other visual symptoms such as glare or haloes will improve.
- It is also important to note that no laser company has presented enough evidence for the U.S. Food and Drug Administration (FDA) to make conclusions about the safety or effectiveness of enhancement surgery.

Contact your eye doctor immediately, if you develop any new, unusual or worsening symptoms at any point after surgery. Such symptoms could signal a problem that, if not treated early enough, may lead to a loss of vision.

KNOW WHAT MAKES YOU A POOR CANDIDATE
- **Career impact**—does your job prohibit refractive surgery?
- **Cost**—can you really afford this procedure?
- **Medical conditions**—e.g., do you have an autoimmune disease or other major illness? Do you have a chronic illness that might slow or alter healing?
- **Eye conditions**—do you have or have you ever had any problems with your eyes other than needing glasses or contacts?
- **Medications**—do you take steroids or other drugs that might prevent healing?
- **Stable refraction**—has your prescription changed in the last year?

- **High or Low refractive error**—do you use glasses/ contacts only some of the time? Do you need an unusually strong prescription?
- **Pupil size**—are your pupils extra large in dim conditions?
- **Corneal thickness**—do you have thin corneas?
- **Tear production**—do you have dry eyes?

KNOW ALL THE RISKS AND PROCEDURE LIMITATIONS

- **Over-treatment or under-treatment**—are you willing and able to have more than one surgery to get the desired result?
- **May still need reading glasses**—do you have presbyopia?
- **Results may not be lasting**—do you think this is the last correction you will ever need? Do you realize that long-term results are not known?
- **May permanently lose vision**—do you know some patients may lose some vision or experience blindness?
- **Dry eyes**—do you know that if you have dry eyes they could become worse, or if you do not have dry eyes before you could develop chronic dry eyes as a result of surgery?
- **Development of visual symptoms**—do you know about glare, halos, starbursts, etc., and that night driving might be difficult?
- **Contrast sensitivity**—do you know your vision could be significantly reduced in dim light conditions?
- **Bilateral treatment**—do you know the additional risks of having both eyes treated at the same time?
- **Patient information**—have you read the patient information booklet about the laser being used for your procedure?

Section 27.5 | Phakic Intraocular Lens Implantation Surgery

This section contains text excerpted from the following sources: Text in this section begins with excerpts from "Before, during and after Surgery," U.S. Food and Drug Administration (FDA), January 8, 2018; Text beginning with the heading "Know What Makes You a Poor Candidate" is excerpted from "Checklist of Questions for Your Doctor," U.S. Food and Drug Administration (FDA), January 8, 2018.

It gives you a general idea of what you might expect if you decide to have phakic intraocular lens implantation surgery. What to expect before, during and after surgery will vary according to:

- The type of phakic lens implanted
- The practices of the medical facility where the surgery will be performed and of the doctor who will be providing your care
- Your unique health circumstances and body's response

WHAT SHOULD YOU EXPECT BEFORE SURGERY?
Initial Visit

Before deciding to have phakic intraocular lens implantation surgery, you will need an initial examination to make sure your eye is healthy and suitable for surgery. Your doctor will take a complete history about your medical and eye health and perform a thorough examination of both eyes, which will include measurements of your pupils, anterior chamber depth (the distance between your cornea and iris), and endothelial cell counts (the number of cells on the back of your cornea).

If you wear contact lenses, your doctor may ask you to stop wearing them before your initial examination (from the day of to a few weeks before), so that your refraction (measure of how much your eye bends light) and central keratometry readings (measure of how much the cornea curves) are more accurate.

At this time, you should tell your doctor if you:

- Take any medications, including over-the-counter medications, vitamins and other supplements
- Have any allergies
- Have had any eye conditions
- Have undergone any previous eye surgery
- Have had any medical conditions

Deciding to Have Surgery

To help you decide whether phakic lenses are right for you, talk to your doctor about your expectations and whether there are elements of your medical history, eye history, or eye examination that might increase your risk or prevent you from having the outcome you expect (Are Phakic Lenses for you?) For ideas of what to ask your doctor, see Questions for Your Doctor. Before you sign an informed consent document (a form giving permission to your doctor to operate on your eye), you should discuss with your doctor:

- Whether you are a good candidate
- What are the risks, benefits and alternatives of the surgery
- What you should expect before, during and after surgery, and
- What your responsibilities will be before, during and after surgery

You should have the opportunity to ask your doctor questions during this discussion. Ask your doctor for the Patient Labeling of the lens that she or he recommends for you. Give yourself plenty of time to think about the risk/benefit discussion, to review any informational literature provided by your doctor, and to have any additional questions answered by your doctor before deciding to go through with surgery and before signing the informed consent document. You should not feel pressured by anyone to make a decision about having surgery. Carefully consider the pros and cons.

PREPARING FOR SURGERY
Within Weeks of Surgery

About one to two weeks before surgery, your eye doctor may schedule you for a laser iridotomy to prepare your eye for implantation of the phakic lens. Before the procedure, your eye doctor may put drops in your eye to make the pupil small and to numb the eye. While you are seated, you doctor will rest a large lens on your eye. She or he will then make a small hole (or holes) in the extreme outer edge of the iris (the colored part of your eye) with a laser.

This hole (holes) are to prevent fluid buildup and pressure in the back chamber of your eye after phakic lens implantation surgery. This procedure is usually performed in an office or clinic setting, not in an operating room, and usually only takes a few minutes.

After the iridotomy procedure, the doctor may have you wait around awhile before checking your eye pressure and letting you go home. The procedure should not prevent you from driving home, but you should check with your eye doctor when you schedule your appointment. You will be given a prescription for steroid drops to put in your eye at home for several days to reduce inflammation from the iridotomy procedure. It is important that you follow all instructions your doctor gives you after the iridotomy procedure.

Possible Complications of Laser Iridotomy Include:

- Iritis (inflammation in the front part of the eye)
- Increase in eye pressure (usually within 1 to 4 hours after the procedure)
- Cataract (clouding of the natural lens) from the laser
- Hyphema (bleeding into the anterior chamber of the eye, behind the cornea and in front of the iris, that can cause high pressure inside the eye)
- Injury to the cornea from the laser that can result in clouding of the cornea
- Incomplete opening of the hole all the way through the iris
- Closure of the new opening
- Rarely, retinal burns
- Your doctor may ask you to stop wearing contact lenses before your surgery (anywhere from the day of the surgery to a few weeks before)

Before your surgery, your eye doctor may ask you to temporarily stop taking certain medications that increase the risk of bleeding during surgery. How long before surgery you may need to stop these medications depends upon which medications you are using and the conditions they are treating. You and your eye doctor may need to discuss stopping certain medications with the doctor who prescribed them, since you may need some of these medications to prevent life-threatening events. For example, you may need medications that stop blood clotting to keep from having a stroke.

Within Days of Surgery

Your doctor may give you prescriptions for antibiotic drops to prevent infection and/or anti-inflammatory drops to prevent inflammation to put in your eye for a few days before surgery.

Arrange for transportation to and from surgery and to your follow-up doctor's appointment the day after surgery, since you will be unable to drive. Your doctor will let you know when it is safe for you to drive again.

Your eye doctor will probably tell you not to eat or drink anything after midnight the night before your surgery.

WHAT SHOULD YOU EXPECT DURING SURGERY?
The Day of Surgery

Just before surgery, drops will be put in your eye. You will have to lie down for the surgery and remain still. If you cannot lie down flat on your back, you may not be a good candidate for this surgery. Usually, patients are not put to sleep for this type of surgery, but you may be given a sedative or other medication to make you relax and an i.v. may be started. Your doctor may inject medication around the eye to numb the eye. The doctor also may give you an injection around the eye to also prevent you from being able to move your eye or see out of your eye. You will have to ask your doctor to find out exactly which of these types of anesthesia will be used in your case. Your eye and the surrounding area will be cleaned and an instrument known as "lid speculum" will be used to hold your eyelids open.

The doctor will make an incision in your cornea, sclera (the white part of your eye), or limbus (where the cornea meets the sclera). She or he will place a lubricant into your eye to help protect the back of the cornea (the endothelial cells) during the insertion of the phakic lens. The doctor will insert the phakic lens through the incision in the eye into the anterior chamber, behind the cornea and in front of the iris. Depending upon the type of phakic lens, the doctor will either attach the lens to the front of the iris in the anterior chamber of the eye or move it through the pupil into position behind the iris and in front of the lens in the posterior chamber of the eye. The doctor will remove the lubricant and may close the incision with tiny stitches, depending upon the type of incision. Your doctor will place some eye drops or ointment in your eye and cover your eye with a patch and/or a shield. The surgery will probably take around 30 minutes.

After the surgery is over, you may be brought to a recovery room for a couple of hours before you will be allowed to go home. You will be given prescriptions for antibiotic and anti-inflammatory drops to use at home as directed. You will be given an Implant Identification Card, which you should keep as a permanent record of the lens that was implanted in your eye. Make sure you show this card to anyone who takes care of your eyes in the future. You will be asked to go home and take it easy for the rest of the day.

KNOW WHAT MAKES YOU A POOR CANDIDATE
- Do you have any conditions that would increase your risks?
- Are the size of the pupils under low lighting conditions bigger than the size of the lens? If so, what are the additional risks?
- Is your anterior chamber shallow? If so, what are the additional risks?

KNOW ALL THE BENEFITS, RISKS, AND ALTERNATIVES
- What are the benefits of the phakic lens for the amount of nearsightedness?
- What are the risks of having the phakic lens implanted?
- What is the risk of needing a corneal transplant in the future, if you have the phakic lens implanted, based on the age and the endothelial cell count?
- What could happen if you get hit in the eye or head after phakic lens implantation that might be different from what could happen if you did not have the lens implanted?

286

- Are the chances greater for a more severe injury after phakic lens implantation?
- Can the phakic lens be removed? What are the risks of removing the phakic lens?
- What other options are available for correcting the nearsightedness?

Chapter 28 | Dental Implants

Dental implants are metal posts or frames that are surgically implanted in the gums. They fuse to the jawbone and serve as permanent anchors or roots for dental prosthetics—including crowns, bridges, and dentures—that replace missing natural teeth.

Dental implants offer many advantages over conventional tooth-replacement techniques. Most patients find that bridges and dentures placed on implants fit securely, feel comfortable and natural, and do not shift while eating or speaking. Ordinary dentures that rest on top of the gums, in contrast, often affect speech, create problems while eating, or cause sore gums by moving around. An advantage over ordinary bridges is that dental implants do not require adjacent teeth to be ground down in order to provide an attachment point to hold the replacement teeth in place.

Dental implants also play an important role in stabilizing and preserving the alveolar bone in the jaw. When teeth are missing, the underlying bone that once connected and supported them breaks down as part of a natural process called "resorption." Studies have shown that the bone width can decrease by 25 percent in the first year after a tooth is lost. As the bone loss progresses, it can lead to aesthetic and functional problems in the mouth. Dental implants fuse to the bone and provide stimulation that helps to keep the bone healthy and strong.

The main disadvantage of dental implants is their cost, which is generally higher than other methods of tooth replacement and not as likely to be covered by insurance. In addition, to be eligible to receive dental implants, a patient must be in good health and

"Dental Implants," © 2017 Omnigraphics. Reviewed April 2020.

have adequate bone to support the implants. Medical conditions such as uncontrolled gum disease, diabetes, or cancer—as well as lifestyle factors, such as smoking or alcoholism—can prevent dental implants from fusing to the bone. Finally, patients who receive dental implants must commit to practicing good oral hygiene and making regular dental visits to keep the structures healthy.

GETTING DENTAL IMPLANTS

Getting dental implants is a multi-step process that involves a team of specialists. The implant dentistry team is likely to include a periodontist, oral surgeon, or general dentist with training in implant surgery; a dental laboratory technician with training in fabrication of crowns, bridgework, and dentures that attach to implants; and a restorative dentist with training in planning and placing tooth restorations. The team works together to assess and plan the placement of the dental implants and the design of the tooth restorations.

To begin the process, the team will typically conduct a detailed assessment of the patient's teeth, jaws, and bite to determine the exact positioning of the dental implants. This assessment will likely involve specialized x-rays and computerized tomography (CT) scans to create a three-dimensional model of the patient's mouth. Once the assessment is complete, the periodontist uses the information to guide the precise surgical placement of the implants. Channels are created in the jawbone, and metal posts are fitted into the sites. In cases where resorption of the bone has occurred, additional surgery may be needed to graft bone into tooth sockets or regenerate bone that has been lost in order to provide a sufficient base for anchoring the implants.

The bone will generally fuse with the implants within two to six months of the surgery. Temporary healing caps may be placed on the implants until they are fully fused. At that point, tooth restorations are fabricated in a dental laboratory to match the patient's existing teeth. Finally, the artificial teeth are screwed or cemented onto the implants. Once the restorations are attached, they are virtually indistinguishable in appearance and function from the patient's original teeth.

TYPES OF DENTAL IMPLANTS

There are two main types of dental implants: endosteal implants and subperiosteal implants. Endosteal implants are artificial roots or anchors that are surgically placed into the jawbone. Once they fuse with the bone and the surrounding gum tissue heals, metal posts are connected to the implants to hold tooth restorations. Subperiosteal implants consist of a metal frame that is surgically fitted on the jawbone beneath the gum tissue. Once the frame fuses with the jawbone, metal posts are attached to it to hold tooth restorations.

Dental implants can be used to replace a single tooth, multiple teeth, or an entire upper or lower set of teeth. In single-tooth replacement, a single implant serves as the anchor for a custom-made, artificial tooth form called a "crown." In multiple-tooth replacement, multiple implants serve as the anchors for a permanent, custom-made bridge that contains several artificial teeth. For patients who are missing all of their upper or lower teeth, four to six implants may be used to support a removable denture that snaps or clips into place.

Since dental implants are made of metal, they are not subject to dental decay in the same way as the roots of natural teeth. In addition, crowns, bridges, and other prosthetic tooth restorations can be replaced by a dentist if they suffer excessive wear or damage without affecting the implants supporting them. However, people with dental implants must commit to practicing good oral hygiene to control bacterial biofilm on the tissues surrounding the implants. Otherwise, the patient may develop an inflammatory response called "peri-implantitis," which can cause disintegration of the bone surrounding the implant. Finally, people with dental implants must visit a dentist regularly to ensure the continued stability and function of the implants.

References

1. "Understanding Dental Implants," International Congress of Oral Implantologists (ICOI), 2016.
2. "What Are Dental Implants?" Colgate Oral Care Center, 2016.
3. "What Types of Dental Implants Are Available?" Gordon West, DDS, 2013.

Chapter 29 | Breast Surgeries

Section 29.1 | Surgery Choices for Women

This section includes text excerpted from "Surgery Choices for Women with DCIS or Breast Cancer," National Cancer Institute (NCI), January 19, 2015. Reviewed April 2020.

ARE YOU FACING A DECISION ABOUT SURGERY FOR DCIS OR BREAST CANCER?

Do you have ductal carcinoma in situ (DCIS) or breast cancer that can be removed with surgery? If so, you may be able to choose which type of breast surgery to have. Often, your choice is between breast-sparing surgery (surgery that takes out the cancer and leaves most of the breast) and a mastectomy (surgery that removes the whole breast).

Once you are diagnosed, treatment will usually not begin right away. There should be enough time for you to meet with breast cancer surgeons, learn the facts about your surgery choices, and think about what is important to you. Learning all you can will help you make a choice you can feel good about.

TALK WITH YOUR DOCTOR

Talk with a breast cancer surgeon about your choices. Find out:
- What happens during surgery
- The types of problems that sometimes occur
- Any treatment you might need after surgery

Be sure to ask a lot of questions and learn as much as you can. You may also wish to talk with family members, friends, or others who have had surgery.

Get a Second Opinion

After talking with a surgeon, think about getting a second opinion. A second opinion means getting the advice of another surgeon. This surgeon might tell you about other treatment options. Or, she or he may agree with the advice you got from the first doctor.

Some people worry about hurting their surgeon's feelings if they get a second opinion. But, it is very common and good surgeons do not mind. Also, some insurance companies require it. It is better to get a second opinion than worry that you made the wrong choice.

If you think you might have a mastectomy, this is also a good time to learn about breast reconstruction. Think about meeting with a reconstructive plastic surgeon to learn about this surgery and if it seems like a good option for you.

Check with Your Insurance Company

Each insurance plan is different. Knowing how much your plan will pay for each type of surgery, including reconstruction, special bras, prostheses, and other needed treatments can help you decide which surgery is best for you.

LEARN ABOUT THE TYPES OF BREAST SURGERY

Most women with DCIS or breast cancer that can be treated with surgery have three surgery choices.

Breast-Sparing Surgery, Followed by Radiation Therapy

Breast-sparing surgery means the surgeon removes only the DCIS or cancer and some normal tissue around it. If you have cancer, the surgeon will also remove one or more lymph nodes from under your arm. Breast-sparing surgery usually keeps your breast looking much like it did before surgery. Other words for breast-sparing surgery include:

- Lumpectomy
- Partial mastectomy
- Breast-conserving surgery
- Segmental mastectomy

After breast-sparing surgery, most women also receive radiation therapy. The main goal of this treatment is to keep cancer from coming back in the same breast. Some women will also need chemotherapy, hormone therapy, and/or targeted therapy.

Mastectomy
In a mastectomy, the surgeon removes the whole breast that contains the ductal carcinoma in situ (DCIS) or cancer. There are two main types of mastectomy. They are:
- **Total mastectomy.** The surgeon removes your whole breast. Sometimes, the surgeon also takes out one or more of the lymph nodes under your arm. This procedure is also called "simple mastectomy."
- **Modified radical mastectomy.** The surgeon removes your whole breast, many of the lymph nodes under your arm, and the lining over your chest muscles. Some women will also need radiation therapy, chemotherapy, hormone therapy, and/or targeted therapy.

If you have a mastectomy, you may choose to wear a prosthesis (breast-like form) in your bra or have breast reconstruction surgery.

MASTECTOMY WITH BREAST RECONSTRUCTION SURGERY
You can have breast reconstruction at the same time as the mastectomy, or anytime after. This type of surgery is done by a plastic surgeon with experience in reconstruction surgery. The surgeon uses an implant or tissue from another part of your body to create a breast-like shape that replaces the breast that was removed. The surgeon may also make the form of a nipple and add a tattoo that looks like the areola (the dark area around your nipple).

There are two main types of breast reconstruction surgery:

Breast Implant
Breast reconstruction with an implant is often done in steps. The first step is called "tissue expansion." This is when the plastic surgeon places a balloon expander under the chest muscle. Over many weeks, saline (salt water) will be added to the expander to stretch the chest muscle and the skin on top of it. This process makes a pocket for the implant.

Once the pocket is the correct size, the surgeon will remove the expander and place an implant (filled with saline or silicone gel) into the pocket. This creates a new breast-like shape. Although this shape looks like a breast, you will not have the same feeling in it because nerves were cut during your mastectomy.

Breast implants do not last a lifetime. If you choose to have an implant, chances are you will need more surgery later on to remove or replace it. Implants can cause problems such as breast hardness, pain, and infection. The implant may also break, move, or shift. These problems can happen soon after surgery or years later.

Tissue Flap

In tissue flap surgery, a reconstructive plastic surgeon builds a new breast-like shape from muscle, fat, and skin taken from other parts of your body (usually your belly, back, or buttock). This new breast-like shape should last the rest of your life. Women who are very thin or obese, smoke, or have serious health problems often cannot have tissue flap surgery.

Healing after tissue flap surgery often takes longer than healing after breast implant surgery. You may have other problems, as well. For example, if you have a muscle removed, you might lose strength in the area from which it was taken. Or, you may get an infection or have trouble healing. Tissue flap surgery is best done by a reconstructive plastic surgeon who has special training in this type of surgery and has done it many times before.

STAGES AND TYPES OF BREAST SURGERY
Before Breast Surgery
IS THIS SURGERY RIGHT FOR YOU?

Breast-sparing surgery. Most women with DCIS or breast cancer can choose to have breast-sparing surgery, usually followed by radiation therapy.

Mastectomy. Most women with DCIS or breast cancer can choose to have a mastectomy.

A mastectomy may be a better choice for you if:
- You have small breasts and a large area of DCIS or cancer.
- You have DCIS or cancer in more than one part of your breast.

- The DCIS or cancer is under the nipple.
- You are not able to receive radiation therapy.

Mastectomy with reconstruction. If you have a mastectomy, you might also want breast reconstruction surgery.

You can choose to have reconstruction surgery at the same time as your mastectomy or wait and have it later.

Recovering from Breast Surgery
WILL YOU HAVE PAIN?

Most people have some pain after surgery.

Talk with your doctor or nurse before surgery about ways to control pain after surgery. Also, tell them if your pain control is not working.

How Long before You Can Return to Normal Activities?

Breast-sparing surgery. Most women are ready to return to most of their usual activities within 5 to 10 days.

Mastectomy. It may take 3 to 4 weeks to feel mostly normal after a mastectomy.

Mastectomy with reconstruction. Your recovery will depend on the type of reconstruction you have. It can take 6 to 8 weeks or longer to fully recover from breast reconstruction.

What Other Problems You Might Have?

Breast-sparing surgery. You may feel very tired and have skin changes from radiation therapy.

Mastectomy. You may feel out of balance if you had large breasts and do not have reconstruction surgery. This may also lead to neck and shoulder pain.

Mastectomy with reconstruction. You may not like how your breast-like shape looks.

If you have an implant:

- Your breast may harden and can become painful.
- You will likely need more surgery if your implant breaks or leaks.

If you have flap surgery, you may lose strength in the part of your body where a muscle was removed.

What Other Types of Treatment Might You Need?

If you chose to have breast-sparing surgery, you will usually need radiation therapy. Radiation treatments are usually given 5 days a week for 5 to 8 weeks.

If you have a mastectomy, you may still need radiation therapy. No matter which surgery you choose, you might need:

- Chemotherapy
- Hormone therapy
- Targeted therapy

Life after Breast Surgery
WHAT WILL YOUR BREAST LOOK LIKE?

Breast-sparing surgery. Your breast should look a lot like it did before surgery.

But, if your tumor is large, your breast may look different or smaller after breast-sparing surgery.

You will have a small scar where the surgeon cut to remove the DCIS or cancer. The length of the scar will depend on how large an incision the surgeon needed to make.

Mastectomy. Your breast and nipple will be removed. You will have a flat chest on the side of your body where the breast was removed.

You will have a scar over the place where your breast was removed. The length of the scar will depend on the size of your breast. If you have smaller breasts, your scar is likely to be smaller than if you have larger breasts.

Mastectomy with reconstruction. You will have a breast-like shape, but your breast will not look or feel like it did before surgery. And, it will not look or feel like your other breast.

You will have scars where the surgeon stitched skin together to make the new breast-like shape.

If you have tissue flap reconstruction, you will have scars around the new breast, as well as the area where the surgeon removed the muscle, fat, and skin to make the new breast-like shape.

To get a better idea of what to expect, ask your surgeon if you can see before and after pictures of other women who have had different types of surgery.

Remember, even though surgery leaves scars where the surgeon cut the skin and stitched it back together, they tend to fade over time.

Will your Breast Have Feeling?

Breast-sparing surgery. Yes. You should still have feeling in your breast, nipple, and areola (the dark area around your nipple).

Mastectomy. Maybe. After surgery, the skin around where the surgeon cut and maybe the area under your arm will be numb (have no feeling).

This numb feeling may improve over 1 to 2 years, but it will never feel like it once did. Also, the skin where your breast was may feel tight.

Mastectomy with reconstruction. No. The area around your breast will not have feeling.

Will You Need More Surgery?

Breast-sparing surgery. If the surgeon does not remove all the DCIS or cancer the first time, you may need more surgery.

Mastectomy. If you have problems after your mastectomy, you may need more surgery.

Mastectomy with reconstruction. You will need more than one surgery to build a new breast-like shape. The number of surgeries you need will depend on the type of reconstruction you have and if you choose to have a nipple or areola added.

Some women may also decide to have surgery on the opposite breast to help it match the new breast-like shape better.

If you have an implant, you are likely to need surgery many years later to remove or replace it.

With all three surgeries, you may need more surgery to remove lymph nodes from under your arm. Having your lymph nodes removed can cause lymphedema.

Will the Type of Breast Surgery You Have Affect How Long You Live?

No. Research has shown that women who have breast-sparing surgery live as long as women who have a mastectomy. This does not change if you also have reconstruction.

What Are the Chances That Breast Cancer Will Return in the Same Area?

Breast-sparing surgery. There is a chance that your cancer will come back in the same breast. But, if it does, it is not likely to affect how long you live. About 10 percent of women (1 in every 10) who have breast-sparing surgery along with radiation therapy get cancer in the same breast within 12 years. If this happens, you can be effectively treated with a mastectomy.

Mastectomy. There is a smaller chance that your cancer will return in the same area than if you have breast-sparing surgery. About 5 percent of women (1 in every 20) who have a mastectomy will get cancer on the same side of their chest within 12 years.

Mastectomy with reconstruction. Your chances are the same as mastectomy, since breast reconstruction surgery does not affect the chances of the cancer returning.

THINK ABOUT WHAT IS IMPORTANT TO YOU

After you have talked with a breast cancer surgeon and learned the facts, you may also want to talk with your spouse or partner, family, friends, or other women who have had breast cancer surgery.

Then, think about what is important to you. Thinking about these questions and talking them over with others might help:

About Breast Surgery Choices

- If you have breast-sparing surgery, are you willing and able to have radiation therapy 5 days a week for 5 to 8 weeks?
- If you have a mastectomy, do you also want breast reconstruction surgery?

- If you have breast reconstruction surgery, do you want it at the same time as mastectomy?
- What treatment does the insurance cover? What do you have to pay for?

Life after Breast Surgery

- How important is it to you how the breast looks after cancer surgery?
- How important is it to you how the breast feels after cancer surgery?
- If you have a mastectomy and do not have reconstruction, will the insurance cover the prostheses and special bras?
- Where can you find breast prostheses and special bras?

Section 29.2 | Breast Biopsy

This section includes text excerpted from "Breast Biopsy," MedlinePlus, National Institutes of Health (NIH), July 24, 2018.

WHAT IS A BREAST BIOPSY?

A breast biopsy is a procedure that removes a small sample of breast tissue for testing. The tissue is looked at under a microscope to check for breast cancer. There are different ways to do a breast biopsy procedure. One method uses a special needle to remove tissue. Another method removes tissue in a minor, outpatient surgery.

A breast biopsy can determine whether you have breast cancer. But, most women who have a breast biopsy do not have cancer.

WHAT IS BREAST BIOPSY USED FOR?

A breast biopsy is used to confirm or rule out breast cancer. It is done after other breast tests, such as a mammogram, or a physical breast exam, show there might be a chance of breast cancer.

WHY DO YOU NEED A BREAST BIOPSY?

You may need a breast biopsy if:

- You or your healthcare provider felt a lump in your breast.
- Your mammogram, magnetic resonance imaging (MRI), or ultrasound tests show a lump, shadow, or other area of concern.
- You have changes in your nipple, such as bloody discharge.

If your healthcare provider has ordered a breast biopsy, it does not necessarily mean you have breast cancer. The majority of breast lumps that are tested are benign, which means noncancerous.

WHAT HAPPENS DURING A BREAST BIOPSY?

There are three main types of breast biopsy procedures:

- **Fine needle aspiration biopsy,** which uses a very thin needle to remove a sample of breast cells or fluid
- **Core needle biopsy,** which uses a larger needle to remove a sample
- **Surgical biopsy,** which removes a sample in a minor, outpatient procedure

Fine needle aspiration and **core needle biopsies** usually include the following steps.

- You will lay on your side or sit on an exam table.
- A healthcare provider will clean the biopsy site and inject it with an anesthetic, so you would not feel any pain during the procedure.
- Once the area is numb, the provider will insert either a fine aspiration needle or core biopsy needle into the biopsy site and remove a sample of tissue or fluid.
- You may feel a little pressure when the sample is withdrawn.
- Pressure will be applied to the biopsy site until the bleeding stops.
- Your provider will apply a sterile bandage at the biopsy site.

Breast Surgeries

In a **surgical biopsy,** a surgeon will make a small cut in your skin to remove all or part of a breast lump. A surgical biopsy is sometimes done if the lump cannot be reached with a needle biopsy. Surgical biopsies usually include the following steps.

- You will lie on an operating table. An IV (intravenous line) may be placed in your arm or hand.
- You may be given medicine, called a "sedative," to help you relax.
- You will be given local or general anesthesia, so you would not feel pain during the procedure.
    - For local anesthesia, a healthcare provider will inject the biopsy site with medicine to numb the area.
    - For general anesthesia, a specialist called an "anesthesiologist" will give you medicine, so you will be unconscious during the procedure.
- When the biopsy area is numb or you are unconscious, the surgeon will make a small cut into the breast and remove part or all of a lump. Some tissue around the lump may also be removed.
- The cut in your skin will be closed with stitches or adhesive strips.

The type of biopsy you have will depend on different factors, including the size of the lump and what the lump or area of concern looks like on a breast test.

WILL YOU NEED TO DO ANYTHING TO PREPARE FOR THE TEST?

You would not need any special preparations if you are getting local anesthesia (numbing of the biopsy site). If you are getting general anesthesia, you will probably need to fast (not eat or drink) for several hours before surgery. Your surgeon will give you more specific instructions. Also, if you are getting a sedative or general anesthesia, be sure to arrange for someone to drive you home. You may be groggy and confused after you wake up from the procedure.

ARE THERE ANY RISKS TO THE TEST?

You may have a little bruising or bleeding at the biopsy site. Sometimes the site gets infected. If that happens, you will be treated with antibiotics. A surgical biopsy may cause some additional pain and discomfort. Your healthcare provider may recommend or prescribe medicine to help you feel better.

WHAT DO THE RESULTS MEAN?

It may take several days to a week to get your results. Typical results may show:

- **Normal.** No cancer or abnormal cells were found.
- **Abnormal, but benign.** These show breast changes that are not cancer. These include calcium deposits and cysts. Sometimes more testing and/or follow-up treatment may be needed.
- **Cancer cells found.** Your results will include information about the cancer to help you and your healthcare provider develop a treatment plan that best meets your needs. You will probably be referred to a provider who specializes in breast cancer treatment.

IS THERE ANYTHING ELSE YOU NEED TO KNOW ABOUT A BREAST BIOPSY?

In the United States, tens of thousands of women and hundreds of men die of breast cancer every year. A breast biopsy, when appropriate, can help find breast cancer at an early stage, when it is most treatable. If breast cancer is found early, when it is confined to the breast only, the five-year survival rate is 99 percent. This means, on average, that 99 in 100 people with breast cancer that was detected early are still alive 5 years after being diagnosed. If you have questions about breast cancer screening, such as mammograms or a breast biopsy, talk to your healthcare provider.

Section 29.3 | **Breast Reconstruction**

This section includes text excerpted from "Breast Reconstruction after Mastectomy," National Cancer Institute (NCI), February 24, 2017.

WHAT IS BREAST RECONSTRUCTION?

Many women who have a mastectomy—surgery to remove an entire breast to treat or prevent breast cancer—have the option of having the shape of the removed breast rebuilt.

Women who choose to have their breasts rebuilt have several options for how it can be done. Breasts can be rebuilt using implants (saline or silicone). They can also be rebuilt using autologous tissue (that is, tissue from elsewhere in the body). Sometimes both implants and autologous tissue are used to rebuild the breast.

Surgery to reconstruct the breasts can be done (or started) at the time of the mastectomy (which is called "immediate reconstruction") or it can be done after the mastectomy incisions have healed and breast cancer therapy has been completed (which is called "delayed reconstruction"). Delayed reconstruction can happen months or even years after the mastectomy.

In a final stage of breast reconstruction, a nipple and areola may be re-created on the reconstructed breast, if these were not preserved during the mastectomy.

Sometimes breast reconstruction surgery includes surgery on the other, or contralateral, breast so that the two breasts will match in size and shape.

HOW DO SURGEONS USE IMPLANTS TO RECONSTRUCT A WOMAN'S BREAST?

Implants are inserted underneath the skin or chest muscle following the mastectomy. (Most mastectomies are performed using a technique called "skin-sparing mastectomy," in which much of the breast skin is saved for use in reconstructing the breast.)

Implants are usually placed as part of a two-stage procedure.

- **In the first stage,** the surgeon places a device, called a "tissue expander," under the skin that is left after the mastectomy or under the chest muscle. The expander is slowly filled with saline during periodic visits to the doctor after surgery.

- **In the second stage,** after the chest tissue has relaxed and healed enough, the expander is removed and replaced with an implant. The chest tissue is usually ready for the implant two to six months after mastectomy.

In some cases, the implant can be placed in the breast during the same surgery as the mastectomy—that is, a tissue expander is not used to prepare for the implant.

Surgeons are increasingly using material called "acellular dermal matrix" as a kind of scaffold or "sling" to support tissue expanders and implants. Acellular dermal matrix is a kind of mesh that is made from donated human or pig skin that has been sterilized and processed to remove all cells to eliminate the risks of rejection and infection.

HOW DO SURGEONS USE TISSUE FROM A WOMAN'S OWN BODY TO RECONSTRUCT THE BREAST?

In autologous tissue reconstruction, a piece of tissue containing skin, fat, blood vessels, and sometimes muscle is taken from elsewhere in a woman's body and used to rebuild the breast. This piece of tissue is called a "flap."

Different sites in the body can provide flaps for breast reconstruction. Flaps used for breast reconstruction most often come from the abdomen or back. However, they can also be taken from the thigh or buttocks.

Depending on their source, flaps can be pedicled or free.

- **With a pedicled flap,** the tissue and attached blood vessels are moved together through the body to the breast area. Because the blood supply to the tissue used for reconstruction is left intact, blood vessels do not need to be reconnected once the tissue is moved.
- **With free flaps,** the tissue is cut free from its blood supply. It must be attached to new blood vessels in the

breast area, using a technique called "microsurgery." This gives the reconstructed breast a blood supply.

Abdominal and back flaps include:
- **DIEP flap.** Tissue comes from the abdomen and contains only skin, blood vessels, and fat, without the underlying muscle. This type of flap is a free flap.
- **Latissimus dorsi (LD) flap.** Tissue comes from the middle and side of the back. This type of flap is pedicled when used for breast reconstruction. (LD flaps can be used for other types of reconstruction as well.)
- **SIEA flap (also called "SIEP flap").** Tissue comes from the abdomen as in a DIEP flap, but includes a different set of blood vessels. It also does not involve cutting of the abdominal muscle and is a free flap. This type of flap is not an option for many women because the necessary blood vessels are not adequate or do not exist.
- **Transverse rectus abdominis myocutaneous (TRAM) flap.** Tissue comes from the lower abdomen as in a DIEP flap, but includes muscle. It can be either pedicled or free.

Flaps taken from the thigh or buttocks are used for women who have had previous major abdominal surgery or who do not have enough abdominal tissue to reconstruct a breast. These types of flaps are free flaps. With these flaps an implant is often used as well to provide sufficient breast volume.
- **IGAP flap.** Tissue comes from the buttocks and contains only skin, blood vessels, and fat.
- **PAP flap.** Tissue, without muscle, that comes from the upper inner thigh.
- **SGAP flap.** Tissue comes from the buttocks as in an IGAP flap, but includes a different set of blood vessels and contains only skin, blood vessels, and fat.
- **TUG flap.** Tissue, including muscle, that comes from the upper inner thigh.

In some cases, an implant and autologous tissue are used together. For example, autologous tissue may be used to cover an implant when there is not enough skin and muscle left after mastectomy to allow for expansion and use of an implant.

HOW DO SURGEONS RECONSTRUCT THE NIPPLE AND AREOLA?

After the chest heals from reconstruction surgery and the position of the breast mound on the chest wall has had time to stabilize, a surgeon can reconstruct the nipple and areola. Usually, the new nipple is created by cutting and moving small pieces of skin from the reconstructed breast to the nipple site and shaping them into a new nipple. A few months after nipple reconstruction, the surgeon can re-create the areola. This is usually done using tattoo ink. However, in some cases, skin grafts may be taken from the groin or abdomen and attached to the breast to create an areola at the time of the nipple reconstruction.

Some women who do not have surgical nipple reconstruction may consider getting a realistic picture of a nipple created on the reconstructed breast from a tattoo artist who specializes in 3D nipple tattooing.

A mastectomy that preserves a woman's own nipple and areola, called "nipple-sparing mastectomy," may be an option for some women, depending on the size and location of the breast cancer and the shape and size of the breasts.

WHAT FACTORS CAN AFFECT THE TIMING OF BREAST RECONSTRUCTION?

One factor that can affect the timing of breast reconstruction is whether a woman will need radiation therapy. Radiation therapy can sometimes cause wound healing problems or infections in reconstructed breasts, so some women may prefer to delay reconstruction until after radiation therapy is completed. However, because of improvements in surgical and radiation techniques, immediate reconstruction with an implant is usually still an option for women who will need radiation therapy. Autologous tissue breast reconstruction is usually reserved for after radiation therapy, so that the breast and chest wall tissue damaged by radiation can be replaced with healthy tissue from elsewhere in the body.

Another factor is the type of breast cancer. Women with inflammatory breast cancer usually require more extensive skin removal. This can make immediate reconstruction more challenging, so it may be recommended that reconstruction be delayed until after completion of adjuvant therapy.

Even if a woman is a candidate for immediate reconstruction, she may choose delayed reconstruction. For instance, some women prefer not to consider what type of reconstruction to have until after they have recovered from their mastectomy and subsequent adjuvant treatment. Women who delay reconstruction (or choose not to undergo the procedure at all) can use external breast prostheses, or breast forms, to give the appearance of breasts.

WHAT FACTORS CAN AFFECT THE CHOICE OF BREAST RECONSTRUCTION METHOD?

Several factors can influence the type of reconstructive surgery a woman chooses. These include the size and shape of the breast that is being rebuilt, the woman's age and health, her history of past surgeries, surgical risk factors (for example, smoking history and obesity), the availability of autologous tissue, and the location of the tumor in the breast. Women who have had past abdominal surgery may not be candidates for an abdominally based flap reconstruction.

Each type of reconstruction has factors that a woman should think about before making a decision. Some of the more common considerations are listed below.

Reconstruction with Implants
SURGERY AND RECOVERY

- Enough skin and muscle must remain after mastectomy to cover the implant.
- Shorter surgical procedure than for reconstruction with autologous tissue; little blood loss.
- Recovery period may be shorter than with autologous reconstruction.

- Many follow-up visits may be needed to inflate the expander and insert the implant.

POSSIBLE COMPLICATIONS

- Infection
- Accumulation of clear fluid causing a mass or lump (seroma) within the reconstructed breast
- Pooling of blood (hematoma) within the reconstructed breast
- Blood clots
- Extrusion of the implant (the implant breaks through the skin)
- Implant rupture (the implant breaks open and saline or silicone leaks into the surrounding tissue)
- Formation of hard scar tissue around the implant (known as a "contracture")
- Obesity, diabetes, and smoking may increase the rate of complications
- Possible increased risk of developing a very rare form of immune system cancer called "anaplastic large cell lymphoma"

OTHER CONSIDERATIONS

- May not be an option for patients who have previously undergone radiation therapy to the chest
- May not be adequate for women with very large breasts
- Will not last a lifetime; the longer a woman has implants, the more likely she is to have complications and to need to have her implants removed or replaced
- Silicone implants may feel more natural than saline implants to the touch
- The U.S. Food and Drug Administration (FDA) recommends that women with silicone implants undergo periodic MRI screenings to detect possible "silent" rupture of the implants

Reconstruction with Autologous Tissue
SURGERY AND RECOVERY
- Longer surgical procedure than for implants.
- The initial recovery period may be longer than for implants.
- Pedicled flap reconstruction is usually a shorter operation than free flap reconstruction and usually requires a shorter hospitalization.
- Free flap reconstruction is a longer, highly technical operation compared with pedicled flap reconstruction that requires a surgeon who has experience with microsurgery to re-attach blood vessels.

POSSIBLE COMPLICATIONS
- Necrosis (death) of the transferred tissue
- Blood clots may be more frequent with some flap sources.
- Pain and weakness at the site from which the donor tissue was taken
- Obesity, diabetes, and smoking may increase the rate of complications.

OTHER CONSIDERATIONS
- May provide a more natural breast shape than implants
- May feel softer and more natural to the touch than implants
- Leaves a scar at the site from which the donor tissue was taken
- Can be used to replace tissue that has been damaged by radiation therapy

All women who undergo mastectomy for breast cancer experience varying degrees of breast numbness and loss of sensation (feeling) because nerves that provide sensation to the breast are cut when breast tissue is removed during surgery. However, a woman may regain some sensation as the severed nerves grow

313

and regenerate, and breast surgeons continue to make technical advances that can spare or repair damage to nerves.

Any type of breast reconstruction can fail if healing does not occur properly. In these cases, the implant or flap will have to be removed. If an implant reconstruction fails, a woman can usually have a second reconstruction using an alternative approach.

WILL HEALTH INSURANCE PAY FOR BREAST RECONSTRUCTION?

The Women's Health and Cancer Rights Act of 1998 (WHCRA) is a federal law that requires group health plans and health insurance companies that offer mastectomy coverage to also pay for reconstructive surgery after mastectomy. This coverage must include all stages of reconstruction and surgery to achieve symmetry between the breasts, breast prostheses, and treatment of complications that result from the mastectomy, including lymphedema. More information about WHCRA is available from the U.S. Department of Labor (DOL) and the Centers for Medicare & Medicaid Services (CMS).

Some health plans sponsored by religious organizations and some government health plans may be exempt from WHCRA. Also, WHCRA does not apply to Medicare and Medicaid. However, Medicare may cover breast reconstruction surgery as well as external breast prostheses (including a postsurgical bra) after a medically necessary mastectomy.

Medicaid benefits vary by state; a woman should contact her state Medicaid office for information on whether, and to what extent, breast reconstruction is covered.

A woman considering breast reconstruction may want to discuss costs and health insurance coverage with her doctor and insurance company before choosing to have the surgery. Some insurance companies require a second opinion before they will agree to pay for a surgery.

WHAT TYPE OF FOLLOW-UP CARE AND REHABILITATION IS NEEDED AFTER BREAST RECONSTRUCTION?

Any type of reconstruction increases the number of side effects a woman may experience compared with those after a mastectomy alone.

A woman's medical team will watch her closely for complications, some of which can occur months or even years after surgery.

Women who have either autologous tissue or implant-based reconstruction may benefit from physical therapy to improve or maintain shoulder range of motion or help them recover from weakness experienced at the site from which the donor tissue was taken, such as abdominal weakness. A physical therapist can help a woman use exercises to regain strength, adjust to new physical limitations, and figure out the safest ways to perform everyday activities.

DOES BREAST RECONSTRUCTION AFFECT THE ABILITY TO CHECK FOR BREAST CANCER RECURRENCE?

Studies have shown that breast reconstruction does not increase the chances of breast cancer coming back or make it harder to check for recurrence with mammography.

Women who have one breast removed by mastectomy will still have mammograms of the other breast. Women who have had a skin-sparing mastectomy or who are at high risk of breast cancer recurrence may have mammograms of the reconstructed breast if it was reconstructed using autologous tissue. However, mammograms are generally not performed on breasts that are reconstructed with an implant after mastectomy.

A woman with a breast implant should tell the radiology technician about her implant before she has a mammogram. Special procedures may be necessary to improve the accuracy of the mammogram and to avoid damaging the implant.

WHAT ARE SOME NEW DEVELOPMENTS IN BREAST RECONSTRUCTION AFTER MASTECTOMY?

Oncoplastic surgery. In general, women who have lumpectomy or partial mastectomy for early-stage breast cancer do not have reconstruction. However, for some of these women the surgeon may use plastic surgery techniques to reshape the breast at the time of cancer surgery. This type of breast-conserving surgery, called "oncoplastic surgery," may use local tissue rearrangement, reconstruction through breast reduction surgery, or transfer of tissue flaps. Long-term outcomes of this type of surgery are comparable to those for standard breast-conserving surgery.

Autologous fat grafting. A newer type of breast reconstruction technique involves the transfer of fat tissue from one part of the body (usually the thighs, abdomen, or buttocks) to the reconstructed breast. The fat tissue is harvested by liposuction, washed, and liquified so that it can be injected into the area of interest. Fat grafting is mainly used to correct deformities and asymmetries that may appear after breast reconstruction. It is also sometimes used to reconstruct an entire breast. Although concern has been raised about the lack of long-term outcome studies, this technique is considered safe.

Section 29.4 | Breast Implant Surgery

This section includes text excerpted from "Breast Implant Surgery," U.S. Food and Drug Administration (FDA), October 23, 2019.

Breast implant surgery can be performed in a hospital or surgery center. Breast implant surgery patients may have to stay overnight in the hospital (inpatient surgery) or may be able to go home afterward (outpatient surgery). The surgery can be done under local anesthesia, where the patient remains awake and only the breast is numbed to block the pain, or under general anesthesia, where medicine is given to make the patient sleep. Most women receive general anesthesia for this surgery. Breast implant surgery can last from one to several hours depending on the procedure and personal circumstances.

If the surgery is done in a hospital, the length of the hospital stay will vary based on the type of surgery, any complications after surgery, and your general health. The length of the hospital stay may also depend on the type of coverage your insurance provides.

SURGICAL MESH AND BREAST SURGERY

Surgical mesh is typically a flexible, thin flat sheet, usually made of nondegradable synthetic materials, biodegradable synthetic materials, or from animal- or human-derived tissues called "acellular dermal matrices" (ADM). Surgical mesh is a medical device, regulated by the U.S. Food and Drug Administration (FDA).

The FDA has not cleared or approved any surgical mesh for use with breast implants or in breast reconstruction, and thus has not reviewed potential benefits and risks for these uses. The FDA recommends that patients discuss the benefits and risks of mesh with their healthcare providers.

SURGICAL CONSULTATION

Before surgery you should have a consultation with your surgeon. Be prepared to ask questions about the surgeon's experience, your surgery and expected outcomes. The FDA has provided a list of questions that may help guide your discussion. The surgeon should be able to discuss whether you are a good candidate for breast implants, the different types of implants, options for size, shape, surface texture, and placement based on your particular circumstances, as well as the risks and benefits of implant surgery. The surgeon should also be able to provide you with before and after pictures of other patients to help you better understand your expectations and potential outcomes from surgery.

During the consultation you will need to discuss your medical history, including any medical conditions or drug allergies you may have. You should also discuss any previous surgeries you have had, especially to the breast, and what drugs you are currently taking, including supplements, herbal and over-the-counter (OTC) medications. It is important to tell the surgeon if you think you may be pregnant.

If you are undergoing breast implant surgery for reconstruction, you will also need to speak with your surgeon about your personal circumstances, including being treated with chemotherapy and/or radiation therapy, as these can affect your risks of complication and the appearance of the reconstructed breast. The surgeon should also speak to you about the amount of breast tissue that will remain after surgery and future screening for breast implant ruptures and breast cancer.

During the consultation be sure to ask the surgeon for a copy of the patient labeling for the breast implant she or he plans to use. You have the right to request this information, and your physician is expected to provide it. Be sure to read the patient labeling entirely prior to surgery. It will provide you with information specific to your breast implants, including how to take care of them. Make sure you read and understand the informed consent form before you sign it.

Breast implant manufacturers are currently conducting clinical studies to evaluate new types of breast implants and to understand the long term experiences of women who receive breast implants. If you are interested in participating in a clinical study, be sure to ask your surgeon what specific steps you will need to take.

QUESTIONS TO ASK YOUR DOCTOR BEFORE HAVING BREAST IMPLANT SURGERY

When choosing a surgeon for a breast implant procedure, you may want to consider their years of experience, their board certification, their patient follow-up, and your own comfort level with the surgeon. Most breast implant procedures are performed by board-certified plastic and reconstructive surgeons.

Section 29.5 | Surgery to Reduce the Risk of Breast Cancer

This section includes text excerpted from "Surgery to Reduce the Risk of Breast Cancer," National Cancer Institute (NCI), August 12, 2013. Reviewed April 2020.

WHAT KINDS OF SURGERY CAN REDUCE THE RISK OF BREAST CANCER?

Two kinds of surgery can be performed to reduce the risk of breast cancer in a woman who has never been diagnosed with breast cancer, but is known to be at very high risk of the disease.

A woman can be at very high risk of developing breast cancer if she has a strong family history of breast and/or ovarian cancer, a deleterious (disease-causing) mutation in the *BRCA1* gene or the

BRCA2 gene, or a high-penetrance mutation in one of several other genes associated with breast cancer risk, such as *TP53* or *PTEN*.

The most common risk-reducing surgery is bilateral prophylactic mastectomy (also called "bilateral risk-reducing mastectomy"). Bilateral prophylactic mastectomy may involve complete removal of both breasts, including the nipples (total mastectomy), or it may involve removal of as much breast tissue as possible while leaving the nipples intact (subcutaneous or nipple-sparing mastectomy). Subcutaneous mastectomies preserve the nipple and allow for more natural-looking breasts if a woman chooses to have breast reconstruction surgery afterward. However, total mastectomy provides the greatest breast cancer risk reduction because more breast tissue is removed in this procedure than in a subcutaneous mastectomy.

Even with total mastectomy, not all breast tissue that may be at risk of becoming cancerous in the future can be removed. The chest wall, which is not typically removed during a mastectomy, may contain some breast tissue, and breast tissue can sometimes be found in the armpit, above the collarbone, and as far down as the abdomen—and it is impossible for a surgeon to remove all of this tissue.

The other kind of risk-reducing surgery is bilateral prophylactic salpingo-oophorectomy, which is sometimes called "prophylactic oophorectomy." This surgery involves removal of the ovaries and fallopian tubes and may be done alone or along with bilateral prophylactic mastectomy in premenopausal women who are at very high risk of breast cancer. Removing the ovaries in premenopausal women reduces the amount of estrogen that is produced by the body. Because estrogen promotes the growth of some breast cancers, reducing the amount of this hormone in the body by removing the ovaries may slow the growth of those breast cancers.

HOW EFFECTIVE ARE RISK-REDUCING SURGERIES?
Bilateral prophylactic mastectomy has been shown to reduce the risk of breast cancer by at least 95 percent in women who have a deleterious (disease-causing) mutation in the *BRCA1* gene or the *BRCA2* gene and by up to 90 percent in women who have a strong family history of breast cancer.

Bilateral prophylactic salpingo-oophorectomy has been shown to reduce the risk of ovarian cancer by approximately 90 percent and the risk of breast cancer by approximately 50 percent in women at very high risk of developing these diseases.

WHICH WOMEN MIGHT CONSIDER HAVING SURGERY TO REDUCE THEIR RISK OF BREAST CANCER?

Women who inherit a deleterious mutation in the *BRCA1* gene or the *BRCA2* gene or mutations in certain other genes that greatly increase the risk of developing breast cancer may consider having bilateral prophylactic mastectomy and/or bilateral prophylactic salpingo-oophorectomy to reduce this risk.

In two studies, the estimated risks of developing breast cancer by age 70 years were 55 to 65 percent for women who carry a deleterious mutation in the *BRCA1* gene and 45 to 47 percent for women who carry a deleterious mutation in the *BRCA2* gene. Estimates of the lifetime risk of breast cancer for women with Cowden syndrome, which is caused by certain mutations in the *PTEN* gene, range from 25 to 50 percent or higher, and for women with Li-Fraumeni syndrome, which is caused by certain mutations in the *TP53* gene, from 49 to 60 percent. (By contrast, the lifetime risk of breast cancer for the average American woman is about 12 percent.)

Other women who are at very high risk of breast cancer may also consider bilateral prophylactic mastectomy, including:

- Those with a strong family history of breast cancer (such as having a mother, sister, and/or daughter who was diagnosed with bilateral breast cancer or with breast cancer before 50 years of age or having multiple family members with breast or ovarian cancer).
- Those with lobular carcinoma in situ (LCIS) plus a family history of breast cancer (LCIS is a condition in which abnormal cells are found in the lobules of the breast. It is not cancer, but women with LCIS have an increased risk of developing invasive breast cancer in either breast. Many breast surgeons consider prophylactic mastectomy to be an overly aggressive

approach for women with LCIS who do not have a strong family history or other risk factors).

- Those who have had radiation therapy to the chest (including the breasts) before the age of 30 years—for example, if they were treated with radiation therapy for Hodgkin lymphoma (Such women are at high risk of developing breast cancer throughout their lives).

CAN A WOMAN HAVE RISK-REDUCING SURGERY IF SHE HAS ALREADY BEEN DIAGNOSED WITH BREAST CANCER?

Yes. Some women who have been diagnosed with cancer in one breast, particularly those who are known to be at very high risk, may consider having the other breast (called "the contralateral breast") removed as well, even if there is no sign of cancer in that breast. Prophylactic surgery to remove a contralateral breast during breast cancer surgery (known as "contralateral prophylactic mastectomy") reduces the risk of breast cancer in that breast, although it is not yet known whether this risk reduction translates into longer survival for the patient.

However, doctors often discourage contralateral prophylactic mastectomy for women with cancer in one breast who do not meet the criteria of being at very high risk of developing a contralateral breast cancer. For such women, the risk of developing another breast cancer, either in the same or the contralateral breast, is very small, especially if they receive adjuvant chemotherapy or hormone therapy as part of their cancer treatment.

Given that most women with breast cancer have a low risk of developing the disease in their contralateral breast, women who are not known to be at very high risk, but who remain concerned about cancer development in their other breast may want to consider options other than surgery to further reduce their risk of a contralateral breast cancer.

WHAT ARE THE POTENTIAL HARMS OF RISK-REDUCING SURGERIES?

As with any other major surgery, bilateral prophylactic mastectomy and bilateral prophylactic salpingo-oophorectomy have potential complications or harms, such as bleeding or infection. Also, both surgeries are irreversible.

Bilateral prophylactic mastectomy can also affect a woman's psychological well-being due to a change in body image and the loss of normal breast functions. Although most women who choose to have this surgery are satisfied with their decision, they can still experience anxiety and concerns about body image. The most common psychological side effects include difficulties with body appearance, with feelings of femininity, and with sexual relationships. Women who undergo total mastectomies lose nipple sensation, which may hinder sexual arousal.

Bilateral prophylactic salpingo-oophorectomy causes a sudden drop in estrogen production, which will induce early menopause in a premenopausal woman (this is also called "surgical menopause"). Surgical menopause can cause an abrupt onset of menopausal symptoms, including hot flashes, insomnia, anxiety, and depression, and some of these symptoms can be severe. The long-term effects of surgical menopause include decreased sex drive, vaginal dryness, and decreased bone density.

Women who have severe menopausal symptoms after undergoing bilateral prophylactic salpingo-oophorectomy may consider using short-term menopausal hormone therapy after surgery to alleviate these symptoms. The increase in breast cancer risk associated with certain types of menopausal hormone therapy is much less than the decrease in breast cancer risk associated with bilateral prophylactic salpingo-oophorectomy.

WHAT ARE THE CANCER RISK REDUCTION OPTIONS FOR WOMEN WHO ARE AT INCREASED RISK OF BREAST CANCER, BUT NOT AT THE HIGHEST RISK?

Risk-reducing surgery is not considered an appropriate cancer prevention option for women who are not at the highest risk of breast cancer (that is, for those who do not carry a high-penetrance gene mutation that is associated with breast cancer or who do not have a clinical or medical history that puts them at very high risk). However, some women who are not at very high risk of breast cancer, but are, nonetheless, considered as being at increased risk of the disease may choose to use drugs to reduce their risk.

Healthcare providers use several types of tools, called "risk assessment models," to estimate the risk of breast cancer for women who do not have a deleterious mutation in *BRCA1*, *BRCA2*, or another gene associated with breast cancer risk. One widely used tool is the Breast Cancer Risk Assessment Tool (BCRAT), a computer model that takes a number of factors into account in estimating the risks of breast cancer over the next 5 years and up to age 90 years (lifetime risk). Women who have an estimated 5-year risk of 1.67 percent or higher are classified as "high-risk," which means that they have a higher than average risk of developing breast cancer. This high-risk cutoff (that is, an estimated 5-year risk of 1.67 percent or higher) is widely used in research studies and in clinical counseling.

Two drugs, tamoxifen and raloxifene hydrochloride, are approved by the U.S. Food and Drug Administration (FDA) to reduce the risk of breast cancer in women who have a 5-year risk of developing breast cancer of 1.67 percent or more. Tamoxifen is approved for risk reduction in both premenopausal and post-menopausal women, and raloxifene is approved for risk reduction in postmenopausal women only. In large randomized clinical trials, tamoxifen, taken for 5 years, reduced the risk of invasive breast cancer by about 50 percent in high-risk postmenopausal women; raloxifene, taken for 5 years, reduced breast cancer risk by about 38 percent in high-risk postmenopausal women. Both drugs block the activity of estrogen, thereby inhibiting the growth of some breast cancers. The U.S. Preventive Services Task Force (USPSTF) recommends that women at increased risk of breast cancer talk with their healthcare professional about the potential benefits and harms of taking tamoxifen or raloxifene to reduce their risk.

Another drug, exemestane, was recently shown to reduce the incidence of breast cancer in postmenopausal women who are at increased risk of the disease by 65 percent. Exemestane belongs to a class of drugs called "aromatase inhibitors," which block the production of estrogen by the body. It is not known, however, whether any of these drugs reduces the very high risk of breast cancer for women who carry a known mutation that is strongly associated with an increased risk of breast cancer, such as deleterious mutations in *BRCA1* and *BRCA2*.

Some women who have undergone breast cancer surgery, regardless of their risk of recurrence, may be given drugs to reduce the likelihood that their breast cancer will recur. (This additional treatment is called "adjuvant therapy.") Such treatment also reduces the already low risks of contralateral and second primary breast cancers. Drugs that are used as adjuvant therapy to reduce the risk of breast cancer after breast cancer surgery include tamoxifen, aromatase inhibitors, traditional chemotherapy agents, and trastuzumab.

WHAT CAN WOMEN AT VERY HIGH RISK DO IF THEY DO NOT WANT TO UNDERGO RISK-REDUCING SURGERY?

Some women who are at very high risk of breast cancer (or of contralateral breast cancer) may undergo more frequent breast cancer screening (also known as "enhanced screening"). For example, they may have yearly mammograms and yearly magnetic resonance imaging (MRI) screening—with these tests staggered so that the breasts are imaged every six months—as well as clinical breast examinations performed regularly by a healthcare professional. Enhanced screening may increase the chance of detecting breast cancer at an early stage, when it may have a better chance of being treated successfully.

Women who carry mutations in some genes that increase their risk of breast cancer may be more likely to develop radiation-associated breast cancer than the general population because those genes are involved in the repair of DNA breaks, which can be caused by exposure to radiation. Women who are at high risk of breast cancer should ask their healthcare provider about the risks of diagnostic tests that involve radiation (mammograms or x-rays). Ongoing clinical trials are examining various aspects of enhanced screening for women who are at high risk of breast cancer.

Chemoprevention (the use of drugs or other agents to reduce cancer risk or delay its development) may be an option for some women who wish to avoid surgery. Tamoxifen and raloxifene have both been approved by the FDA to reduce the risk of breast cancer in women at increased risk. Whether these drugs can be used to prevent breast cancer in women at much higher risk, such as women with harmful mutations in *BRCA1* or *BRCA2* or other breast cancer susceptibility genes, is not yet clear, although tamoxifen may be able to help lower the risk of contralateral breast cancer among *BRCA1* and *BRCA2* mutation carriers previously diagnosed with breast cancer.

DOES HEALTH INSURANCE COVER THE COST OF RISK-REDUCING SURGERIES?

Many health insurance companies have official policies about whether and under what conditions they will pay for prophylactic mastectomy (bilateral or contralateral) and bilateral prophylactic salpingo-oophorectomy for breast and ovarian cancer risk reduction. However, the criteria used for considering these procedures as medically necessary may vary among insurance companies. Some insurance companies may require a second opinion or a letter of medical necessity from the healthcare provider before they will approve coverage of any surgical procedure. A woman who is considering prophylactic surgery to reduce her risk of breast and/or ovarian cancer should discuss insurance coverage issues with her doctor and insurance company before choosing to have the surgery.

The Women's Health and Cancer Rights Act (WHCRA), enacted in 1999, requires most health plans that offer mastectomy coverage to also pay for breast reconstruction surgery after mastectomy.

WHO SHOULD A WOMAN TALK TO WHEN CONSIDERING SURGERY TO REDUCE HER RISK OF BREAST CANCER?

The decision to have any surgery to reduce the risk of breast cancer is a major one. A woman who is at high risk of breast cancer may wish to get a second opinion on risk-reducing surgery as well as on alternatives to surgery.

A woman who is considering prophylactic mastectomy may also want to talk with a surgeon who specializes in breast reconstruction. Other healthcare professionals, including a breast health specialist, medical social worker, or cancer clinical psychologist

325

or psychiatrist, can also help a woman consider her options for reducing her risk of breast cancer.

Many factors beyond the risk of disease itself may influence a woman's decision about whether to undergo risk-reducing surgery. For example, for women who have been diagnosed with cancer in one breast, these factors can include distress about the possibility of having to go through cancer treatment a second time and the worry and inconvenience associated with long-term breast surveillance. For this reason, women who are considering risk-reducing surgery may want to talk with other women who have considered or had the procedure. Support groups can help connect women with others who have had similar cancer experiences. The searchable NCI database national organizations that offer cancer-related services has listings for many support groups.

Finally, if a woman has a strong family history of breast cancer, ovarian cancer, or both, she and other members of her family may want to obtain genetic counseling services. A genetic counselor or other healthcare provider trained in genetics can review the family's risks of disease and help family members obtain genetic testing for mutations in cancer-predisposing genes, if appropriate.

Chapter 30 | Respiratory Tract and Lung Surgeries

Chapter Contents

Section 30.1 | Treating Recurrent Respiratory Papillomatosis (RRP)

This section includes text excerpted from "Recurrent Respiratory Papillomatosis or Laryngeal Papillomatosis," National Institute on Deafness and Other Communication Disorders (NIDCD), November 28, 2017.

WHAT IS RECURRENT RESPIRATORY PAPILLOMATOSIS?

Recurrent respiratory papillomatosis (RRP) is a disease in which benign (noncancerous) tumors called "papillomas" grow in the air passages leading from the nose and mouth into the lungs (respiratory tract). Although the tumors can grow anywhere in the respiratory tract, they most commonly grow in the larynx (voice box)—a condition called "laryngeal papillomatosis." The papillomas may vary in size and grow very quickly. They often grow back after they have been removed.

HOW IS RECURRENT RESPIRATORY PAPILLOMATOSIS PREVENTED OR TREATED?

Vaccination with the human papillomavirus (HPV) vaccine could prevent the development of RRP. The Centers for Disease Control and Prevention (CDC) currently recommends that all children (both boys and girls) receive the HPV vaccine at ages 11 or 12. Ask your child's doctor whether the type of HPV vaccine your child will receive will protect against HPV 6 and 11. As more young people receive the vaccine, future research will reveal its effectiveness in preventing HPV-associated diseases, such as RRP.

Once RRP develops, there is currently no cure. Surgery is the primary method for removing tumors from the larynx or airway. Because traditional surgery can cause problems due to scarring of the larynx tissue, many surgeons now use laser surgery. Carbon dioxide (CO_2) or potassium titanyl phosphate (KTP) lasers are frequently used for this purpose. Surgeons also commonly use a device called a "microdebrider," which uses suction to hold the tumor in place while a small internal rotary blade removes the growth.

Once the tumors have been removed, they can still return. It is common for patients to require multiple surgeries. With some patients, surgery may be required every few weeks in order to keep the breathing passage open, while others may require surgery only once a year or even less frequently.

In the most extreme cases of aggressive tumor growth, a tracheotomy may be performed. A tracheotomy is a surgical procedure in which an incision is made in the front of the patient's neck and a breathing tube (trach tube) is inserted through an opening, called a "stoma," into the trachea (windpipe). Rather than breathing through the nose and mouth, the patient will now breathe through the trach tube. Although the trach tube keeps the breathing passage open, doctors try to remove it as soon as possible.

Some patients may be required to keep a trach tube indefinitely in order to keep the breathing passage open. Because the trach tube re-routes all or some of the exhaled air away from the vocal folds, the patient may find it difficult to use her or his voice. With the help of a voice specialist or speech-language pathologist who specializes in voice, the patient can learn to use her or his voice with the use of a speaking valve.

In severe cases of RRP, therapies in addition to surgery may be used. Drug treatments may include antivirals, such as interferon and cidofovir, which block the virus from making copies of itself; indole-3-carbinol, a cancer-fighting compound found in cruciferous vegetables, such as broccoli and brussels sprouts; or bevacizumab, which targets the blood vessel growth of papilloma. To date, the results of these and other nonsurgical therapies have been mixed or not yet fully proven.

Section 30.2 | **Tracheostomy**

This section contains text excerpted from the following sources: Text under the heading "The Surgery" is excerpted from "Tracheostomy," National Heart, Lung, and Blood Institute (NHLBI), December 10, 2016. Reviewed April 2020; Text beginning the heading "Indications" is excerpted from "Breathe Easy: Safe Tracheostomy Management," Agency for Healthcare Research and Quality (AHRQ), U.S. Department of Health and Human Services (HHS), August 1, 2015. Reviewed April 2020.

THE SURGERY

A tracheostomy is a surgically made hole that goes through the front of your neck into your trachea, or windpipe. A breathing tube, called a "trach tube," is placed through the hole and directly into your windpipe to help you breathe. A tracheostomy may be used to help people who need to be on ventilators for more than a couple of weeks or who have conditions that block the upper airways.

A surgeon can make a tracheostomy in a hospital operating room when you are asleep from general anesthesia. A doctor or emergency medical technician can make a tracheostomy safely at a patient's bedside, such as in the intensive care unit (ICU), or elsewhere in a life-threatening situation. A tracheostomy usually takes 20 to 45 minutes to perform. The surgeon or other healthcare professional will make a cut through the lower front part of your neck and then cut into your windpipe. Cuffed trach tubes may be used. These tubes use air to widen or narrow the tube to fit the hole. After inserting and placing the trach tube into the windpipe, the surgeon or other healthcare professional will use stitches, surgical tape, or a velcro band to hold the tube in place.

After getting the tracheostomy, you may stay in the hospital to recover depending on your health. It can take up to two weeks for a tracheostomy to fully form, or mature. During this time, you will not be able to eat normally and will likely receive nutrients through a feeding tube. You may have difficulty talking after your tracheostomy. A speech therapist can help you to regain normal swallowing ability and use your voice to speak clearly. Your trach tube will be removed when you no longer need it. The hole usually closes on its own, but surgery can close the hole if needed.

Tracheostomy is a fairly common and simple procedure, especially for critical care patients in hospitals. Soon after the procedure, it is possible to have bleeding, infection, pneumothorax or collapsed lung, or subcutaneous emphysema. Over time, complications may include windpipe scarring or an abnormal connection, called a "fistula," between the windpipe and esophagus that causes food and saliva to enter your lungs. It is also possible to have complications that affect the function of the trach tube, such as the tube slipping or falling out of place, or that affect the windpipe or other airway structures. Proper care and handling of the tracheostomy, the tubes, and other related supplies can help reduce risks.

INDICATIONS

Prolonged respiratory failure is the most common indication for tracheostomy in the United States. The purported benefits of tracheostomy include enhanced weaning off the ventilator, improved pulmonary hygiene, greater patient comfort, facilitation of speech and swallowing, and earlier transition out of the ICU. Relative contraindications to tracheostomy placement include an existing coagulopathy, a high level of dependence on the ventilator (e.g., PEEP [positive end-expiratory pressure] greater than 16 cm H_2O, FiO_2 [fraction of inspired oxygen] greater than 0.60), and a high-riding innominate artery (owing to its proximity to the procedure location). It is also important to recognize that goals of care discussions frequently occur contemporaneously with the decision for tracheostomy, especially in cases where the decision to place a tracheostomy implies the need for prolonged mechanical ventilation due to poor clinical prognosis. This approach is contrasted with clinical situations where patients require prolonged tracheostomy use and the benefits are for airway protection rather than mechanical ventilation (e.g., head and neck cancers causing airway obstruction).

There is no consensus on the ideal timing of tracheostomy placement in prolonged ventilator dependence. Tracheostomy should be considered around 14 days of intubation in an adult population to avoid laryngotracheal injury from prolonged intubation. Some healthcare providers promote early tracheostomy (for patients with more than 4 days of intubation) to reduce sedation requirements, ventilator-associated pneumonia, and length of stay, though this remains controversial and cannot be considered standard of care.

Finally, tracheostomy may be performed via an open surgical approach or by percutaneous dilatational technique. Factors that determine the approach are beyond the scope of this review, but with appropriate patient selection, both are safe procedures.

MANAGEMENT

Tracheostomy care is an interdisciplinary effort. Physicians, nurses, respiratory therapists, speech-language pathologists, and family caregivers all play a crucial role in posttracheostomy care. Each institution should develop and maintain policies and procedures to define and standardize tracheostomy care.

Care and maintenance of a tracheostomy involves routine cleaning of the device and surrounding skin, regular suctioning of secretions, inner cannula maintenance, and oral care. Tracheostomy devices can cause pressure ulcers, particularly along the inferior aspect of the tracheostomy faceplate. Standardized processes for skincare, including removing sutures at 5 to 7 days and placement of a skin-barrier dressing under the tracheostomy faceplate, can reduce the incidence of tracheostomy-related pressure ulcers.

The tracheostomy device should also be changed at regular intervals. The first change is typically performed by the proceduralist. Tracheostomy changes are relatively safe when accomplished by trained providers. All tracheostomy changes within 5 days of insertion should be performed with surgical equipment available, as the stoma is not yet well-formed.

For many patients, a tracheostomy does not preclude the ability to communicate. Tracheostomy speaking valves are one-way valves placed on the tracheostomy tube connector. The valve opens during inspiration and closes during exhalation. During the expiratory phase, airflow is redirected to the upper airway, passing through the larynx, allowing for phonation. Anecdotally, tracheostomy speaking valves can improve quality of life (QOL) by restoring verbal communication. However, not all tracheostomy patients are candidates for speaking valve use. These valves may only be used in patients with patent upper airways. Placement of a tracheostomy speaking valve in a patient who is unable to pass air around the tracheostomy tube (i.e., inflated cuff or upper airway obstruction) may result in asphyxiation and death. Candidacy for speaking valve use should be determined through an evaluation by the proceduralist or speech-language pathologist.

Although some patients have lifelong tracheostomies, many can have their tracheostomy weaned as their underlying condition improves. Steps for tracheostomy wean include: i) wean from positive pressure ventilation, ii) demonstrate that the patient can tolerate cuff deflation, iii) perform sequential downsizing of tracheostomy tube, and iv) perform a capping trial. Cuff deflation requires restoration of airway protection and cough reflexes. Sequential downsizing to smaller tubes may follow as tolerated. With a small, cuffless tube in place, a capping trial can be performed, whereby the inner cannula is replaced with a plug. If the cap is tolerated for at least one wake-sleep cycle (approximately 24 hours), the tracheostomy is removed (decannulation) and the wound closes by secondary intention. An occlusive dressing is placed to prevent air escape during wound healing. The weaning process may be managed by trained providers, including physicians and respiratory therapists, in the rehabilitation setting.

COMPLICATIONS

Tracheostomy-related complications are uncommon (3.2% in an analysis of the National Inpatient Sample (NIS)). Most complications carry low morbidity, including minor bleeding, crepitus, cellulitis, and granulation. Major complications occur in less than 1 percent of patients and include major hemorrhage, airway obstruction, accidental decannulation, pneumothorax, tracheal stenosis, and tracheoesophageal fistula (TEF). Although inpatient mortality is high in this cohort (20%) it is generally from the underlying disease. Tracheostomy-specific mortality is rare (0.4%).

Most bleeding after tracheostomy is manageable with topical hemostatic agents. Rarely, prolonged tracheostomy can lead to erosion of the anterior tracheal wall adjacent to the innominate artery and cause life-threatening hemorrhage from tracheo-innominate fistula (TIF). TIF may be preceded by a sentinel bleed, with the patient presenting with brisk peristomal bleeding. Such bleeding mandates evaluation by the proceduralist to rule out TIF.

Accidental decannulation may occur in the early or late postoperative period. Signs of this complication include: gross device dislodgement, airway obstruction not relieved by suctioning or inner cannula replacement, or inability to pass a flexible suction catheter. Presentation may be subtle in a stable patient. During the first 5 to 7 days after tracheostomy, before the stoma is well-formed, dislodgement of the tube carries a greater risk of erroneous replacement into the paratracheal soft tissues and mediastinum (false passage). Until maturation, the tracheostomy tube should be secured by sutures and collar ties; torque on the device should be minimized. It is unclear what the root cause of the dislodgement was, but it is possible that the initial attempts to replace the tracheostomy were directed into a false passage.

Replacement of a dislodged tracheostomy tube should be accomplished by a trained provider with appropriate lighting and visualization to prevent a false passage. Standard airway management, including mask ventilation and trans-oral intubation, should be undertaken in cases of respiratory distress, except in cases of glottic obstruction, severe subglottic stenosis, or in patients following laryngectomy.

Pneumothorax is another uncommon early postoperative complication of tracheostomy (0.26%). Breath sounds should be auscultated in any patient with respiratory distress following tracheostomy. Chest radiograph is prudent if respiratory distress and asymmetric breath sounds are present.

The TEF occurs in approximately 1 in 1250 patients following tracheostomy. This complication results from posterior tracheal wall erosion. The hallmark of TEF is an air-leak despite a functional, fully inflated cuff. This complication may lead to aspiration and pneumonia, and these complications should prompt the clinician to rule out TEF.

Finally, laryngotracheal stenosis occurs in approximately 1.7 percent of patients following tracheostomy, though many of these cases may be related to preceding intubation, particularly with a large (more than 7.5 mm) endotracheal tube.

CREATING SAFE SYSTEMS

Tracheostomy management is largely based on clinical algorithms and lends itself well to standardized care pathways. While many aspects of tracheostomy care are not evidence-based, practice variability within a healthcare system may lead to communication breakdown and inefficient or unsafe care. It is, therefore, incumbent upon healthcare systems to develop standardized care pathways that facilitate coordinated and safe care. Our anecdotal experience suggests that implementation of standardized protocols minimizes confusion among the multiple services who provide tracheostomy care and allows for safe and streamlined delivery of care.

TAKE-HOME POINTS

- Tracheostomy is a safe and beneficial tool in critically ill patients when managed appropriately.
- Each institution should develop standard tracheostomy management protocols to enhance patient safety.
- If unable to replace the tracheostomy tube, standard airway management algorithms can be utilized to secure the airway.

Chapter 31 | **Heart and Vascular Surgery**

Chapter Contents

Section 31.1 | An Overview of Heart Surgery

This section includes text excerpted from "Heart Surgery," National Heart, Lung, and Blood Institute (NHLBI), September 7, 2012. Reviewed April 2020.

WHAT IS HEART SURGERY?

Heart surgery is done to correct problems with the heart. Many heart surgeries are done each year in the United States for various heart problems.

Heart surgery is used for both children and adults. The most common type of heart surgery for adults is coronary artery bypass grafting (CABG). During CABG, a healthy artery or vein from the body is connected, or grafted, to a blocked coronary (heart) artery.

The most common type of heart surgery for adults is CABG. During CABG, a healthy artery or vein from the body is connected, or grafted, to a blocked coronary (heart) artery.

The grafted artery or vein bypasses (that is, goes around) the blocked portion of the coronary artery. This creates a new path for oxygen-rich blood to flow to the heart muscle. CABG can relieve chest pain and may lower your risk of having a heart attack.

Doctors also use heart surgery to:
- Repair or replace heart valves, which control blood flow through the heart
- Repair abnormal or damaged structures in the heart
- Implant medical devices that help control the heartbeat or support heart function and blood flow
- Replace a damaged heart with a healthy heart from a donor

TRADITIONAL HEART SURGERY

Traditional heart surgery, often known as "open-heart surgery," is done by opening the chest wall to operate on the heart. The surgeon cuts through the patient's breastbone (or just the upper part of it) to open the chest.

Once the heart is exposed, the patient is connected to a heart-lung bypass machine. The machine takes over the heart's pumping action and moves blood away from the heart. This allows the surgeon to operate on a heart that is not beating and that does not have blood flowing through it.

Another type of heart surgery is called "off-pump," or beating heart surgery. It is like traditional open-heart surgery because the chest bone is opened to access the heart. However, the heart is not stopped, and a heart-lung bypass machine is not used. Off-pump heart surgery is limited to CABG.

Surgeons can now make small incisions (cuts) between the ribs to do some types of heart surgery. The breastbone is not opened to reach the heart. This is known as "minimally invasive heart surgery." This type of heart surgery may or may not use a heart-lung bypass machine.

Newer methods of heart surgery (such as off-pump and minimally invasive) may reduce risks and speed up recovery time. Studies are underway to compare these types of heart surgery with traditional open-heart surgery.

The results of these studies will help doctors decide the best surgery to use for each patient.

The results of heart surgery in adults often are excellent. Heart surgery can reduce symptoms, improve quality of life, and improve the chances of survival.

TYPES OF HEART SURGERY
Coronary Artery Bypass Grafting

Coronary artery bypass grafting is the most common type of heart surgery. CABG improves blood flow to the heart. Surgeons use CABG to treat people who have severe coronary heart disease (CHD).

Coronary heart disease is a disease in which a waxy substance called "plaque" builds up inside the coronary arteries—the arteries that supply oxygen-rich blood to your heart.

Over time, plaque can harden or rupture (break open). Hardened plaque narrows the coronary arteries and reduces the flow of oxygen-rich blood to the heart. This can cause chest pain or discomfort called "angina."

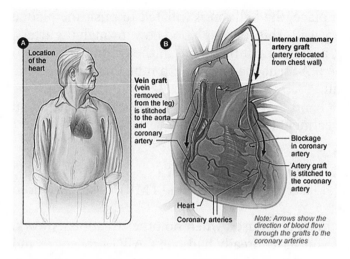

Figure 31.1. Grafting of Coronary Artery Bypass

Figure A shows the location of the heart. Figure B shows how vein and artery bypass grafts are attached to the heart.

If the plaque ruptures, a blood clot can form on its surface. A large blood clot can mostly or completely block blood flow through a coronary artery. This is the most common cause of a heart attack. Over time, ruptured plaque also hardens and narrows the coronary arteries.

During CABG, a healthy artery or vein from the body is connected, or grafted, to the blocked coronary artery. The grafted artery or vein bypasses (that is, goes around) the blocked portion of the coronary artery. This creates a new path for oxygen-rich blood to flow to the heart muscle.

Surgeons can bypass multiple blocked coronary arteries during one surgery.

Coronary artery bypass grafting is not the only treatment for CHD. A nonsurgical procedure that opens blocked or narrow coronary arteries is percutaneous coronary intervention (PCI), also known as "coronary angioplasty."

During PCI, a thin, flexible tube with a balloon at its tip is threaded through a blood vessel to the narrow or blocked coronary artery. Once in place, the balloon is inflated to push the plaque against the artery wall. This restores blood flow through the artery.

During PCI, a stent might be placed in the coronary artery to help keep it open. A stent is a small mesh tube that supports the inner artery wall.

If both CABG and PCI are options, your doctor can help you decide which treatment is right for you.

Transmyocardial Laser Revascularization

Transmyocardial laser revascularization (TMR), is surgery used to treat angina.

The TMR is most often used when no other treatments work. For example, if you have already had one CABG procedure and cannot have another one, TMR might be an option. For some people, TMR is combined with CABG.

If TMR is done alone, the procedure may be performed through a small opening in the chest.

During TMR, a surgeon uses lasers to make small channels through the heart muscle and into the heart's lower left chamber (the left ventricle).

It is not fully known how TMR relieves angina. The surgery may help the heart grow tiny new blood vessels. Oxygen-rich blood may flow through these vessels into the heart muscle, which could relieve angina.

Heart Valve Repair or Replacement

For the heart to work well, blood must flow in only one direction. The heart's valves make this possible. Healthy valves open and close in a precise way as the heart pumps blood.

Each valve has a set of flaps called "leaflets." The leaflets open to allow blood to pass from one heart chamber into another or into the arteries. Then the leaflets close tightly to stop blood from flowing backward.

Heart surgery is used to fix leaflets that do not open as wide as they should. This can happen if they become thick or stiff or fuse together. As a result, not enough blood flows through the valve.

Heart surgery also is used to fix leaflets that do not close tightly. This problem can cause blood to leak back into the heart chambers, rather than only moving forward into the arteries as it should.

To fix these problems, surgeons either repair the valve or replace it with a human-made or biological valve. Biological valves are made from pig, cow, or human heart tissue and may have human-made parts as well.

To repair a mitral or pulmonary valve that is too narrow, a cardiologist (heart specialist) will insert a catheter (a thin, flexible tube) through a large blood vessel and guide it to the heart.

The cardiologist will place the end of the catheter inside the narrow valve. She or he will inflate and deflate a small balloon at the tip of the catheter. This widens the valve, allowing more blood to flow through it. This approach is less invasive than open-heart surgery.

Researchers also are testing new ways to use catheters in other types of valve surgeries. For example, catheters might be used to place clips on the mitral valve leaflets to hold them in place.

Catheters also might be used to replace faulty aortic valves. For this procedure, the catheter usually is inserted into an artery in the groin (upper thigh) and threaded to the heart.

In some cases, surgeons might make a small cut in the chest and left ventricle (the lower left heart chamber). They will thread the catheter into the heart through the small opening.

The catheter has a deflated balloon at its tip with a folded replacement valve around it. The balloon is used to expand the new valve so it fits securely within the old valve.

Surgery to replace the valve is the traditional treatment for reasonably healthy people. However, catheter procedures might be a safer option for patients who have conditions that make open-heart surgery very risky.

Arrhythmia Treatment

An arrhythmia is a problem with the rate or rhythm of the heartbeat. During an arrhythmia, the heart can beat too fast, too slow, or with an irregular rhythm.

Many arrhythmias are harmless, but some can be serious or even life-threatening. If the heart rate is abnormal, the heart may not be able to pump enough blood to the body. Lack of blood flow can damage the brain, heart, and other organs.

Medicine usually is the first line of treatment for arrhythmias. If medicine does not work well, your doctor may recommend surgery. For example, surgery may be used to implant a pacemaker or an implantable cardioverter-defibrillator (ICD).

A pacemaker is a small device that is placed under the skin of your chest or abdomen. Wires connect the pacemaker to your heart chambers. The device uses low-energy electrical pulses to control your heart rhythm. Most pacemakers have a sensor that starts the device only if your heart rhythm is abnormal.

An ICD is another small device that is placed under the skin of your chest or abdomen. This device also is connected to your heart with wires. An ICD checks your heartbeat for dangerous arrhythmias. If the device senses one, it sends an electric shock to your heart to restore a normal heart rhythm.

Another arrhythmia treatment is called "maze surgery." For this surgery, the surgeon makes new paths for the heart's electrical signals to travel through. This type of surgery is used to treat atrial fibrillation, the most common type of serious arrhythmia.

Simpler, less invasive procedures also are used to treat atrial fibrillation. These procedures use high heat or intense cold to prevent abnormal electrical signals from moving through the heart.

Aneurysm Repair

An aneurysm is a balloon-like bulge in the wall of an artery or the heart muscle. This bulge can occur if the artery wall weakens. Pressure from blood moving through the artery or heart causes the weak area to bulge.

Over time, an aneurysm can grow and burst, causing dangerous, often fatal bleeding inside the body. Aneurysms also can develop a split in one or more layers of the artery wall. The split causes bleeding into and along the layers of the artery wall.

Aneurysms in the heart most often occur in the heart's lower left chamber (the left ventricle). Repairing an aneurysm involves surgery to replace the weak section of the artery or heart wall with a patch or graft.

Heart Transplant

A heart transplant is surgery to remove a person's diseased heart and replace it with a healthy heart from a deceased donor. Most heart transplants are done on patients who have end-stage heart failure.

Heart failure is a condition in which the heart is damaged or weak. As a result, it cannot pump enough blood to meet the body's needs. "End-stage" means the condition is so severe that all treatments, other than heart transplant, have failed.

Patients on the waiting list for a donor heart receive ongoing treatment for heart failure and other medical conditions. Ventricular assist devices (VADs) or total artificial hearts (TAHs) might be used to treat these patients.

SURGERY TO PLACE VENTRICULAR ASSIST DEVICES OR TOTAL ARTIFICIAL HEARTS

A VAD is a mechanical pump that is used to support heart function and blood flow in people who have weak hearts.

Your doctor may recommend a VAD if you have heart failure that is not responding to treatment or if you are waiting for a heart transplant. You can use a VAD for a short time or for months or years, depending on your situation.

A TAH is a device that replaces the two lower chambers of the heart (the ventricles). You may benefit from a TAH if both of your ventricles do not work well due to end-stage heart failure.

Placing either device requires open-heart surgery.

SURGICAL APPROACHES

Surgeons can use different approaches to operate on the heart, including open-heart surgery, off-pump heart surgery, and minimally invasive heart surgery.

The surgical approach will depend on the patient's heart problem, general health, and other factors.

Open-Heart Surgery

Open-heart surgery is any kind of surgery in which a surgeon makes a large incision (cut) in the chest to open the rib cage and operate on the heart. "Open" refers to the chest, not the heart. Depending on the type of surgery, the surgeon also may open the heart.

Once the heart is exposed, the patient is connected to a heart-lung bypass machine. The machine takes over the heart's pumping action and moves blood away from the heart. This allows the surgeon to operate on a heart that is not beating and that does not have blood flowing through it.

Open-heart surgery is used to do CABG, repair or replace heart valves, treat atrial fibrillation, do heart transplants, and place VADs and TAHs.

Off-Pump Heart Surgery

Surgeons also use off-pump, or beating heart, surgery to do CABG. This approach is like traditional open-heart surgery because the chest bone is opened to access the heart. However, the heart is not stopped, and a heart-lung bypass machine is not used.

Off-pump heart surgery is not right for all patients. Work with your doctor to decide whether this type of surgery is an option for you. Your doctor will carefully consider your heart problem, age, overall health, and other factors that may affect the surgery.

Minimally Invasive Heart Surgery

For minimally invasive heart surgery, a surgeon makes small incisions (cuts) in the side of the chest between the ribs. This type of surgery may or may not use a heart-lung bypass machine.

Minimally invasive heart surgery is used to do some bypass and maze surgeries. It is also used to repair or replace heart valves, insert pacemakers or ICDs, or take a vein or artery from the body to use as a bypass graft for CABG.

One type of minimally invasive heart surgery that is becoming more common is robotic-assisted surgery. For this surgery, a surgeon uses a computer to control surgical tools on thin robotic arms.

The tools are inserted through small incisions in the chest. This allows the surgeon to do complex and highly precise surgery. The surgeon is always in total control of the robotic arms; they do not move on their own.

Section 31.2 | Angioplasty and Stent Placement

This section contains text excerpted from the following sources: Text in this section begins with excerpts from "Percutaneous Coronary Intervention," National Heart, Lung, and Blood Institute (NHLBI), November 14, 2011, Reviewed April 2020; Text beginning with the heading "Coronary Artery Stent, Carotid Artery Stent, Airway Stent " is excerpted from "Stents," National Heart, Lung, and Blood Institute (NHLBI), November 4, 2012. Reviewed April 2020.

Percutaneous coronary intervention (PCI) requires cardiac catheterization, which is the insertion of a catheter tube and injection of contrast dye, usually iodine-based, into your coronary arteries. Doctors use PCI to open coronary arteries that are narrowed or blocked by the buildup of atherosclerotic plaque. PCI may be used to relieve symptoms of coronary heart disease or to reduce heart damage during or after a heart attack.

A cardiologist, or doctor who specializes in the heart, will perform PCI in a hospital cardiac catheterization laboratory. You will stay awake, but you will be given medicine to relax you. Before your procedure, you will receive medicines through an intravenous (IV) line in your arm to prevent blood clots. Your doctor will clean and numb an area on the wrist or groin where your doctor will make a small hole and insert the catheter into your blood vessel. Live x-rays will help your doctor guide the catheter into your heart to inject special contrast dye that will highlight the blockage. To open a blocked artery, your doctor will insert another catheter over a guidewire and inflate a balloon at the tip of that catheter. Your doctor may put a small mesh tube called a "stent" in your artery to help keep the artery open.

After PCI, your doctor will remove the catheters and close and bandage the opening on your wrist or groin. You may develop a bruise and soreness where the catheters were inserted. It also is common to have discomfort or bleeding where the catheters were inserted. You will recover in a special unit of the hospital for a few hours or overnight. You will get instructions on how much activity you can do and what medicines to take. You will need a ride home because of the medicines or anesthesia you received. Your doctor will check your progress during a follow-up visit. If a stent is implanted, you will have to take special anticlotting medicines exactly as prescribed, usually for at least three to 12 months.

Serious complications from PCI do not occur often, but they can happen. These complications may include bleeding, blood vessel damage, a treatable allergic reaction to the contrast dye, the need for emergency coronary artery bypass grafting during the procedure, arrhythmias, damaged arteries, kidney damage, heart attack, stroke, or blood clots. Sometimes chest pain can occur during PCI because the balloon briefly blocks blood supply to the heart. Restenosis, or tissue regrowth in the treated portion of the artery, may occur in the following months and cause the artery to become narrow or blocked again. The risk of complications is higher if you are older, have chronic kidney disease, are experiencing heart failure at the time of the procedure, or have extensive heart disease and multiple blockages in your coronary arteries.

CORONARY ARTERY STENT, CAROTID ARTERY STENT, AIRWAY STENT

A stent is a small mesh tube that holds open passages in the body, such as weak or narrow arteries. Stents are often used to treat narrowed coronary arteries that supply the heart with oxygen-rich blood. The stent holds open the narrowed arteries to allow adequate blood to flow to the heart. Stents are also sometimes used to treat the aorta if it has an aneurysm or bulge in it. The aorta carries blood from the left side of the heart to the body. Stents can also be used in the carotid arteries in the neck to prevent or treat stroke, or sometimes to treat narrowed airways in the lungs.

Stenting is a minimally invasive procedure. Stents can be made of metal mesh, fabric, silicone, or combinations of materials. Stents used for coronary arteries have a base of metal mesh. Fabric stents, also called "stent grafts," are used in larger arteries, such as the aorta. Stents used in the airways of the lungs are often made of silicone.

You may need to take certain medicines, such as aspirin and other antiplatelet medicines, for a year or longer after receiving a stent in your artery to prevent serious complications, such as blood clots. The most common complication after a stenting procedure is a blockage or blood clot in the stent. Complications from placing an airway stent include the stent moving out of place or becoming blocked.

TYPES OF STENTS

There are different types of stents such as bare-metal stents, drug-eluting stents, or stent grafts, that may be used for different purposes. Stents used in the airways of the lungs include silicone stents and metal stents.

Airway Stents

Stents used in airways include:
- **Metal stents.** These stents may be made of bare metal or covered with another material, such as silicone. Metal stents that are covered with another material are also known as "hybrid stents," meaning they contain a mixture of materials.
- **Silicone stents.** These stents are made of a material that can be molded to a certain shape. They are used more often if the stent is temporary.

Aortic Aneurysm Stents

Stent grafts are used to treat aortic aneurysms. The stent graft is typically a tube made of leak-proof polyester with a metal mesh backbone. Stent grafts are used in larger arteries, such as the aorta, and provide a stable channel to support blood flow.

Coronary or Carotid Artery Stents

The stents used in coronary or carotid arteries include:
- **Bare-metal stents.** These simple tubes are made of metal mesh and can be used in both the coronary and carotid arteries.

349

- **Drug-eluting stents.** These are the most common type of stents used in the coronary arteries. They are coated with medicine, which is released into the artery over time to prevent the artery from narrowing again. Different types of drug-eluting stents are coated with different medicines.

WHO NEEDS STENTS

Your doctor may recommend a stent to provide support inside an artery that has become narrowed by plaque buildup from atherosclerosis, or for lung airways that have narrowed due to other medical conditions. Your doctor will discuss the risks and benefits of the procedure with you. Sometimes, a stenting procedure is not recommended or another procedure is recommended instead.

Aortic Aneurysm or Dissection

Your doctor may use a stent graft to treat an aneurysm or dissection, or tear, of the aorta. The stent graft supports the weak area of the aorta and helps to prevent the aneurysm or dissection from bursting. Stent grafts can also help to treat injuries that have weakened the aorta. Blood flows through the stent graft and prevents blood from leaking into the body.

Carotid Artery Disease

The carotid arteries are found in the neck and supply oxygen-rich blood to the brain. Plaque can build up in the carotid arteries, causing carotid artery disease and an increased risk of stroke and other complications.

Ischemic Heart Disease

Stents are often used to treat coronary arteries, which supply oxygen-rich blood to the heart, when they become narrow. A stent may be recommended to treat the symptoms that come with this narrowing, such as chest pain from angina that occur from lack of blood flow to the heart. A stent can also reduce damage to the heart muscle immediately after a heart attack, which is a complication of ischemic heart disease.

Lung Conditions

A stent may be used to treat narrowed airways in the lungs. Conditions that may lead to this include:

- **A congenital problem.** A problem at birth can cause the airways to be too narrow.
- **Infections or diseases.** Infections, inflammatory diseases such as sarcoidosis, or any problem in the body that presses on the lungs can narrow the airways.
- **Injury.** An airway may become narrowed or blocked from injury. Injuries can include side effects from intubation, which involves having a tube guided down into the lungs, or tracheostomy.
- **Lung transplant complications.** Sometimes after a lung transplant, problems occur within the airways of the new lungs. An airway may collapse, or a hole may form where the transplanted lungs were stitched together.
- **Tumors.** A tumor may block the airways within the lungs. Cancer treatment, such as radiation or chemotherapy, can sometimes damage the connection between an airway and an organ like the trachea. This connection prevents the airway from working correctly. A stent may be used to help open the airway.

Peripheral Artery Disease

A stent may be used as treatment for narrowed arteries caused by peripheral artery disease (PAD), a condition that happens when plaque builds up in the arteries that carry blood to your legs, arms, or abdomen.

Stents may be used to treat PAD symptoms and help prevent future complications caused by reduced blood flow.

When a Stent May Not Be Recommended

An artery stent may not be recommended in the following circumstances:

- Your condition is mild. Your doctor may monitor your condition, start you on medicine, and recommend heart-healthy lifestyle changes.
- You have multiple narrowed coronary arteries, chronic kidney disease, or diabetes. Your doctor may recommend coronary artery bypass graft surgery (CABG) instead of the coronary stent procedure.
- You are older or have certain risk factors for complications. Your doctor may recommend another procedure instead of a carotid stent if you are over 70 years of age, as the risk of complications, including stroke, may be higher. Stent grafts may be riskier for older patients or those with conditions, such as renal failure or heart failure. For all procedures, your doctor will consider your health, talk to you about the risks, and make a decision with you and your family.

An airway stent may not be recommended in the following circumstances:

- You cannot have anesthesia or sedation.
- You need future procedures. Some lung procedures, such as laser therapy, can break or burn the stent. The stent can also get in the way if your lung requires surgery for other reasons.

BEFORE GETTING A STENT

Your doctor and specialists on your healthcare team can determine if you need a stent by using certain tests and procedures. If you need a stent, talk to your doctor about how to prepare for the procedure.

Diagnostic Tests and Procedures

To diagnose narrowed arteries or an aortic aneurysm, your doctor may have you undergo some of the following tests and procedures:

- **Chest magnetic resonance imaging (MRI)** to look for aneurysms in the aorta. This test works well for detecting aneurysms and pinpointing their size and exact location.
- **Computer tomography angiography (CTA)** and **magnetic resonance angiography (MRA)** to take pictures of your blood vessels. These tests may give your doctor more information about the flow of blood and whether arteries are narrowed or have aneurysms.
- **Coronary angiography** to see how blood flows through your coronary arteries. This type of test involves injecting dye into your blood so that your blood vessels can be seen by x-ray.
- **Fractional flow reserve** can help determine how narrow the artery is. This is an added test done during CTA or coronary angiography to check the blood pressure in a specific artery.
- **Ultrasound** to see whether plaque has narrowed or blocked your carotid or peripheral arteries or to see if you have an aneurysm and where it may be located. This painless test uses high-energy sound waves to create pictures of the insides of your blood vessels.
- **Echocardiography (echo)** to evaluate the structure and function of your heart. Echocardiography uses sound waves to create moving pictures of your heart.
- **Nuclear imaging** to see whether the blood is flowing normally to the heart. Your doctor will inject a tracer substance that will show whether the heart is receiving enough blood flow.

To diagnose narrowed airways, your doctor may have you undergo some of the following tests and procedures:
- Bronchoscopy to figure out the location and severity of the narrowed airway
- Chest CT scan to see whether one of your airways is being affected by a tumor, pneumonia, mucus, or other problem

- Pulmonary function tests to measure how well your lungs are working

Preparing for the Stenting Procedure

You may need additional tests such as blood tests, EKG, chest x-ray, or chest CT scan, to prepare you for the procedure. Tell your doctor about any medicines you take, other surgical procedures you have had, and any medical conditions you have such as diabetes, kidney disease, or sleep apnea.

You will be asleep for most stent procedures, so plan to have someone to take you home. You may go home the same day or after a few days, depending on the stent and any other medical conditions you have.

Before your procedure, you will be given detailed information, including:

- When you should stop eating or drinking
- If and when you should start or stop taking medicines
- When to arrive at the hospital and where to go
- How long you should expect to stay
- What happens during the procedure
- What to expect after the procedure, including potential complications, such as bleeding or soreness
- What to do after the procedure, such as what medicines to take
- How to live with your stent

WHAT TO EXPECT WHEN GETTING A STENT

Having a stent placed is a minimally invasive procedure, meaning it is not a major surgery. Stents for coronary arteries and carotid arteries are placed in similar ways. A stent graft is placed to treat an aneurysm in a procedure called "aortic aneurysm repair." Airway stents are placed in a procedure that helps open airways in the lung. For most stents, you will be given medicine to make you sleep during the procedure. The stent procedure may be planned ahead of time or it may be performed in an emergency situation.

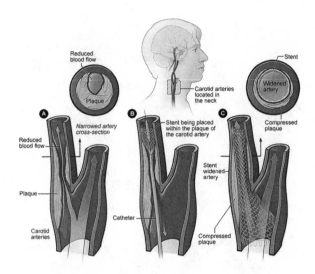

Figure 31.2. Placing a Stent in a Carotid Artery

These images show how a stent is placed in a carotid artery. The top middle inset figure shows the location of carotid arteries in the neck. Figure A shows how plaque can narrow the carotid artery, decreasing blood flow to the brain. Figure B shows how a catheter with a balloon and stent can be inserted into the carotid artery. Figure C shows how the stent is expanded once the artery is opened. The inset image on the left shows a cross-section of an artery containing plaque compared to the inset figure on the right, which shows a cross-section of an artery after a stent is placed.

Coronary and Carotid Artery Stenting

The procedures to place a stent to treat coronary and carotid arteries are similar. In both procedures, a thin tube with a deflated balloon on the end is threaded through a blood vessel to the narrowed or blocked artery. Once in place, the balloon is inflated and the stent is opened and placed in the artery.

- The procedure to place a coronary stent is known as "percutaneous coronary intervention" (PCI), commonly known as "coronary angioplasty." Sometimes the procedure is done in an emergency, such as during a heart attack. The stent provides support to the artery after the artery is reopened.

355

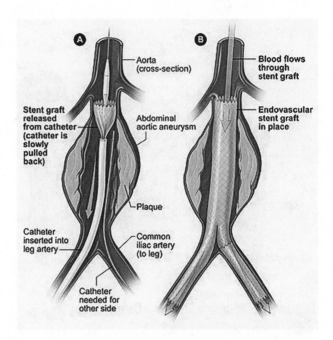

Figure 31.3. Aortic Aneurysm Repair

Figure 31.3 shows the placement of a stent graft in an abdominal aortic aneurysm. In figure A, a catheter is inserted into an artery in the upper thigh. The catheter is threaded to the abdominal aorta, and the stent graft is released from the catheter. In figure B, the stent graft is placed and allows blood to flow through the aorta.

- The procedure to place a stent in the carotid artery is called "carotid artery stenting." This is a minimally invasive treatment for severe carotid artery disease.

Aortic Aneurysm Stenting

After an incision is made in your upper thigh, your doctor will insert a stent graft through a large blood vessel using a catheter. Your doctor will guide the catheter and stent graft through the arteries to the aorta, where the aneurysm is located. The stent graft is opened up and placed in the aorta once it is in the right place.

Dye may be injected into the blood after the stent graft is placed to make sure the stent graft is working correctly and blood is not leaking into the aneurysm. The dye can be seen on an x-ray.

Airway Stenting

An airway stent is placed using a bronchoscope, a small camera on the end of a long tube. The doctor will slide the bronchoscope through your nose or mouth and then down through your throat into the trachea and the airways.

The stent will be placed by sliding a guide wire along the side of the bronchoscope, then sliding a thin tube along the guide wire that carries the stent. Using the bronchoscope to watch, the doctors will open the stent in the narrowed airway. Fluoroscopy, a type of x-ray imaging, or ultrasound may also be used to help guide the stent placement. Afterward, the doctors may check your lungs by using chest x-ray.

AFTER GETTING A STENT

After the procedure to place a coronary stent, carotid stent, or airway stent, you will recover in the hospital for a few hours or overnight. For stent grafts, you may be in the hospital for a longer time. Although not common, you may also experience complications from the stenting procedure.

Recovery

Before you leave the hospital, you will be given instructions that include:

- **Which medicines to take.** You will need to take medicine to prevent a blood clot from forming in the stent. You may need to take other medicines for different reasons. Follow your doctor's instructions carefully.
- **When to resume normal physical activity.** Most people are able to return to work within a few days to a week.
- **When to make a follow-up appointment.** Your doctor will need to check on your progress and make sure there are no complications.

Possible Complications of the Stenting Procedure

Sometimes there are complications from a stenting procedure in an artery. These complications may include:

- Allergic reaction to the dye used to show the blood vessels by x-ray
- Arrhythmia, or an irregular heartbeat
- Bleeding or discomfort where the catheter was inserted
- Damage to blood vessels from the catheter
- Infection
- Rarely, damage to the kidney from the contrast dye

More serious or life-threatening complications may occur during a stenting procedure, but these are rare. People who have had other procedures to treat blocked arteries or who have congestive heart failure, chronic kidney disease, or diabetes, are usually at higher risk for complications, which may include:
- Blood flow being cut off from the gut or the lower part of the body during an aortic aneurysm repair
- Heart attack
- Rupture of the aortic aneurysm
- Stroke
- Tear in the artery

Possible complications from a stenting procedure in an airway may include:
- Coughing up blood
- Sore mouth, sore throat, or hoarse voice

Less common, but serious complications may include:
- Arrhythmia
- Needing a tracheostomy
- Pneumothorax
- Respiratory failure
- Sudden cardiac arrest

LIVING WITH A STENT
It is important to follow your treatment plan, including taking medicines prescribed by your doctor, making healthy lifestyle choices, and getting regular medical checkups. It is also important to know

your risk of and what to do if you experience complications that are specific to the stent in your body.

Receive Routine Follow-Up Care

It is important to get routine medical care if you have a stent. Talk with your doctor about how often you should schedule office visits and blood tests.

- Discuss when you should follow up with specialists, such as a cardiologist or pulmonologist.
- Take medicines to prevent complications. If you have a stent in your artery, take all medicines regularly, as your doctor prescribes. Do not change the amount of your medicine or skip a dose unless your doctor tells you to. You will need to take antiplatelet medicines, or blood thinners, to prevent blood clots from forming in the stents in your arteries. Your doctor may prescribe these medicines for one year or more after getting a coronary stent, while it may be one month or more for carotid or peripheral artery stents. Antiplatelet medicines include aspirin, clopidogrel, dipyridamole, and ticlopidine. Bleeding is a possible side effect, which can make it much riskier to have surgery.
- Talk with your doctor about when you can resume normal physical activity. It will depend on the stent and your condition before the stent procedure.

Monitor Your Condition

Stents serve as treatment, but cannot cure an underlying condition. Some types of stents need to be checked by your doctor to make sure they have not moved and are functioning properly. The different types of tests may include:

- **Bronchoscopy** to check an airway stent about four to six weeks after placement
- **Chest x-ray** or **CT scan** to look for signs of any complications from an airway stent

- **CT angiography (CTA)** or **ultrasound** to make sure a stent graft placed to treat an aortic aneurysm is not leaking or has moved. You will likely need imaging about one month after your procedure. If a leak or other problem is detected, you may need imaging tests again after six months or one year to check it. If there is a bad leak, more surgery may be needed. Your stent graft will need to be monitored by imaging throughout your life.
- **Referring you to a specialist** if you have signs or symptoms related to your condition.
- **Regular general exams** to check overall physical and mental health.

Make Healthy Lifestyle Changes

Your doctor may recommend the following healthy lifestyle changes to reduce the chance of needing more procedures in the future or experiencing a heart attack or stroke:
- Aiming for a healthy weight
- Being physically active
- Heart-healthy eating
- Managing stress
- Quitting smoking

Learn the Warning Signs of Coronary or Carotid Stent Complications and Have a Plan

Watch for signs or symptoms of complications from a coronary stent, carotid stent, or stent graft, including:
- **Blood clotting.** A blood clot is an uncommon, but serious complication that can occur within the stent. Your risk of getting a blood clot is much higher if you stop taking your blood thinners before your doctor says to do so. Blood clots can lead to life-threatening conditions such as heart attack, stroke, and venous thromboembolism.
- **Chest pain.** This can be a symptom of restenosis, in which the artery where a stent is located closes up

again. Restenosis is a common complication because of too much tissue growth within the portion of the artery where the stent is placed. It can lead to a heart attack if your stent is in a coronary artery. In this case, a symptom of restenosis may be chest pain. If it happens in other arteries, restenosis may or may not cause symptoms. If restenosis occurs, you will need another procedure, such as one that involves both angioplasty and possibly placing another drug-eluting stent.

- **Stent or stent graft failure.** Occasionally stents may break within a peripheral artery. Rarely, a stent graft used to repair an aortic aneurysm or dissection may move from where it was placed. Blood may also leak out of the graft. Symptoms may be similar to those you experienced before getting a stent, or you may have no symptoms. Your doctor will use imaging to monitor the stent graft.

If you have a stent because of ischemic heart disease or carotid artery disease, you are still at risk for complications related to those diseases, such as heart attack or stroke. If you think you are or someone else is having the following symptoms, call 911 immediately.

Heart attack signs and symptoms include:

- **Mild or severe chest pain or discomfort** in the center of the chest or upper abdomen that lasts for more than a few minutes or goes away and comes back. It can feel like pressure, squeezing, fullness, heartburn, or indigestion.
- **Nausea, vomiting, light-headedness or fainting**, or breaking out in a cold sweat. These symptoms of a heart attack are more common in women.
- **Shortness of breath**, which may occur with or before chest discomfort
- **Upper body discomfort** in one or both arms, the back, neck, jaw, or upper part of the stomach

If you think someone may be having a stroke, act F.A.S.T. and perform the following simple test:

- **F—Face.** Ask the person to smile. Does one side of the face droop?
- **A—Arms.** Ask the person to raise both arms. Does one arm drift downward?
- **S—Speech.** Ask the person to repeat a simple phrase. Is their speech slurred or strange?
- **T—Time.** If you observe any of these signs, call for help immediately. Early treatment is essential.

Learn the Warning Signs of Airway Stent Complications and Have a Plan

Complications of an airway stent procedure may happen soon after the procedure or later. You should call your doctor right away if you experience any of the following signs or symptoms:

- Changes in your cough
- Coughing up blood
- High fever
- Persistent bad breath
- Problems breathing

These signs and symptoms may be caused by one of the following complications of your airway stenting procedure:

- Changes in stent placement, which can happen if the stent moves out of place. You may need another procedure to fix or remove the stent. This occurs more often with silicone stents. In rare cases, stents can become fractured or distorted.
- Lung infection
- Mucus caught in the stent
- Tissue growing into the stent, which can happen if the condition that caused a narrowed airway also causes it to become blocked again, such as in the case of a tumor growing through the stent. This occurs most often in the spaces in metal stents.

Section 31.3 | **Coronary Artery Bypass Grafting Surgery**

This section includes text excerpted from "Coronary Artery Bypass Grafting Surgery," National Heart, Lung, and Blood Institute (NHLBI), April 3, 2016. Reviewed April 2020.

Coronary artery bypass grafting (CABG) is a procedure to improve poor blood flow to the heart. It may be needed when the arteries supplying blood to heart tissue, called "coronary arteries," are narrowed or blocked. This surgery may lower the risk of serious complications for people who have obstructive coronary artery disease, a type of ischemic heart disease. The CABG may also be used in an emergency, such as a severe heart attack.

The CABG uses blood vessels from another part of the body and connects them to blood vessels above and below the narrowed artery, bypassing the narrowed or blocked coronary arteries. One or more blood vessels may be used, depending on the severity and number of blockages. The blood vessels are usually arteries from the arm or chest, or veins from the legs. Risks and possible complications may occur with this procedure. After CABG, your doctor may recommend medicines and heart-healthy lifestyle changes to further reduce your symptoms, treat your disease, and help prevent complications, such as blood clots.

WHO MAY BENEFIT?

People who have certain conditions may benefit from CABG, such as those who have obstructive coronary artery disease, a type of ischemic heart disease. Obstructive coronary artery disease occurs when plaque builds up in the coronary arteries that supply the heart with oxygen-rich blood.

Your heart care team will work with you to decide if CABG is right for you. Your team includes your heart doctor, called a "cardiologist," and a cardiothoracic surgeon, who specializes in heart, lung, and chest surgeries.

During an emergency, such as a heart attack or sudden cardiac arrest, CABG or another procedure may be performed with consent from a heart care team. If it is not an emergency, the team will evaluate your symptoms, medical history, the severity of your condition, your overall health, and how treatment will help you. The team will also consider your preferences after discussing the risks and benefits of CABG with you and your family.

When Is Coronary Artery Bypass Grafting Recommended?

The heart care team may recommend CABG to relieve symptoms and to improve your chance of living longer. Surgery is not always the best option for everyone. Depending on your overall health and other conditions, your care team may recommend an alternative procedure called "percutaneous coronary intervention" (PCI), which may include placing a stent. This procedure is also known as "coronary angioplasty."

CABG may be recommended when you have:

- **A need for open-heart surgery** for other reasons
- Diabetes
- **Heart attack due to coronary artery disease** that cannot be treated properly with PCI
- **Ischemic heart disease with angina** that has not gone away with medicine, or with a history of sudden cardiac arrest related to heart arrhythmia
- **Multiple blocked coronary arteries** or large amounts of plaque in the left main coronary artery that would be difficult to treat with PCI
- **Severe or advanced heart failure** that affects your heart's ability to pump blood

BEFORE SURGERY

Your doctor may use diagnostic tests or procedures before CABG to determine how serious your ischemic heart disease is and where the coronary arteries are narrowed. If you need CABG, talk to your doctor about how to prepare for the procedure.

Diagnostic Tests and Procedures

Tests and procedures may include the following:

- **Electrocardiogram (ECG or EKG)** to record the electrical activity of the heart. An EKG can show signs of heart damage.

- **Stress tests** to measure how well your heart works during physical stress. The stress may be physical exercise, such as walking on a treadmill, or it may be a medicine given to have the same effect.
- **Echocardiogram** to assess heart function. This includes whether the valves or pumping is abnormal.
- **Coronary angiography** to see how blood flows through your arteries. It is performed along with cardiac catheterization. The angiogram shows how severe the disease is, which arteries are affected, and the location of the affected arteries.
- **CT angiography** to take pictures of your blood vessels. This is an alternative to cardiac catheterization that uses an injection of dye in the arm along with computed tomography (CT) imaging. Because it does not involve threading a catheter into the heart as cardiac catheterization does, CT angiography may be safer for some patients.
- **Coronary calcium scan** to get images of the calcium in the walls of your coronary arteries, which is linked to coronary artery disease. This test uses CT imaging.

Preparing for Surgery

Coronary artery bypass grafting may be planned ahead of time, or it may be performed in an emergency situation, such as after a heart attack that leads to severe heart failure. If your surgery is scheduled, talk to your doctor about what to expect and how to prepare, such as:

- Which medicines you should stop taking and when to stop. Ask about all the medicines you take, even if they are not prescription, as well as supplements.
- Which medicines you should begin taking and when to start them.
- How to bathe before surgery. You may be told to use a special soap to wash your body.
- When to stop eating and drinking before surgery.
- When to arrive at the hospital and where to go.

- What to expect after surgery and during the recovery period.

Your doctor will also discuss treatment options with you, including the risks and possible complications during and after surgery. Ask your doctor any questions you have so you can make the best decision about your treatment.

DURING SURGERY

During CABG, a surgical team will take one or more blood vessels from another part of your body and connect it to the blocked artery in your heart. CABG may be performed in one of three ways. In traditional CABG, the chest is cut open and a machine pumps your blood. In "off-pump" CABG, the chest is opened, but a machine for pumping blood is not used. With minimally invasive CABG methods, only small cuts are made in the chest, and a machine is not used.

Surgical Team

Your surgical team will include a cardiothoracic surgeon, who will work on your heart. An anesthesiologist will give you medicine to make you sleep before the surgery, connect you to a breathing machine, and monitor your vital signs throughout the procedure. A perfusionist will manage the heart-lung pump, and nurses and other surgeons may help throughout the surgery.

Traditional Coronary Artery Bypass Grafting surgery

Traditional CABG is the most common type of CABG surgery. This surgery takes about three to six hours, depending on how many arteries need to be bypassed.

You will be given an intravenous (IV) line for fluids and medicines that will make you sleep before the surgery. You will be connected to a ventilator to support your breathing. The surgeon makes a cut down the middle of the chest, through the breastbone. The bone is split and the rib cage separated so the surgeon can reach the heart.

You will receive medicines to temporarily stop your heart from beating. This makes it easier for the surgeon to connect the healthy blood vessels, called "grafts," into the coronary arteries. This requires a heart-lung bypass machine, which adds oxygen to your blood and pumps it throughout your body during surgery while your heart is not beating.

The surgeon will then take an artery or a vein from your leg, arm, stomach, or chest. The graft is connected to the blocked coronary artery. The new blood vessel bypasses the blocked portion to create a new path for blood flow to the heart muscle. The number of grafts depends on how many coronary arteries need to be bypassed.

When the grafting is finished, the surgeon will restart the heart and restore blood flow. The heart usually starts beating on its own, but sometimes mild shocks are used to start it. Surgeons will sew the breastbone back together with a wire.

Off-Pump Coronary Artery Bypass Grafting

Sometimes CABG can be done without stopping the heart and using a heart-lung bypass machine. This is called "off-pump CABG" because the heart-lung bypass machine, or pump, is not used. The heart is steadied with a mechanical device. It is more difficult for surgeons because the heart is beating, and surgeons do not have easy access to blood vessels. However, it may be safer for certain people, such as those who have a higher risk of complications from using a heart-lung bypass machine. These include older adults and people who have ventricular dysfunction, diabetes, kidney disease, and chronic lung disease. This type of surgery is also sometimes called "beating-heart bypass grafting."

Minimally Invasive Coronary Artery Bypass Grafting

Sometimes, CABG surgery may not be done as open heart surgery. There are less-invasive methods, including:

- **Minimally invasive direct coronary artery bypass (MIDCAB).** MIDCAB is a modified version of CABG where the chest bone is not cut open. Instead, the surgeon makes a smaller cut on the left side of the chest over the artery that needs to be bypassed and enters in between the ribs. It is also usually an off-pump procedure.

- **Robotic.** Sometimes CABG surgery can be done using a robot to surgically place the graft. This is called "robotic-assisted" or "robotic surgery." The surgeon controls the robot instead of doing the work by hand, and the machinery only needs small openings in the chest. A heart-lung bypass machine is sometimes used.
- **Hybrid.** During a hybrid bypass surgery, the robotic bypass is done for one of the main arteries, but a stent is used for other blocked arteries. The stent is a rolled-up mesh tube-like structure that goes inside the blocked artery to hold it open. This procedure is typically used only if your doctor is unable to perform the traditional bypass procedure.

AFTER SURGERY

After CABG surgery, you will need time to recover. There are also potential complications from surgery.

Recovery in the Hospital

You will stay in the hospital for about one week. You may stay longer if you had other procedures done as well or if you have a complication. You will stay in an intensive care unit (ICU) for a day or two, where medical staff may do the following:

- **Apply bandages** on your chest and wherever the graft was removed
- **Attach tubes to drain fluid** from your chest and urine from your bladder
- **Connect you to an electrocardiogram (ECG)** to monitor your heart rhythm
- **Implant a temporary pacemaker**, and, in some cases, an implantable cardioverter defibrillator (ICD), while you are recovering in the ICU
- **Give you compression stockings** to wear on your legs to help maintain proper blood flow and avoid venous thromboembolism

- **Give you medicines.** Some medicines you may take for only a short time, while others you may need to keep taking. These medicines may help with pain during recovery, prevent blood clots or irregular heart rhythms, control cholesterol and fats in the blood, and lower your risk of complications.
- **Give you oxygen therapy**, which delivers oxygen into your nose through nasal prongs or a mask
- **Monitor your vital signs** such as your heart rate, blood pressure, and oxygen levels

Recovery at Home

After you leave the hospital, you will need to continue taking medicines. Some common side effects from surgery, which should go away in four to six weeks, include the following:

- **Chest pain** around the site of the surgical cut
- Constipation
- **Discomfort or itching** from healing cuts
- **Fatigue**, mood swings, or depression
- **Muscle pain or tightness** in the shoulders and upper back
- **Problems sleeping** or loss of appetite
- **Swelling** of the area where an artery or vein was removed for grafting

After you leave the hospital, you will need about six to 12 weeks to recover completely. People who undergo minimally invasive CABG need less time to recover than for traditional CABG.

Possible Surgery-Related Complications

All surgeries have risks. The risk is generally higher for certain people such as those who get CABG in an emergency situation, have plaque in other arteries throughout the body, or have other medical conditions such as major heart failure, or lung or kidney disease. Potentially serious complications may include:

- **Arrhythmia, or irregular heartbeat.** The most common type is called "atrial fibrillation," which may occur after the surgery, but usually goes away on its own.
- **Bleeding,** which may require more surgery to control it.
- **Confusion or problems thinking clearly,** temporary memory loss, vision problems, and slurred speech can occur for a short time right after surgery. This is also known as "postoperative cognitive decline" (POCD). Delirium, or intense confusion, is rare. The exact cause of POCD is not known. Many factors, including the health of the patient before surgery, likely play a role.
- Heart attack.
- **Infection,** which can occur where the surgical cut was made or inside the chest where the surgery was performed. This may require additional surgeries.
- Kidney failure
- Stroke

LIFE AFTER CORONARY ARTERY BYPASS GRAFTING

Coronary artery bypass grafting is a treatment, but not a cure for ischemic heart disease. It is important to work with your doctor after CABG to help you stay healthy. This may include taking medicines prescribed by your doctor, making healthy lifestyle changes, getting regular medical checkups, and participating in cardiac rehabilitation.

Take Your Medicines as Directed

Your doctor will likely discuss medicines with you shortly after your surgery. Some of them are important to start right away. You may need to take them for up to one year or even continuously throughout your life. These medicines may include:

- **Angiotensin-converting enzyme (ACE)** inhibitors to treat high blood pressure, and for people who have had a heart attack, have diabetes or kidney disease, or whose heart does not pump properly.

- **Angiotensin receptor blockers (ARBs)** to treat high blood pressure and for people who have had a heart attack or have diabetes or kidney disease. Your doctor may recommend an ARB if you cannot take an ACE inhibitor or for other reasons.
- **Beta-blockers** to decrease the chance of irregular heart rhythms after CABG, as well as to treat high blood pressure and other heart conditions. These medicines slow your heart rate and lower your blood pressure to decrease the amount of stress on your heart.
- **Blood thinners, or antiplatelet medicines**, to keep your graft from developing a blockage and help prevent blood clots. One type is aspirin. Your doctor will likely start you on aspirin right away, even before you get CABG surgery. Your doctor may prescribe other types of anticlotting medicines, such as clopidogrel. Possible side effects of this medicine can include bleeding, especially if you are taking other medicines that also thin your blood, such as aspirin.
- **Calcium channel blockers** to treat high blood pressure when beta blockers and ACE inhibitors do not control it.
- **Diuretics**, or medicines to reduce the amount of fluid in your body or to treat high blood pressure when beta blockers and ACE inhibitors do not control it.
- **Statins** to lower the amount of lipids in your blood and manage the cholesterol levels that can cause plaque. If you do not already take statins for your coronary artery disease, your doctor may recommend that you take statins before and after surgery.

Monitor Your Condition

After surgery and after recovery, your doctor will want to schedule checkups to look for common complications of CABG or further problems from ischemic heart disease.

Even if you do not experience any signs or symptoms, you may need testing about five years after CABG surgery, or sooner if you have new symptoms or have other risk factors. You may take a stress test with an electrocardiogram or echocardiogram, or other heart and lung imaging. If you have symptoms, such as chest pain, especially before or during the stress test, your doctor will likely recommend coronary angiography to check on the graft and other arteries.

Make Healthy Lifestyle Changes

Your doctor will discuss heart-healthy lifestyle habits and changes that are important to maintaining your health and controlling risk factors, such as hypertension and diabetes. These include:

- Aiming for a healthy weight
- Being physically active
- Heart-healthy eating
- Managing stress
- Quitting smoking

Enroll in Cardiac Rehabilitation

Your doctor may refer you to cardiac rehabilitation to improve your heart health after a heart-related procedure or heart condition. Cardiac rehabilitation helps you maintain or adopt heart-healthy lifestyle practices to lower your risk for cardiovascular diseases. This program includes exercise training, education on heart-healthy living, and counseling to reduce stress and help you return to an active life. These rehabilitation programs are supervised by doctors and are usually offered in hospitals or community facilities.

Monitor Your Emotional Health

Your doctor will likely ask if you have had any changes in your mood or other aspects of your well-being. It is important to be treated for depression to increase your chance of full recovery.

If you have symptoms of depression, your doctor may refer you to a mental health specialist. Treatment may include counseling and medicine.

Learn the Warning Signs of Complications and Have a Plan

Complications can occur quickly or years after CABG. One possible complication is that the graft will become blocked with plaque and limit or stop blood flow to the heart. If your graft stops working, this may cause a heart attack or other problem with your heart, and you may need additional surgery or PCI.

- **Heart attack.** Signs of heart attack include mild or severe chest pain or discomfort in the center of the chest or upper abdomen that lasts for more than a few minutes or goes away and comes back. It can feel like pressure, squeezing, fullness, heartburn, or indigestion. There may also be pain down the left arm. For those who have had a heart attack in the past, the symptoms may be similar to the previous heart attack.
- **Stroke.** If you think someone may be having a stroke, act F.A.S.T. and do the following simple test:
  - **F—Face.** Ask the person to smile. Does one side of the face droop?
  - **A—Arms.** Ask the person to raise both arms. Does one arm drift downward?
  - **S—Speech.** Ask the person to repeat a simple phrase. Is their speech slurred or strange?
  - **T—Time.** If you observe any of these signs, call for help immediately. Early treatment is essential.

Section 31.4 | Valve Repair and Replacement

This section includes text excerpted from "Heart Valve Disease," National Heart, Lung, and Blood Institute (NHLBI), June 12, 2019.

REPAIRING OR REPLACING HEART VALVES

Your doctor may recommend repairing or replacing your heart valve(s), even if your heart valve disease is not causing symptoms. Repairing or replacing a valve can prevent lasting damage to your heart and sudden death.

The decision to repair or replace heart valves depends on many factors, including:
- The severity of your valve disease
- Whether you need heart surgery for other conditions, such as bypass surgery to treat coronary heart disease. Bypass surgery and valve surgery can be performed at the same time.
- Your age and general health

When possible, heart valve repair is preferred over heart valve replacement. Valve repair preserves the strength and function of the heart muscle. People who have valve repair also have a lower risk of infective endocarditis after the surgery, and they do not need to take blood-thinning medicines for the rest of their lives.

However, heart valve repair surgery is harder to do than valve replacement. Also, not all valves can be repaired. Mitral valves often can be repaired. Aortic and pulmonary valves often have to be replaced.

Repairing Heart Valves

Heart surgeons can repair heart valves by:
- Adding tissue to patch holes or tears or to increase the support at the base of the valve
- Removing or reshaping tissue so the valve can close tighter
- Separating fused valve flaps

Sometimes cardiologists repair heart valves using cardiac catheterization. Although catheter procedures are less invasive than surgery, they may not work as well for some patients. Work with your doctor to decide whether repair is appropriate. If so, your doctor can advise you on the best procedure.

Heart valves that cannot open fully (stenosis) can be repaired with surgery or with a less invasive catheter procedure called "balloon valvuloplasty." This procedure is also called "balloon valvotomy."

During the procedure, a catheter (thin tube) with a balloon at its tip is threaded through a blood vessel to the faulty valve in your heart. The balloon is inflated to help widen the opening of the valve. Your doctor then deflates the balloon and removes both, the catheter and the tube. You will be awake during the procedure, and it usually requires an overnight stay in a hospital.

Balloon valvuloplasty relieves many symptoms of heart valve disease, but may not cure it. The condition can worsen over time. You still may need medicines to treat symptoms or surgery to repair or replace the faulty valve. Balloon valvuloplasty has a shorter recovery time than surgery. The procedure may work as well as surgery for some patients who have mitral valve stenosis. For these people, balloon valvuloplasty often is preferred over surgical repair or replacement.

Balloon valvuloplasty does not work as well as surgery for adults who have aortic valve stenosis. Doctors often use balloon valvuloplasty to repair valve stenosis in infants and children.

Replacing Heart Valves

Sometimes heart valves cannot be repaired and must be replaced. This surgery involves removing the faulty valve and replacing it with a human-made or biological valve.

Biological valves are made from pig, cow, or human heart tissue and may have man-made parts as well. These valves are specially treated, so you would not need medicines to stop your body from rejecting the valve.

Human-made valves last longer than biological valves and usually do not have to be replaced. Biological valves usually have to be replaced after about 10 years, although newer ones may last 15 years or longer. Unlike biological valves, however, human-made valves require you to take blood-thinning medicines for the rest of your life. These medicines prevent blood clots from forming on the valve. Blood clots can cause a heart attack or stroke. Human-made valves also raise your risk of infective endocarditis.

You and your doctor will decide together whether you should have a human-made or biological replacement valve.

375

If you are a woman of childbearing age or if you are athletic, you may prefer a biological valve so you do not have to take blood-thinning medicines. If you are elderly, you also may prefer a biological valve, as it will likely last for the rest of your life.

Ross Procedure

Doctors also can treat faulty aortic valves with the Ross procedure. During this surgery, your doctor removes your faulty aortic valve and replaces it with your pulmonary valve. Your pulmonary valve is then replaced with a pulmonary valve from a deceased human donor.

This is more involved surgery than typical valve replacement, and it has a greater risk of complications. The Ross procedure may be especially useful for children because the surgically replaced valves continue to grow with the child. Also, lifelong treatment with blood-thinning medicines is not required. But, in some patients, one or both valves fail to work well within a few years of the surgery.

Other Approaches for Repairing and Replacing Heart Valves

Some forms of heart valve repair and replacement surgery are less invasive than traditional surgery. These procedures use smaller incisions (cuts) to reach the heart valves. Hospital stays for these newer types of surgery usually are three to five days, compared with a five-day stay for traditional heart valve surgery.

New surgeries tend to cause less pain and have a lower risk of infection. Recovery time also tends to be shorter—two to four weeks versus six to eight weeks for traditional surgery.

TRANSCATHETER VALVE THERAPY

Interventional cardiologists perform procedures that involve threading clips or other devices to repair faulty heart valves using a catheter (tube) inserted through a large blood vessel. The clips or devices are used to reshape the valves and stop the backflow of blood. People who receive these clips recover more easily than people who have surgery. However, the clips may not treat backflow as well as surgery.

Doctors also may use a catheter to replace faulty aortic valves. This procedure is called "transcatheter aortic valve replacement" (TAVR). For this procedure, the catheter usually is inserted into an artery in the groin (upper thigh) and threaded to the heart. A deflated balloon with a folded replacement valve around it is at the end of the catheter.

Once the replacement valve is placed properly, the balloon is used to expand the new valve so it fits securely within the old valve. The balloon is then deflated, and the balloon and catheter are removed.

A replacement valve also can be inserted in an existing replacement valve that is failing. This is called a "valve-in-valve" procedure.

Section 31.5 | Carotid Endarterectomy

This section includes text excerpted from "Carotid Endarterectomy," National Heart, Lung, and Blood Institute (NHLBI), December 10, 2016. Reviewed April 2020.

Carotid endarterectomy surgery is done to restore normal blood flow to the brain to prevent a stroke if you already have symptoms of reduced blood flow. Carotid endarterectomy also may be performed preventively if a diagnostic test, such as carotid ultrasound shows significant blockage that is likely to trigger a stroke. Carotid endarterectomy is not a cure. Your arteries can become blocked again if your underlying condition, such as high blood cholesterol, is not controlled and causes new plaque buildup.

Carotid endarterectomy is done in a hospital. You may have general anesthesia and will not be awake or feel pain during the surgery. Your surgeon instead may decide to use local anesthesia to numb only the part of your body being worked on so that she or he can check your brain's reaction to the decreased blood flow during surgery. You also will be given medicine to relax you during the surgery. Your vital signs will be monitored during surgery. You will lie on your back on an operating table with your head turned to one side. Your surgeon will make an incision, or cut, on your neck to expose the blocked section of the carotid artery. Your surgeon will cut into the affected artery and remove the plaque through this cut. A temporary flexible tube may be inserted so blood can flow around the blocked area as the plaque is cleared. After removing the plaque from your artery, the surgeon will close the artery and neck incisions with stitches.

After surgery, you will recover in the hospital for one to two days. Your neck may hurt for a few days, and you may find it hard to swallow. Your doctor may prescribe medicine to prevent clots and suggest steps to keep your carotid arteries healthy.

Carotid endarterectomy is fairly safe when performed by experienced surgeons. However, serious complications such as clotting, stroke, or death may occur. Taking anticlotting medicines before and after surgery can reduce this risk. Other complications may include a reaction to anesthesia, short-term nerve injury that causes temporary numbness in your face or tongue, bleeding, infection, high blood pressure, heart attack, and seizure. The risk of complications is higher in women, older people, those with certain conditions, such as chronic kidney disease or diabetes, and those with other serious medical conditions.

Section 31.6 | Aneurysm Repair

This section contains text excerpted from the following sources: Text beginning with the heading "What Is Aortic Aneurysm?" is excerpted from "Aortic Aneurysm," Centers for Disease Control and Prevention (CDC), December 9, 2019; Text under the heading "Treatment" is excerpted from "Aortic Aneurysm," National Heart, Lung, and Blood Institute (NHLBI), March 29, 2012. Reviewed April 2020.

WHAT IS AORTIC ANEURYSM?

An aortic aneurysm is a balloon-like bulge in the aorta, the large artery that carries blood from the heart through the chest and torso.

Aortic aneurysms can dissect or rupture:
- The force of blood pumping can split the layers of the artery wall, allowing blood to leak in between them. This process is known as "dissection."

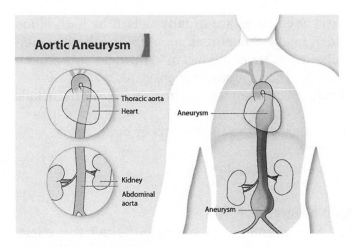

Figure 31.4. Aortic Aneurysm

- The aneurysm can burst completely, causing bleeding inside the body. This is known as "rupture."

Dissections and ruptures are the cause of most deaths from aortic aneurysms.

FACTS ABOUT AORTIC ANEURYSM IN THE UNITED STATES
- Aortic aneurysms were the cause of 9,928 deaths in 2017.
- About 60 percent of deaths due to aortic rupture or aortic dissection happen among men.
- A history of smoking accounts for about 75 percent of all abdominal aortic aneurysms.
- The U.S. Preventive Services Task Force recommends that men 65 to 75 years old who have ever smoked should get an ultrasound screening for abdominal aortic aneurysms, even if they have no symptoms.

WHAT ARE THE TYPES OF AORTIC ANEURYSM?
Thoracic Aortic Aneurysm
A thoracic aortic aneurysm happens in the chest. Men and women are equally likely to get thoracic aortic aneurysms, which become more common with increasing age.

Thoracic aortic aneurysms are usually caused by high blood pressure or sudden injury. Sometimes people with inherited connective tissue disorders, such as Marfan syndrome and Ehlers-Danlos syndrome, get thoracic aortic aneurysms.

Signs and symptoms of thoracic aortic aneurysm can include the following:

- Sharp, sudden pain in the chest or upper back
- Shortness of breath
- Trouble breathing or swallowing

Abdominal Aortic Aneurysm

An abdominal aortic aneurysm happens below the chest. Abdominal aortic aneurysms happen more often than thoracic aortic aneurysms.

Abdominal aortic aneurysms are more common in men and among people 65 years of age and older. Abdominal aortic aneurysms are more common among white people than among black people.

Abdominal aortic aneurysms are usually caused by atherosclerosis (hardened arteries), but infection or injury can also cause them.

Abdominal aortic aneurysms often do not have any symptoms. If an individual does have symptoms, they can include the following:

- Throbbing or deep pain in the back or side.
- Pain in the buttocks, groin, or legs.

Other Types of Aneurysms

Aneurysms can happen in other parts of your body. A ruptured aneurysm in the brain can cause a stroke. Peripheral aneurysms—those found in arteries other than the aorta—can happen in the neck, in the groin, or behind the knees. These aneurysms are less likely to rupture or dissect than aortic aneurysms, but they can form blood clots. These clots can break away and block blood flow through the artery.

WHAT ARE THE RISK FACTORS FOR AORTIC ANEURYSM?

Diseases and unhealthy behaviors that damage your heart and blood vessels also increase your risk for aortic aneurysm. Smoking is the most important unhealthy behavior related to aortic aneurysm.

Other factors include:
- High blood pressure
- High blood cholesterol
- Atherosclerosis (hardened arteries)

Some inherited connective tissue disorders, such as Marfan syndrome and Ehlers-Danlos syndrome, can also increase your risk for aortic aneurysm. Your family may also have a history of aortic aneurysms that can increase your risk.

HOW ARE AORTIC ANEURYSMS TREATED?

The two main treatments for aortic aneurysms are medicines and surgery. Medicines can lower blood pressure and reduce risk for an aortic aneurysm. Surgery can repair or replace the affected section of the aorta.

TREATMENT
Procedures or Surgery

Depending on the cause or size of an aortic aneurysm or how quickly it is growing, your doctor may recommend surgery to repair it. Rupture or dissection of an aneurysm may require immediate surgical repair.

- **Open surgical repair** is the most common type of surgery. You will be asleep during the procedure. Your surgical team first makes a large incision, or cut, in your abdomen or chest, depending on the location of the aneurysm, then removes the aneurysm and sews a graft in its place. This graft is typically a tube made of leak-proof polyester. Recovery time for open surgical repair is about a month.
- **Endovascular aneurysm repair (EVAR)** is less invasive than open surgical repair. This is because the surgical cut is smaller, and you usually need less recovery time. EVAR is used to repair abdominal aortic aneurysms

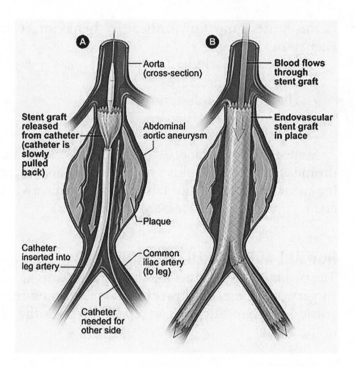

Figure 31.5. Aneurysm—Endo-Repair

The illustration shows the placement of a stent graft in an abdominal aortic aneurysm. In figure A, a catheter is inserted into an artery in the groin. The catheter is threaded to the abdominal aorta, and the stent graft is released from the catheter. In figure B, the stent graft is expanded and allows blood to flow through the aorta.

more often than to repair thoracic aortic aneurysms. During the procedure, your surgical team makes a small cut, usually in the groin, then guides a stent graft—a tube covered with fabric—through your blood vessels up to the aorta. The stent graft then expands and attaches to the aortic walls. A seal forms between the stent graft and the vessel wall to prevent blood from entering the aortic aneurysm.

Possible Surgery-Related Complications

Complications of both types of aortic aneurysm repair can occur, and they may be life-threatening. These include:

- Bleeding and blood loss
- Blood clots in blood vessels leading to the bowel, kidneys, legs, or in the graft
- Damage to blood vessels or walls of the aorta when placing the stent graft. The stent graft may also move after it is placed.
- Endoleak, which is a blood leak around the stent graft into the aneurysm. Endoleak may cause rupture of the aneurysm if not treated.
- Gastrointestinal bleeding, which rarely occurs if an abnormal connection forms between the aorta and your intestines after the repair. Blood may show up in your stool, or your stool may be black.
- Heart complications, such as heart attack or arrhythmia
- Decreased blood flow to the bowels, legs, kidneys, or other organs during surgery. This may lead to injury to these organs.
- Infection of the incision or the graft
- Kidney damage
- Spinal cord injury which may cause paralysis
- Stroke

Chapter 32 | Arrhythmia-Related Surgery and Devices

Chapter Contents

Section 32.1 | **Radiofrequency Ablation**

This section includes text excerpted from "Catheter Ablation," National Heart, Lung, and Blood Institute (NHLBI), March 15, 2019.

Radiofrequency (RF) ablation uses high-energy, locally delivered RF signals to make the scars. Cryoablation uses extremely cold temperatures to make the scars. Sometimes, laser light energy is used. Catheter ablation is used to treat certain types of arrhythmias, or irregular heartbeats, that cannot be controlled by medicine or if you have a high risk for ventricular fibrillation (v-fib), sudden cardiac arrest, or atrial fibrillation.

Cardiologists, or doctors who specialize in the heart, will perform catheter ablation in a hospital. You will be awake, but you will receive medicine through an IV line in your arm to relax you during the procedure. Machines will measure your heart's activity. All types of ablation require cardiac catheterization to place flexible tubes, or catheters, inside your heart to make the scars. Your doctor will clean and numb an area on your arm, groin or upper thigh, or neck before making a small hole in a blood vessel. Your doctor will thread a series of catheters through the blood vessel to the correct place in your heart. An x-ray imaging method called "fluoroscopy" will let your doctor see the catheters as they are moved into your heart. Some catheters have wire electrodes that record and locate the source of your abnormal heartbeats. Your doctor will aim the tip of a special catheter at the small area of heart tissue. A machine will send either RF waves, extremely cold temperatures, or laser light through the catheter to create a scar called the "ablation line." This scar forms a barrier that prevents electrical impulses from crossing between the damaged heart tissue to the surrounding healthy tissue. This will stop abnormal electrical signals from traveling to the rest of the heart and causing arrhythmias.

After catheter ablation, your doctor will remove the catheters and close and bandage the opening on your arm, groin, or neck. You may develop a bruise and soreness where the catheters were inserted. You will stay in the hospital for a few hours or overnight.

During this time, your heart rate and blood pressure will be monitored. Your movement will be limited to prevent bleeding in the area where the catheters were inserted. You will need a ride home after the procedure because of the medicines or anesthesia you received.

Catheter ablation has some risks, including bleeding, infection, blood vessel damage, heart damage, arrhythmias, and blood clots. There also may be a very slight risk of cancer from radiation used during catheter ablation. Talk to your doctor and the technicians performing the test about whether you are or could be pregnant. If the procedure is not urgent, they may have you wait until after your pregnancy. If it is urgent, the technicians will take extra steps to protect your baby during catheter ablation.

Section 32.2 | Implantable Cardioverter Defibrillator

This section includes text excerpted from "Defibrillators," National Heart, Lung, and Blood Institute (NHLBI), June 30, 2018.

DEFIBRILLATORS

Defibrillators are devices that restore a normal heartbeat by sending an electric pulse or shock to the heart. They are used to prevent or correct an arrhythmia, a heartbeat that is uneven or that is too slow or too fast. Defibrillators can also restore the heart's beating if the heart suddenly stops.

Different types of defibrillators work in different ways. Automated external defibrillators (AEDs), which are in many public spaces, were developed to save the lives of people experiencing sudden cardiac arrest. Even untrained bystanders can use these devices in an emergency.

Other defibrillators can prevent sudden death among people who have a high risk of a life-threatening arrhythmia. They include implantable cardioverter defibrillators (ICDs)—which are surgically placed inside your body, and wearable cardioverter defibrillators (WCDs)—which rest on the body. It can take time and effort to get used to living with a defibrillator, and it is important to be aware of possible risks and complications.

HOW DEFIBRILLATORS WORK

There are three types of defibrillators: AEDs, ICDs, and WCDs. Each type works by checking for arrhythmias, or irregular heart rhythms. Once detected, each defibrillator will send a shock to restore a normal rhythm.

How Do Automated External Defibrillators Work?

An AED is a lightweight, battery-operated, portable device that checks the heart's rhythm and sends a shock to the heart to restore a normal rhythm. The device is used to help people having sudden cardiac arrest.

Sticky pads with sensors, called "electrodes," are attached to the chest of someone who is having cardiac arrest. The electrodes send information about the person's heart rhythm to a computer in the AED. The computer analyzes the heart rhythm to find out whether an electric shock is needed. If needed, the electrodes deliver the shock.

How Do Implantable Cardioverter Defibrillators Work?

The ICDs are placed surgically in the chest or abdomen, where it checks for arrhythmias. Arrhythmias can interrupt the flow of blood from your heart to the rest of your body or cause your heart to stop. The ICD sends a shock to correct the arrhythmia.

An ICD can give off a low-energy shock—to speed up or slow down an abnormal heart rate or a high-energy shock—which can correct a fast or irregular heartbeat. If the low-energy shocks do not restore your normal heart rhythm, the device will switch to high-energy shocks for defibrillation. The device also will switch to high-energy shocks if your ventricles start to quiver rather than contract strongly. ICDs are similar to pacemakers, but pacemakers deliver only low-energy electrical shocks.

The ICDs have a generator connected to wires to detect your heart's pulses and deliver a shock when needed. Some models have

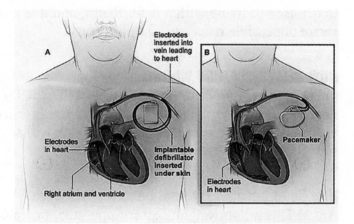

Figure 32.1. Comparison of an Implantable Cardioverter-Defibrillator and a Pacemaker

The image compares an ICD with a pacemaker. Figure A shows the location and general size of an ICD in the upper chest. The wires with electrodes on the ends are inserted into the heart through a vein in the upper chest. Figure B shows the location and general size of a pacemaker in the upper chest. The wires with electrodes on the ends are inserted into the heart through a vein in the upper chest.

wires that rest in one or two chambers of the heart. Others do not have wires threaded into the heart chambers but rest on the heart to monitor its rhythm.

The ICD can also record the heart's electrical activity and heart rhythms. The recordings can help your doctor fine-tune the programming of your device so it works better to correct irregular heartbeats. Your device will be programmed to respond to the type of arrhythmia you are most likely to have.

How Do Wearable Cardioverter Defibrillators Work?

The WCDs have sensors that attach to the skin. They are connected by wires to a unit that checks your heart's rhythm and delivers shocks when needed. Like an ICD, the WCD can deliver low- and high-energy shocks. The device has a belt attached to a vest and is worn under your clothes. Your doctor will fit the device to your size. The device is programmed to detect a particular heart rhythm.

The sensors detect when an arrhythmia occurs and notifies you with an alert. You can turn off the alert to prevent a shock if not needed, but if you do not respond, the device will administer a shock to correct the rhythm. Typically, this happens within one minute. The device can deliver repeated shocks during an episode. After each episode, the sensors must be replaced.

The device can also send a record of your heart's activity to your doctors.

WHO NEEDS DEFIBRILLATORS

Defibrillators can be used in children, teens, and adults. AEDs are used to treat sudden cardiac arrest. Your doctor may recommend an ICD or WCD to treat arrhythmia and prevent new or repeated sudden cardiac arrests.

Who Needs an Implantable Cardioverter Defibrillators

The ICDs can correct a dangerous arrhythmia or keep an irregular heartbeat from triggering sudden cardiac arrest. Life-threatening arrhythmias can develop for many reasons and can affect people of any age, from newborns to older adults. Your doctor may recommend an ICD if you have a type of arrhythmia that causes your heart's ventricles to quiver instead of pumping blood. This type of arrhythmia is most likely to cause sudden cardiac arrest.

If you have the following conditions, you may be at risk for a life-threatening arrhythmia and your doctor may recommend an ICD:

- You survived sudden cardiac arrest
- You developed an arrhythmia during or after treatment for a heart attack
- You have a genetic condition that causes arrhythmia. This includes having congenital heart disease or an inherited conduction disorder.
- You have a neuromuscular disorder. For example, the progression of muscular dystrophy can damage the heart and cause unpredictable heart rhythms. This can lead to unexplained fainting and a high risk of death.

- You have an abnormally slow heart rate or other problem with the heart's electrical signals
- You have cardiac sarcoidosis
- You have poor heart function following a procedure to improve blood flow
- Your doctor detected an arrhythmia during an electrocardiogram (EKG) or stress test. If this happened several times, you may be at increased risk.

Who Needs a Wearable Cardioverter Defibrillators?

The WCDs are used to protect against sudden cardiac arrest in certain circumstances, such as if you are at risk of arrhythmia for just a short time. This might occur under these conditions:

- You are recovering from a heart attack
- You are waiting for a heart transplant
- You are fighting an infection
- You are removing or waiting to replace your ICD

SURGERY FOR IMPLANTABLE CARDIOVERTER DEFIBRILLATORS

If your doctor recommends an ICD to treat an arrhythmia, your healthcare team will help you prepare for surgery. Learn about what to expect from the surgery and during the early days of your recovery. As with any surgery, there are risks involved.

Before and during Surgery

You may have questions about your condition and whether an ICD is right for you. Discuss them with your doctor. You may be able to choose between different ICD models with different benefits and risks. Your doctor will help you make the decision that is right for you.

Placing an ICD requires minor surgery, which usually is done in a hospital. Your doctor will discuss the procedure with you. This is a good time to ask questions.

Before the surgery, members of your healthcare team will give you medicines to relax you and to numb the area where the device will go. They may also give you antibiotics to prevent infections.

Typically, the ICD is placed under your breastbone or along your ribs. In infants, it can be placed in the abdomen. With some devices, your doctor may first thread one or two sensor wires through your blood vessels into the chambers of your heart. With others, a single sensor wire is placed along the breastbone. The doctors will use a monitor to guide the wires and put them in the right place.

Once the device is in place, your doctor will test it. Then your doctor will sew up the cut. The entire surgery takes a few hours.

Recovery from Surgery

You may be able to leave the hospital once the medicines you received for the surgery wear off. You can then continue your recovery at home.

Follow the instructions you receive. Your healthcare team may tell you to take these steps:

- Check the cut on your chest often and keep the area clean and dry.
- Call your doctor if any swelling or bleeding occurs or if you develop a fever.
- Take over-the-counter pain medicines, such as acetaminophen if you feel pain. But talk to your doctor first; she or he may tell you to avoid taking ibuprofen or other kinds of pain medicines, for example.
- Ask your doctor when you can resume taking medicines that you took before the surgery, how soon you can take a shower, and when you can return to work. You will probably have to avoid driving for at least a week while you recover from your surgery. Your doctor may also ask you to avoid high-impact activities and heavy lifting for about a month.

At your next scheduled appointment, ask your doctor about living with an ICD and what to do when you feel an electric pulse or shock from your device.

Possible Surgery-Related Complications

As with any surgery, there are some risks related to the surgery used to place an ICD. Although they are rare, possible complications include:

- A bad reaction to the medicine used to make you relax or sleep during the surgery
- A collapsed lung
- A defibrillator wire puncturing the heart or a vessel
- Bleeding from the site where the device was placed
- Blood vessel, heart, or nerve damage
- Swelling, bruising, or infection at the area where the device was placed
- Venous thromboembolism

Some ICD models have a lower risk of clots, puncture, and infection.

What to Expect from Electric Shocks

It takes time to get used to having an ICD or WCD. These devices can deliver electrical energy at different strengths to regulate your heart.

- **Low-energy shocks.** The low-energy electrical shocks your device gives are not painful. You may not notice them, or you may feel a fluttering in your chest.
- **High-energy shocks.** The high-energy shocks last only a fraction of a second, but they can be strong or painful. They may feel like thumping or a kick in the chest, depending on their strength. Before a shock, you may feel arrhythmia symptoms. If you feel one or two strong shocks over a short period and the symptoms go away, it may be a sign that the device is working. Notify your doctor's office and set up an appointment that day or the next day. She or he will want to assess your condition and the device.
- **Unnecessary shocks.** During the adjustment period after your surgery, your device may deliver a shock when it is not needed. A damaged wire or a very fast

heart rate due to extreme physical activity may trigger unnecessary shocks. These shocks can also occur if you forget to take your medicines. Some people also feel phantom shocks, even when the device does not detect an arrhythmia.

Make Sure Your Wearable Cardioverter Defibrillators Is Fitted Properly

You will be wearing it all the time, except when you are taking a shower or bath. Like shocks from ICDs, shocks from WCDs can be painful and sometimes cause burns. Your doctor will explain how to charge and change the batteries in your WCD.

Return to Normal Daily Activities

Talk to your doctor about when you can return to normal activities, such as physical activity and driving.

- **Physical activity.** An ICD usually will not limit you from taking part in sports and exercise, including strenuous activities. You may need to avoid full-contact sports, such as football. Contact sports can damage your ICD or shake loose the wires in your heart. Ask your doctor how much and what types of physical activity are safe for you.
- **Driving.** You probably will be able to resume your typical driving patterns after you recover from surgery. However, if you received an ICD to prevent another sudden cardiac arrest or ventricular arrhythmia, it will probably be several months before your doctor says you are ready to drive again. This is because of the risks of fainting or getting a shock from your device. Your doctor may also suggest driving restrictions based on the activity recorded by your device.

Receive Routine Follow-Up Care

Once you have an ICD, you will visit your doctor at least every six months. At these visits, your doctor will examine the area where the device was implanted and check information about your heart rhythm that was recorded by the device. In between visits, your doctor can monitor data from your device remotely. If it is needed, she or he can adjust the device's settings.

At the follow-up visits, your doctor may also take these steps:

- Prescribe or adjust your medicines to decrease the number of irregular heartbeats you have. Fewer irregular beats will mean fewer high-energy shocks that have to be sent to your heart.

- Check to make sure the device continues to work properly and that it has not shifted in your body or caused irritation or injury. Over time, your ICD may stop working well because its wires get dislodged or broken, its battery fails, your heart disease progresses, or other devices have disrupted its electrical signaling. Your doctor also may recommend an electrocardiogram (EKG) to check for changes in your heart's electrical activity.

- Check to see whether you are at risk of heart failure. If device and medicine adjustments do not reduce your irregular heart rhythms, your doctor may suggest a procedure called "ablation" to stop excess electrical signals in your heart.

- Check to see whether the battery needs to be replaced. Batteries in ICDs last between five and seven years. When the batteries in your device run down, you will need surgery to replace them. Replacing the battery is less involved than the original surgery to implant the ICD. Ask your doctor whether the device generator or its wires need to be replaced, too.

Manage Devices That Can Interfere with Your Implantable Cardioverter Defibrillators

Electrical devices and devices with strong magnetic fields can interfere with your ICD. You may not be able to sense when this happens. If something disrupts your ICD, step away from the disruptive device to help restore its normal working. To be safe, keep your ICD at least six inches away from the following devices, or, when necessary, use them only briefly:

- **Cell phones.** If you have an ICD on the left side of your chest, hold your cell phone to your right ear.
- **Headphones.** Most headphones have a magnetic element in them. Wear them as far away from your ICD as possible, and do not carry your headphones in a chest pocket.
- **Metal detectors,** such as those used for airport security. The risk of harm is low, but you can show your ID card and ask for alternative inspection.

Some medical procedures, including magnetic resonance imaging (MRI), can damage ICDs. This depends on the procedure and your device model. For example, some people with newer models can undergo MRI. Tell your dentist or doctor that you have an ICD and discuss your options with them. You can show them the card with information about your device.

Learn the Warning Signs of Complications and Make a Plan

It is possible for a wire in an ICD to fire at the wrong time or become infected. Call your doctor if you have signs or symptoms that concern you, and if you have these signs in particular:

- Fainting
- Dizziness or feeling out of breath
- Fever
- Heart palpitations or chest pain

Go to a hospital emergency room if you feel many strong shocks from your device in a short time.

Occasionally an ICD does not work properly and cannot be fixed with changes in programming or medicine. If this happens, your doctor might have to replace the ICD. When you visit the doctor, ask whether the manufacturer has announced any problems with your device.

Tend to Your Emotional Health

If you have survived sudden cardiac arrest, you may worry about whether it will happen again. After surgery to implant an ICD or fitting for a WCD, adjusting to the uncertainty of life with the device may cause fear, anxiety, and stress. When your device sends a strong shock, it may startle or distress you or cause you pain. This can make some people stop doing the things they used to do. After having sudden cardiac arrest or getting an ICD, some people report anxiety, depression, or other more serious emotional health concerns.

If you have survived cardiac arrest or are living with an ICD or WCD and experience anxiety or depression, tell your doctor about your concerns.

Section 32.3 | Pacemaker

This section includes text excerpted from "Pacemakers," National Heart, Lung, and Blood Institute (NHLBI), November 1, 2011. Reviewed April 2020.

WHAT IS A PACEMAKER?

A pacemaker is a small device that is placed in the chest or abdomen to help control abnormal heart rhythms. This device uses electrical pulses to prompt the heart to beat at a normal rate.

Pacemakers are used to treat arrhythmias. Arrhythmias are problems with the rate or rhythm of the heartbeat. During an arrhythmia, the heart can beat too fast, too slow, or with an irregular rhythm.

A heartbeat that is too fast is called "tachycardia." A heartbeat that is too slow is called "bradycardia."

During an arrhythmia, the heart may not be able to pump enough blood to the body. This can cause symptoms such as fatigue (tiredness), shortness of breath, or fainting. Severe arrhythmias can damage the body's vital organs and may even cause loss of consciousness or death.

A pacemaker can relieve some arrhythmia symptoms, such as fatigue and fainting. A pacemaker also can help a person who has abnormal heart rhythms resume a more active lifestyle.

Pacemakers can:

- Speed up a slow heart rhythm
- Help control an abnormal or fast heart rhythm
- Make sure the ventricles contract normally if the atria are quivering instead of beating with a normal rhythm (a condition called "atrial fibrillation")
- Coordinate electrical signaling between the upper and lower chambers of the heart
- Coordinate electrical signaling between the ventricles. Pacemakers that do this are called "cardiac resynchronization therapy" (CRT) devices. CRT devices are used to treat heart failure.
- Prevent dangerous arrhythmias caused by a disorder called "long QT syndrome"

Doctors also treat arrhythmias with another device called an "implantable cardioverter-defibrillator" (ICD). An ICD is similar to a pacemaker. However, besides using low-energy electrical pulses, an ICD also can use high-energy pulses to treat life-threatening arrhythmias.

HOW DOES A PACEMAKER WORK?

A pacemaker consists of a battery, a computerized generator, and wires with sensors at their tips. (The sensors are called "electrodes.") The battery powers the generator, and both are surrounded by a thin metal box. The wires connect the generator to the heart.

A pacemaker helps monitor and control your heartbeat. The electrodes detect your heart's electrical activity and send data through the wires to the computer in the generator.

If your heart rhythm is abnormal, the computer will direct the generator to send electrical pulses to your heart. The pulses travel through the wires to reach your heart.

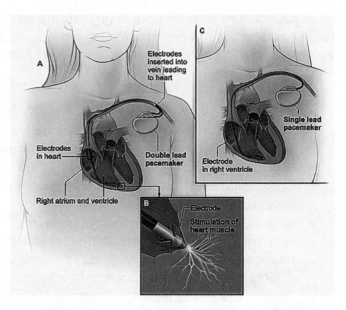

Figure 32.2. Cross-Section of a Chest with a Pacemaker

Figure A shows the location and general size of a double-lead, or dual-chamber, pacemaker in the upper chest. The wires with electrodes are inserted into the hearts right atrium and ventricle through a vein in the upper chest. Figure B shows an electrode electrically stimulating the heart muscle. Figure C shows the location and general size of a single-lead, or single-chamber, pacemaker in the upper chest.

Newer pacemakers can monitor your blood temperature, breathing, and other factors. They also can adjust your heart rate to changes in your activity.

The pacemaker's computer also records your heart's electrical activity and heart rhythm. Your doctor will use these recordings to adjust your pacemaker so it works better for you.

Your doctor can program the pacemaker's computer with an external device. She or he does not have to use needles or have direct contact with the pacemaker.

Pacemakers have one to three wires that are each placed in different chambers of the heart.

- The wires in a single-chamber pacemaker usually carry pulses from the generator to the right ventricle (the lower right chamber of your heart).

- The wires in a dual-chamber pacemaker carry pulses from the generator to the right atrium (the upper right chamber of your heart) and the right ventricle. The pulses help coordinate the timing of these two chambers' contractions.
- The wires in a biventricular pacemaker carry pulses from the generator to an atrium and both ventricles. The pulses help coordinate electrical signaling between the two ventricles. This type of pacemaker also is called a "cardiac resynchronization therapy" (CRT) device.

WHAT TO EXPECT DURING PACEMAKER SURGERY

Placing a pacemaker requires minor surgery. The surgery usually is done in a hospital or special heart treatment laboratory.

Before the surgery, an intravenous (IV) line will be inserted into one of your veins. You will receive medicine through the IV line to help you relax. The medicine also might make you sleepy.

Your doctor will numb the area where she or he will put the pacemaker so you do not feel any pain. Your doctor also may give you antibiotics to prevent infection.

First, the doctor will insert a needle into a large vein, usually near the shoulder opposite your dominant hand. The doctor will then use the needle to thread the pacemaker wires into the vein and to correctly place them in your heart.

An x-ray "movie" of the wires as they pass through your vein and into your heart will help your doctor place them. Once the wires are in place, your doctor will make a small cut into the skin of your chest or abdomen.

She or he will slip the pacemaker's small metal box through the cut, place it just under your skin, and connect it to the wires that lead to your heart. The box contains the pacemaker's battery and generator.

Once the pacemaker is in place, your doctor will test it to make sure it works properly. She or he will then sew up the cut. The entire surgery takes a few hours.

WHAT TO EXPECT AFTER PACEMAKER SURGERY

Expect to stay in the hospital overnight so your healthcare team can check your heartbeat and make sure your pacemaker is working well. You will likely have to arrange for a ride to and from the hospital because your doctor may not want you to drive yourself.

For a few days to weeks after surgery, you may have pain, swelling, or tenderness in the area where your pacemaker was placed. The pain usually is mild; over-the-counter (OTC) medicines often can relieve it. Talk to your doctor before taking any pain medicines.

Your doctor may ask you to avoid vigorous activities and heavy lifting for about a month after pacemaker surgery. Most people return to their normal activities within a few days of having the surgery.

WHAT ARE THE RISKS OF PACEMAKER SURGERY?

Pacemaker surgery generally is safe. If problems do occur, they may include:

- Swelling, bleeding, bruising, or infection in the area where the pacemaker was placed
- Blood vessel or nerve damage
- A collapsed lung
- A bad reaction to the medicine used during the procedure

Talk with your doctor about the benefits and risks of pacemaker surgery.

HOW WILL A PACEMAKER AFFECT YOUR LIFESTYLE?

Once you have a pacemaker, you have to avoid close or prolonged contact with electrical devices or devices that have strong magnetic fields. Devices that can interfere with a pacemaker include:

- Cell phones and MP3 players (for example, iPods)
- Household appliances, such as microwave ovens
- High-tension wires

- Metal detectors
- Industrial welders
- Electrical generators

These devices can disrupt the electrical signaling of your pacemaker and stop it from working properly. You may not be able to tell whether your pacemaker has been affected.

How likely a device is to disrupt your pacemaker depends on how long you are exposed to it and how close it is to your pacemaker.

To be safe, some experts recommend not putting your cell phone or MP3 player in a shirt pocket over your pacemaker (if the devices are turned on).

You may want to hold your cell phone up to the ear that is opposite the site where your pacemaker is implanted. If you strap your MP3 player to your arm while listening to it, put it on the arm that is farther from your pacemaker.

You can still use household appliances, but avoid close and prolonged exposure, as it may interfere with your pacemaker.

You can walk through security system metal detectors at your normal pace. Security staff can check you with a metal detector wand as long as it is not held for too long over your pacemaker site. You should avoid sitting or standing close to a security system metal detector. Notify security staff if you have a pacemaker.

Also, stay at least 2 feet away from industrial welders and electrical generators.

Some medical procedures can disrupt your pacemaker. These procedures include:

- Magnetic resonance imaging, or MRI
- Shockwave lithotripsy to get rid of kidney stones
- Electrocauterization to stop bleeding during surgery

Let all of your doctors, dentists, and medical technicians know that you have a pacemaker. Your doctor can give you a card that states what kind of pacemaker you have. Carry this card in your wallet. You may want to wear a medical ID bracelet or necklace that states that you have a pacemaker.

Physical Activity

In most cases, having a pacemaker would not limit you from doing sports and exercise, including strenuous activities.

You may need to avoid full-contact sports, such as football. Such contact could damage your pacemaker or shake loose the wires in your heart. Ask your doctor how much and what kinds of physical activity are safe for you.

Ongoing Care

Your doctor will want to check your pacemaker regularly (about every three months). Over time, a pacemaker can stop working properly because:

- Its wires get dislodged or broken
- Its battery gets weak or fails
- Your heart disease progresses
- Other devices have disrupted its electrical signaling

To check your pacemaker, your doctor may ask you to come in for an office visit several times a year. Some pacemaker functions can be checked remotely using a phone or the Internet.

Your doctor also may ask you to have an EKG (electrocardiogram) to check for changes in your heart's electrical activity.

Battery Replacement

Pacemaker batteries last between 5 and 15 years (average 6 to 7 years), depending on how active the pacemaker is. Your doctor will replace the generator along with the battery before the battery starts to run down.

Replacing the generator and battery is less-involved surgery than the original surgery to implant the pacemaker. Your pacemaker wires also may need to be replaced eventually.

Your doctor can tell you whether your pacemaker or its wires need to be replaced when you see her or him for follow-up visits.

Chapter 33 | Joint, Bone, and Spine Surgery

Chapter Contents

Section 33.1 | Joint Replacement Surgery Basics

This section includes text excerpted from "Joint Replacement Surgery," National Institute of Arthritis and Musculoskeletal and Skin Diseases (NIAMS), August 30, 2016. Reviewed April 2020.

Joint replacement surgery is removing a damaged joint and putting in a new one. The doctor may suggest a joint replacement to improve how you live. Replacing a joint can relieve pain and help you move and feel better.

Hips and knees are replaced most often. Other joints that can be replaced include the shoulders, fingers, ankles, and elbows.

The new joint can be made of plastic, metal, or ceramic parts. Sometimes, the surgeon will not remove the whole joint, but will only replace or fix the damaged parts. Types of new joints include:

- **Cemented joints.** Used more often in older people who do not move around as much and in people with "weak" bones. The cement holds the new joint to the bone.
- **Uncemented joints.** Often recommended for younger, more active people and those with good bone quality. It may take longer to heal, because it takes longer for bone to grow and attach to it.
- **Hybrid replacements.** Use both methods to keep the new joint in place.

WHY JOINT REPLACEMENT SURGERY MAY BE NEEDED

Pain, stiffness, and swelling may be due to joint damage caused by:

- Arthritis
- Years of use
- Disease

To see if you need a joint replaced, your doctor may:

- Look at your joint with an x-ray or another machine
- Put a small, lighted tube (arthroscope) into your joint to look for damage
- Take a small sample of your tissue for testing

After looking at your joint, the doctor may recommend:
- Exercise
- Walking aids, such as braces or canes
- Physical therapy
- Medicines and vitamin supplements
- Osteotomy, which involves cutting and lining up bone. This may be simpler than replacing a joint, but it may take longer to recover. However, this operation has become less common.

If you still have constant pain and have trouble with things such as walking, climbing stairs, and taking a bath, your doctor may recommend joint replacement.

WHAT TO EXPECT DURING JOINT REPLACEMENT SURGERY

During joint replacement surgery your doctors will:
- Give you medicine so you would not feel pain. The medicine may block the pain only in one part of the body, or it may put your whole body to sleep.
- Replace the damaged joint with a new human-made joint.
- Move you to a recovery room until you are fully awake or the numbness goes away.

COMPLICATIONS OF JOINT REPLACEMENT SURGERY

Technology and advances in surgical techniques have greatly reduced the complications involved with joint replacements. When problems do occur, most are treatable. Possible problems include:
- **Infection.** Areas in the wound or around the new joint may get infected. It may happen while you are still in the hospital or after you go home. It may even occur years later. Minor infections in the wound are usually treated with drugs. Deep infections may need a second operation to treat the infection or replace the joint.
- **Blood clots.** If your blood moves too slowly, it may begin to form lumps of blood parts called "clots." If

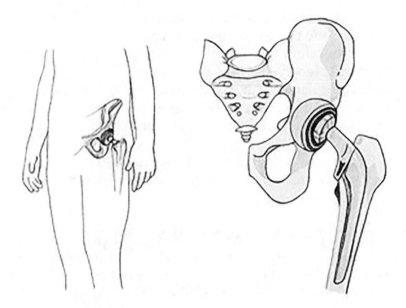

Figure 33.1. Hip Replacement Location

pain and swelling develop in your legs after hip or knee surgery, blood clots may be the cause. The doctor may suggest drugs to make your blood thin or special stockings, exercises, or boots to help your blood move faster. If swelling, redness, or pain occurs in your leg after you leave the hospital, contact your doctor right away.

- **Loosening.** The new joint may loosen, causing pain. If the loosening is bad, you may need another operation to reattach the joint to the bone.
- **Dislocation.** Sometimes after hip or other joint replacement, the ball of the prosthesis can come out of its socket. In most cases, the hip can be corrected without surgery. A brace may be worn for a while if a dislocation occurs.
- **Wear.** Some wear can be found in all joint replacements. Too much wear may help cause loosening. The doctor may need to operate again if

the prosthesis comes loose. Sometimes, the plastic can wear thin, and the doctor may just replace the plastic and not the whole joint.

- **Nerve and blood vessel injury.** Nerves near the replaced joint may be damaged during surgery, but this does not happen often. Over time, the damage often improves and may disappear. Blood vessels may also be injured.

As you move your new joint and let your muscles grow strong again, pain will lessen, flexibility will increase, and movement will improve.

WHAT TO EXPECT AFTER JOINT REPLACEMENT SURGERY

With knee or hip surgery, you will probably need to stay in the hospital for a few days. If you are an older adult or have additional disabilities, you may then need to spend several weeks in an intermediate-care facility before going home. You and your team of doctors will determine how long you stay in the hospital.

After hip or knee replacement, you will often stand or begin walking the day of surgery. First, you will walk with a walker or crutches. You may have some temporary pain in the new joint because your muscles are weak from not being used. Also, your body is healing. The pain can be helped with medicines and should end in a few weeks or months.

Physical therapy can begin the day after surgery to help strengthen the muscles around the new joint and help you regain motion in the joint. If you have your shoulder joint replaced, you can usually begin exercising the same day of your surgery. A physical therapist will help you with gentle, range-of-motion exercises. Before you leave the hospital, your therapist will show you how to use a pulley device to help bend and extend your arm.

RESEARCH PROGRESS RELATED TO JOINT REPLACEMENT SURGERY

Research on joint replacement surgery is exploring:
- The various forms of arthritis to stop or slow joint damage

- New joint materials and other ways to improve surgery and decrease complications
- Why some people who need surgery do not choose it

Section 33.2 | Arthroscopic Surgery

"Arthroscopic Surgery," © 2016 Omnigraphics. Reviewed April 2020.

Arthroscopy is a minimally invasive surgical technique used to evaluate, diagnose, and treat or repair a variety of joint-related conditions. Literally translated, arthroscopy means "looking into the joint." Surgeons insert a tiny, fiberoptic camera through a small incision and use it to examine the interior structure of the joint. Images are greatly magnified and displayed on a television screen.

Initially used as a diagnostic tool prior to performing traditional open surgery, arthroscopy has rapidly gained popularity as a standalone medical procedure. Since it is most often performed on an outpatient basis, it is less stressful for patients and offers faster recovery times than traditional surgeries. In addition, advancements in medical instrumentation and fiberoptic technology have enabled surgeons to use it to treat an expanding array of conditions.

INDICATIONS FOR ARTHROSCOPY

Arthroscopy is one of the final steps in the process of diagnosing and treating joint injuries and diseases. The process begins with a complete medical history and physical examination of the patient, and then it involves noninvasive imaging tests such as X-rays, magnetic resonance imaging (MRI), or computed tomography (CT). After reviewing the results of these tests, an orthopedic surgeon may recommend an arthroscopic procedure for one of the following problems:

- **Unexplained joint pain.** Arthroscopy can be used to determine the causes of joint pain that cannot be explained using conventional diagnostic tools.

- **Synovitis.** This condition, which is characterized by inflammation of the synovial membrane lining the cavities of joints, can often be treated through arthroscopy.
- **Removal of loose pieces of bone or cartilage.** Fragments arising from arthritis, injury, or other causes can be easily removed through arthroscopy.
- **Arthritis.** Arthroscopy cannot completely cure arthritis, but it may be used to repair damaged joints and relieve symptoms associated with it.
- **Biopsies.** Arthroscopy can be used to collect samples and analyze the characteristics of synovial fluid in order to diagnose joint disease. Arthroscopy is also used to obtain cartilage tissue for use in cartilage transplant procedures.
- **Meniscal injury.** The meniscus is a crescent-shaped cartilage that distributes weight and reduces friction in the knee, wrist, and other joints. Damage to the meniscus—which can occur suddenly from a traumatic injury or gradually from normal wear and tear—can result in pain, swelling, and impaired joint function. Meniscal repair is one of the most common types of arthroscopic procedures, and it leads to improvement in symptoms for many patients.
- **Ligament repair.** Arthroscopy is often used to diagnose, repair, or reconstruct torn or damaged ligaments.

THE ARTHROSCOPIC PROCEDURE

Arthroscopy may be performed under general, spinal, or local anesthesia, depending on the joint being treated and the type of problem being investigated. The orthopedic surgeon makes a small incision in the skin of the affected joint and inserts a pencil-sized instrument called an "arthroscope." The arthroscope is fitted with a small lens and a light source to illuminate the interior structure of the joint. The arthroscope is also equipped with a fiberoptic camera that transmits images onto a screen. If the initial examination of the joint reveals the need for a corrective procedure, the surgeon makes additional incisions as needed to insert other miniature medical instruments.

RECOVERY AFTER ARTHROSCOPY

As a minimally invasive procedure, arthroscopic surgery causes significantly less trauma to the soft tissues of the joint than traditional open surgery. As a result, it offers a faster recovery time. The small arthroscopic incisions heal quickly, and the operative dressing is usually removed within a couple of days. The joint itself may take several weeks to recover, depending on the overall health of the patient and the procedure involved. In patients who require complex surgical procedures to correct extensive damage to cartilage and ligaments, recovery may take several months. Prior to discharge from the hospital, the healthcare provider generally provides the patient with explicit instructions on the type of activities to avoid, as well as the rehabilitative activities to undertake in order to speed recovery and improve postoperative joint function.

RISKS INVOLVED IN ARTHROSCOPY

Arthroscopy is generally considered a safe and effective medical procedure. Although most people who undergo it will experience some discomfort and swelling, these symptoms are typically short-lived. Many patients can return to work and resume normal activities within a few weeks. Serious complications are rare, affecting less than one percent of cases, and may include the following:

- **Postoperative infection.** If an infection develops within the joint, the patient will experience swelling, pain, and fever.
- **Nerve damage.** When an arthroscopic procedure damages a nerve, the patient may experience numbness and tingling sensations around the joint.
- **Hemorrhage.** A small amount of bleeding is normal in arthroscopic procedures, but excessive bleeding may require treatment in a hospital setting.

- **Equipment or implant failure.** Arthroscopic instruments are tiny and fragile, and they occasionally break during surgery. In these instances, the procedure may be extended, or a second surgery may be required. Likewise, the implants and components the surgeon uses to hold the joint in place (including pins, screws, rods, plates, and suture anchors) may break, leaving loose pieces floating around inside the joint. Since these fragments can rub against and damage surrounding tissues, they may need to be removed in a second surgery.
- **Deep-vein thrombosis (DVT).** DVT occurs when a blood clot forms in a vein following surgery. In rare cases, the blood clot may break away and pass through the bloodstream to the lungs, where it can obstruct the blood supply and create a dangerous condition called "pulmonary embolism." Most surgeons take precautions to reduce the risk of DVT, such as administering blood thinners and getting the patients up and moving as soon as possible after surgery.

References

1. NHS Choices. "Arthroscopy," Gov.UK, 2015.
2. Waller, C.S. "Knee Arthroscopy," May 2010.
3. Wilkerson, Rick. "Arthroscopy," American Academy of Orthopaedic Surgeons (AAOS), May 2010.

Section 33.3 | Basics of Hip Replacement Surgery

This section includes text excerpted from "Hip Replacement Surgery," National Institute of Arthritis and Musculoskeletal and Skin Diseases (NIAMS), July 30, 2016. Reviewed April 2020.

The hip joint is located where the upper end of the femur (thigh bone) meets the pelvis (hip bone). A ball at the end of the femur, called the "femoral head," fits in a socket (the acetabulum) in the pelvis to allow a wide range of motion.

Hip replacement, or arthroplasty, is a surgical procedure in which the diseased parts of the hip joint are removed and replaced with new, artificial parts. These artificial parts are called the "prosthesis."

The goals of hip replacement surgery include increasing mobility, improving the function of the hip joint, and relieving pain.

TYPES OF HIP REPLACEMENT SURGERY

There are two primary types of hip replacement surgery:

Traditional Surgery

During a traditional hip replacement, which lasts from 1 to 2 hours, the surgeon makes a 6- to 8-inch incision over the side of the hip through the muscles and removes the diseased bone tissue and cartilage from the hip joint, while leaving the healthy parts of the joint intact. Then the surgeon replaces the head of the femur and acetabulum with new, artificial parts. The new hip is made of materials that allow a natural gliding motion of the joint.

Minimally Invasive Surgery

Some surgeons perform what is called a "minimally invasive," or mini-incision, hip replacement, which requires smaller incisions and a shorter recovery time than traditional hip replacement. Candidates for this type of surgery are usually 50 years of age or younger, of normal weight based on body mass index, and healthier than candidates for traditional surgery. Joint resurfacing is also being used.

Regardless of whether you have traditional or minimally invasive surgery, the parts used to replace the joint are the same and come in two general varieties: cemented and uncemented.

- **Cemented replacements,** which fasten artificial parts to healthy bone with a special glue or cement. These replacements are typically used for older, less active people and people with weak bones.
- **Uncemented replacements,** which use artificial parts with a porous surface. This allows bone to grow

into the pores to hold the new parts in place. These replacements are typically used for younger, more active people. Because it takes a long time for the natural bone to grow and attach to the prosthesis, activity must be limited for up to three months to protect the hip joint. Thigh pain may occur while the bone is growing into the prosthesis.

- **Hybrid replacements** use a cemented femur part and uncemented acetabular part.

WHY IS HIP REPLACEMENT SURGERY NEEDED?

Common reasons for hip replacement surgery include damage to the hip joint from:

- Arthritis
- Disease that breaks down the bone in the joint
- Injuries or fractures
- Bone tumors that break down the hip joint

If hip joint damage causes pain and interferes with daily activities, your doctor may try treatments, such as exercise, walking aids (canes and walkers), and medication. If these treatments do not relieve pain and improve joint function, the doctor may suggest either hip replacement surgery or a less complex corrective surgery. One alternative to hip replacement is osteotomy, which involves cutting and realigning bone to shift the weight to a healthier bone surface.

In the past, hip replacement surgery was mostly done in people over 60 years of age. The thinking was that older people are less active, which puts less stress on the artificial hip. However, new technologies have improved artificial parts so that they handle more stress and last longer. This means that hip replacement surgery can also be successful in younger people.

Hip replacement may not be recommended for people with certain health conditions, such as:

- Parkinson disease
- Conditions that result in severe muscle weakness, which increases the risk of damaging or dislocating an artificial hip

- People at high risk for infections or in poor health, since they are less likely to recover successfully

PREPARING FOR HIP REPLACEMENT SURGERY

You can do a number of things before hip replacement surgery to make everyday tasks easier and help speed your recovery.

- Learn what to expect. Request written information from the doctor. Arrange for transportation to and from the hospital.
- Arrange for someone to help you around the house for a week or two after coming home from the hospital.
- Stock up on kitchen supplies and prepare food in advance, such as frozen casseroles or soups that can be reheated and served easily.
- Set up a recovery station at home:
  - Place the television remote control, telephone, medicine, tissues, wastebasket, and pitcher and glass next to the spot where you will spend the most time while you recover.
  - Place other items you use every day at arm's level to avoid reaching up or bending down.

WHAT TO EXPECT DURING HIP REPLACEMENT SURGERY

During hip replacement, which lasts from one to two hours, your doctors:

- Will give you medicine to put your whole body to sleep so that you would not feel pain
- Makes a 6- to 8-inch incision over the side of the hip. Your surgeon may recommend a minimally invasive hip replacement, which requires smaller incisions. Candidates for minimally invasive hip replacement surgery are usually:
  - Age 50 or younger
  - Normal weight based on body mass index
  - Healthier than candidates for traditional surgery
- Removes the diseased bone tissue and cartilage from the hip joint, while leaving the healthy parts of the joint in place

- Replaces the head of the femur and acetabulum with new, artificial parts
- Move you to a recovery room for 1 to 2 hours until you are fully awake or the numbness goes away

WHAT TO EXPECT AFTER HIP REPLACEMENT SURGERY

Immediate. Usually, people do not spend more than one to four days in the hospital after hip replacement surgery. It is important to get instructions from your doctor before leaving the hospital and to follow them carefully once you get home. Doing so will give you the greatest chance of a successful surgery.

- Immediately after your hip surgery:
  - You will be allowed only limited movement.
  - When you are in bed, pillows or a special device will brace the hip in the correct position.
  - You may receive fluids through an intravenous tube to replace fluids lost during surgery.
  - Drains may also be located near the incision to drain fluid, and a catheter may be inserted to remove urine until you can use the bathroom.
  - The doctor will prescribe medicine for pain or discomfort.
- The day of or day after surgery:
  - Therapists will teach you exercises to improve recovery.
  - A respiratory therapist may ask you to breathe deeply, cough, or blow into a simple device that measures lung capacity. These exercises reduce the collection of fluid in the lungs after surgery.
- As early as one to two days after surgery:
  - You may be able to sit on the edge of the bed, stand, and even walk with assistance.
  - A physical therapist may teach you exercises to strengthen the hip. The physical therapist also will teach you how to perform daily activities without injuring your new hip.
- Once you return home you should:

- Follow the doctor's instructions.
- Wear an apron for carrying things around the house. This leaves hands and arms free for balance or to use crutches.
- Use a long-handled "reacher" to turn on lights or grab things that are beyond arm's length. Hospital personnel may provide one of these or suggest where to buy one.
- Work with a physical therapist or other healthcare professional to rehabilitate your hip.

Long term. Full recovery from hip replacement surgery takes about three to six months, depending on the type of surgery, your overall health, and the success of your rehabilitation.

You should talk to your doctor or physical therapist about an appropriate exercise program, which can reduce stiffness, increase flexibility, and strengthen muscles. Most of these programs begin with safe range-of-motion activities and muscle-strengthening exercises. The doctor or therapist will decide when you can move on to more demanding activities.

Revision surgery (replacement of an artificial joint) is becoming more common as more people are having hip replacements at a younger age. This is because wearing away of the joint surface becomes a problem after 15 to 20 years. Doctors consider revision surgery when:

- Medication and lifestyle changes do not relieve pain and disability
- X-rays show bone loss, wearing of the joint surfaces, or joint loosening
- Fracture, dislocation of the artificial parts, or infection occurs

Section 33.4 | **Basics of Knee Replacement Surgery**

This section includes text excerpted from "The NIH Consensus Development Conference on Total Knee Replacement," National Institute of Health (NIH), December 10, 2003. Reviewed April 2020.

Based on research evidence, total knee replacement (TKR) is a safe and cost-effective treatment for alleviating pain and restoring physical function in patients who do not respond to nonsurgical therapies. There are few contraindications to this surgery as it is currently used.

Overall, TKR has been shown to be a very successful, relatively low-risk therapy despite variations in patient health status and characteristics, type of prosthesis implanted, orthopedic surgeons, and surgical facilities. Improvements can be made in the overall success of TKR by addressing each of these areas of variation through further research.

Each year, approximately 300,000 TKR surgeries are performed in the United States for end-stage arthritis of the knee joint. As the number of TKR surgeries performed each year increases and the indications for TKR extend to younger as well as older patients, a review of available scientific information is necessary to enhance clinical decision making and stimulate further research.

First used in the late 1950s, early TKR implants poorly mimicked the natural motion of the knee and resulted in high failure and complication rates. Advances in TKR technology have enhanced the design and fit of knee implants, resulting in improved short- and long-term outcomes.

Despite the increased success of TKR, questions remain concerning which materials and implant designs are most effective for specific patient populations and which surgical approach is optimal for a successful outcome. Physical, social, and psychological issues may influence the success of TKR, and understanding patient differences could facilitate the decision making process before, during, and after surgery, thereby achieving the greatest benefit from TKR. Particular attention also must be given to the treatment and timing options related to the revision of failed TKR surgery.

Primary TKR is most commonly performed for knee joint failure caused by OA; other indications include RA, juvenile RA, osteonecrosis, and other types of inflammatory arthritis. The aims of TKR are relief of pain and improvement in function. Candidates for elective TKR should have radiographic evidence of joint damage, moderate-to-severe persistent pain not adequately relieved by an extended course of nonsurgical management, and clinically significant functional limitation resulting in diminished quality of life.

The success of primary TKR in most patients is strongly supported by more than 20 years of follow-up data. There appears to be a rapid and substantial improvement in the patient's pain, functional status, and overall health-related quality of life in about 90 percent of patients; about 85 percent of patients are satisfied with the results of surgery.

Short-term outcomes, as documented by functional outcome scales, are generally substantially improved after TKR. Functional outcome is improved after TKR for people across the spectrum of disability status. In general, prostheses are durable, but failure does occur.

Age younger than 55 at the time of TKR, male gender, diagnosis of OA, obesity, and presence of comorbid conditions are risk factors for revision.

Factors related to a surgeon's case volume, technique, and choice of the prosthesis may have important influences on surgical outcomes. One of the clearest associations with better outcomes appears to be the procedure volume of the individual surgeon and the hospital.

Technical factors in performing surgery may influence both the short- and long-term success rate. Proper alignment of the prosthesis appears to be critical. Many design features, such as the use of mobile bearings or designs sparing cruciate ligaments, have theoretical advantages, but durability and success rates appear roughly similar to most commonly used designs.

There is consensus regarding the following perioperative interventions that improve TKR outcomes: systemic antibiotic prophylaxis, aggressive postoperative pain management, perioperative risk assessment and management of medical conditions, and pre-operative education.

The effectiveness of anticoagulation for the prevention of pulmonary emboli is unclear. There are insufficient data to support specific perioperative rehabilitation strategies, methods to reduce postoperative anemia, postoperative physical activity recommendations, and the site of post-acute care.

Revision TKR is done to alleviate pain and improve function. Fracture or dislocation of the patella, instability of the components or aseptic loosening, infection, and periprosthetic fractures are common reasons for total knee revision. A painful knee without an identifiable cause is a controversial indication. Contraindications for revision TKR include persistent infection, poor bone quality, highly limited quadriceps or extensor function, poor skin coverage, and poor vascular status. Results are not as good as with primary TKR; outcomes are better for aseptic loosening than for infections. When an infection is involved, successful results occur with a two-stage revision. Failed revisions require a salvage procedure (resection of arthroplasty, arthrodesis, or amputation), with inferior results compared with revision TKR.

There is clear evidence of racial/ethnic and gender disparities in the provision of TKR in the United States. Racial or ethnic differences in the provision of care are not limited to joint replacements. The limited role of economic and other access factors in these racial or ethnic disparities can be demonstrated by significant differences in the rate of procedures in the VA system, where cost and access are assumed equivalent across race or ethnic groups.

The patient's acceptance of physician recommendations varies greatly. Among persons with a potential need for TKR, only 12.7 percent of women and 8.8 percent of men were indefinitely willing to have the procedure. The interaction between the patient and physician affects the final recommendations and the patient's acceptance of those recommendations. Physician's beliefs about their patients, the limited familiarity with these procedures in minority communities, patient's mistrust of the healthcare system, and personal beliefs about the most effective treatment of joint problems may all have a role in these racial or ethnic disparities.

The goal of new population-based observational research is to discover the need for services among persons with knee disability and the extent to which this need is currently being met by resources available within the family and in the community at large (including the healthcare system).

Research into the impact of providers and the healthcare system should be broadened to include all TKR variables related to the surgeon, such as training and experience; surgical technique, including the type of prosthesis and implantation technique; selection and perioperative care of patients; quality and characteristics of the institution, such as infection control methods and surgical volume; preoperative and postoperative modalities, including rehabilitation therapy; and continuity of care, including the pre- and postoperative plan for longer-term followup and physical activity. In addition to broadening the scope of variables studied, the outcomes assessment must include all persons who receive knee surgery, as opposed to a convenience sample of those who return to the surgeon, and the followup must be sufficiently long to encompass the expected life of the prostheses.

Research should identify the extent to which disparities in the use of TKR are the result of subjective differences across groups in the perception of pain or disability and orientation to surgery (risk aversion or cultural affinity with the healthcare providers who might refer to surgery, or both); objective differences in access to care as a result of the potential financial burden and extent and kind of health insurance; or discrimination on the part of healthcare providers. Research also should identify the patient-level factors affecting outcomes after surgery, including medical and sociodemographic characteristics, participation in rehabilitation services, the extent of social support, and the level of a patient's physical activity after the surgery.

Section 33.5 | **Rotator Cuff Repair**

WHAT IS ROTATOR CUFF REPAIR?

In a patient's shoulder joint, a cuff known as a "rotator" helps for movement, rotation, and hand-raising. Like any other joint, the rotator cuff gets deteriorated with time and usage and also opens to the possibility of tendon injury and damage. All these health complications will result in the patient to experience weak shoulders and the best treatment will be surgery to repair and heal them.

In this surgery, the size of the surgical incision will depend on the procedure performed by the surgeon on the patient. Smaller incisions are done to trim or smoothen the tendons with the objective of strengthening the shoulder. While larger incisions are performed to reattach or stitch the injured or damaged tendons and let it heal.

WHY ROTATOR CUFF REPAIR IS PERFORMED?

Rotator cuff repair is suggested as an option on patients:
- Who have undergone nonsurgical methods but still have unmanageable pain
- Who are very active in sports such as swimmers, tennis players, baseball pitchers, etc.
- Who relies heavily in the use of arms for work-related tasks such as carpenters, painters, etc.

Apart from the above underlying conditions, rotator cuff surgery is also recommended when a patient is:
- Having symptoms that have lasted 6 to 12 months
- Having more than an inch tear but the quality of the tissues surrounding the tendon is still good
- Having significant shoulder weakness and loss of function
- Having a large tear due to an injury, trauma, etc.

ROTATOR CUFF INJURY DIAGNOSIS

A rotator cuff injury on a patient is usually diagnosed by palpating the area and doing a series of range-of-motion tests. Normally, a doctor will do a physical examination, such as asking the patient to rotate and raise their arm. In case it causes pain during this type of motion tests, then the rotator cuff may be inflamed.

If a patient has noticeable weakness, then it will need further testing using x-rays or magnetic resonance imaging (MRI) in order to check for a rotator cuff tear.

RISKS FACTORS

The following factors determine whether a patient has an increased risk of having a rotator cuff injury:

- **Age.** Advanced age is associated with a higher incidence of rotator cuff injury. Rotator cuff tears (RCTs) are most common in people above 40 years of age.
- **Certain sports.** Being an athlete, there is greater risk of facing a rotator cuff injury especially for those who use repetitive arm motions frequently such as badminton players, swimmers, cricket players, archers, baseball pitchers, tennis players, etc.
- **Construction jobs.** Rotator cuffs get damaged in people who continuously conduct overhead motions in their occupations. This repetitive overhead activity or heavy lifting, such as carpentry or house painting over a prolonged period of time will lead to rotator cuff tears or injury.
- **Family history.** Getting to know about a family history of rotator cuff injuries can warn patients to take some precautionary actions to protect against their own injuries due to a possibility of an involvement of genetic component with rotator cuff injuries.

COMPLICATIONS

The patients are advised to rest their shoulder for recovery. Keeping the shoulder immobilized for a prolonged time can cause the connective tissue enclosing the joint to become thickened and tight (frozen shoulder). This can cause pain, stiffness, and loss of normal range of motion in the shoulder.

References

1. "Rotator Cuff Repair," URAC, April 21, 2019.
2. "Rotator Cuff Injury," Harvard Health Publishing, December 19, 2018.
3. "Rotator Cuff Injury," Mayo Foundation for Medical Education and Research (MFMER), May 17, 2018.

Section 33.6 | Shoulder Replacement Surgery

"Shoulder Replacement," © 2018 Omnigraphics. Reviewed April 2020.

Shoulder replacement is a surgical procedure to replace the bones of the shoulder with an artificial implant. According to the Agency for Healthcare Research and Quality (AHRQ), more than 53,000 people in the United States have shoulder replacement surgeries each year. Shoulder replacement surgery was first performed to treat shoulder fractures; however, it is also used to treat other painful conditions of the shoulder. Shoulder replacement is an effective procedure to remove pain and improve motion, strength, and function in the shoulder.

CAUSES OF SHOULDER PAIN

There are several causes for shoulder pain, and many reasons why patients should consider a shoulder replacement surgery.

Rheumatoid Arthritis

Rheumatoid arthritis, also called "inflammatory arthritis," affects the shoulders. The synovial membrane that lubricates the cartilage becomes inflamed and causes joint stiffness, eventually resulting in loss of cartilage and shoulder pain.

Osteoarthritis (Degenerative Joint Disease)

Osteoarthritis is one of the most common reasons for shoulder replacement surgery. As people age, their chances of developing osteoarthritis are high. The cartilage wears away and causes stiffness in the shoulder bones. As a result, when the bones rub against one another, there is severe shoulder pain.

Rotator Cuff Tear Arthropathy

When the rotator cuff muscles contract, they put pressure on the humerus, resulting in rotator cuff tears. The sudden changes in the shoulder muscles caused by the rotator cuff damages the joint cartilage. This leads to arthritis of the shoulder.

Posttraumatic Arthritis

Arthritis of the shoulder may lead to fractures that cause tears in the shoulder muscles. After a shoulder injury, the ligaments and tendons damage the cartilage and prevent smooth movement of the shoulder.

Severe Fractures

A doctor may recommend a shoulder replacement in the case of a severe fracture. Blood supply to the bone is stopped because of the fracture. When the humerus is fractured, it is not easy to replace the bones, and therefore, a surgeon may recommend shoulder replacement.

Avascular Necrosis (Osteonecrosis)

Osteonecrosis causes shoulder pain when the bone cells die due to the lack of blood supply. This eventually leads to arthritis. Often, this condition is caused by excessive use of alcohol, steroids, shoulder fractures, and sickle cell disease.

Failed Shoulder Replacement Surgery

Sometimes, shoulder replacements fail because of infection, wear and tear, dislocation, or the loosening of the implant. In such cases, another shoulder replacement surgery might be necessary.

DO YOU NEED A SHOULDER REPLACEMENT SURGERY?

When other treatment options have been considered and there is no relief, the doctor may recommend a shoulder replacement surgery. Often in the case of osteoarthritis, rheumatoid arthritis, and severe trauma caused by a shoulder fracture, complete shoulder replacement enables smooth functioning of the shoulder muscles. It is important to discuss this surgery with your loved ones, your doctor, and your surgeon and to be assured of their cooperation as you decide to undergo the surgery.

Your doctor may recommend shoulder replacement surgery for the following reasons:

- Decreased motion or weakness in the shoulder
- Severe pain while resting, to the extent of robbing you of sleep
- Difficulty in performing everyday activities such as reaching into a cabinet, dressing, and washing because of excess strain in the shoulders
- No improvement after treatments with anti-inflammatory medications, cortisone injections, or physical therapy

You may consider shoulder replacement surgery for the following reasons:

- A torn rotator cuff
- A serious shoulder injury like a broken bone
- Severe arthritis

However, your doctor will recommend surgery only after treating you with drugs and physical therapy and determining that they have not helped alleviate your pain.

TYPES OF SHOULDER REPLACEMENT SURGERIES

There are a few types of shoulder replacement surgeries. Your doctor will determine which one is right for you depending on the condition of your shoulder.

TOTAL SHOULDER REPLACEMENT

Total shoulder replacement surgery is performed by replacing the surface of the affected joint with a metal ball and a plastic socket. They come in all sizes and your surgeon will choose what is necessary for the surgery. Your doctor may use a noncemented humeral component if the quality of the bone is good and bone cement if the bone is soft. However, an all-plastic glenoid substance is inserted with bone cement.

Glenoid component is not recommended when:
- The rotator cuff tendons are torn beyond repair
- The glenoid has good cartilage
- The glenoid bone is severely deficient

Total shoulder replacement surgery is particularly appropriate for patients with osteoarthritis and intact rotator cuff tendons.

STEMMED HEMIARTHROPLASTY

Hemiarthroplasty is the surgical procedure of replacing only the ball in the shoulder. The humeral head is replaced with a metal ball and stem in a traditional hemiarthroplasty, also known as a "stemmed hemiarthroplasty."

Hemiarthroplasty is recommended only when the humeral head is damaged but the socket is intact. A hemiarthroplasty also includes:
- Shoulders with considerable damage to the bone in the glenoid
- Torn rotator cuff tendons and arthritis of the shoulders
- Damage to the humeral head but the glenoid has a healthy cartilage surface

However, there are instances when the surgeons decide to make a call whether to proceed with a total shoulder replacement or a hemiarthroplasty during the surgery.

RESURFACING HEMIARTHROPLASTY

As the name suggests, the surface of the humeral head is replaced with a prosthetic cap. Resurfacing hemiarthroplasty is a procedure that increases bone life, offering patients with arthritis of the shoulder an option to choose between the traditional hemiarthroplasty and resurfacing hemiarthroplasty.

You can choose resurfacing hemiarthroplasty if:
- There is no damage to the humeral neck or head
- The cartilage surface of the glenoid is healthy
- The humeral bone has to be preserved

Resurfacing hemiarthroplasty decreases the risk of wear and tear and loosening of the implant and is highly recommended for young patients. If required, later resurfacing hemiarthroplasty can be converted to a total shoulder replacement.

REVERSE TOTAL SHOULDER REPLACEMENT

In a reverse total shoulder replacement, a metal ball is attached to the shoulder bone and to the upper arm bone—a plastic socket. This allows the patient to use the muscles of the upper arm instead of the torn rotator cuff. Reverse total shoulder replacement is recommended only in the case of:
- Severe arthritis and rotator cuff tearing (cuff tear arthropathy)
- A torn rotator cuff with severe arm weakness
- A previously failed shoulder replacement

Sometimes, patients find it difficult to lift their arms and move them sideways. A reverse shoulder replacement provides relief while a traditional total shoulder replacement can still leave them with pain.

RISK FACTORS

As is the case in most surgeries, your surgeon will describe the potential risks in undergoing a shoulder replacement surgery. Complications can occur after the surgery; however, most of these conditions can be treated:

- Infection or bleeding around the joint
- Allergic reaction to the artificial joint
- Damage to the blood vessel during surgery
- Nerve damage during surgery
- Dislocation of the artificial joint
- Loosening of the implant over time
- Bone break during surgery

PREPARING FOR SURGERY

Preparation for a shoulder replacement surgery involves a full physical exam, x-rays, or other imaging tests to confirm the need for surgery. Your orthopedic surgeon will make a thorough examination to determine your fitness level for the surgery.

The medical examination consists of:

- **A medical history.** In addition to the general health checkup, your doctor will examine the functioning of your affected shoulder.
- **A physical examination.** Shoulder motion, strength, and stability are gauged.
- **X-rays.** The level of damage to the shoulder, spaces between the bones, deformities, or any irregularities in the bone or cartilage can be determined by viewing the images generated by the x-ray.
- **Other tests.** Magnetic resonance imaging (MRI) scans and other blood tests help evaluate the condition of bone and soft tissues of the shoulder.

After reviewing the results of your evaluation, your orthopedic surgeon will determine the need for surgery. However, other options for treatment will also be discussed by the doctor, who will consider whether injections, physical therapy, or another type of treatment may be required. If surgery has been confirmed, it will be explained to you ahead of time. This will give you time to prepare yourself for your stay after the surgery, and also allow time to plan for any help required after your discharge from the hospital.

AFTER THE SURGERY

After you are transported to the postanesthesia recovery unit (PACU), the anesthesiology team will check your vital signs (breathing, pulse, and blood pressure). When you have recovered from the anesthesia, you will be attached to a cooling unit. A large dressing on your shoulder will be covered with an arm sling for protection. After an hour at the PACU, you will be assigned to a hospital room.

- You will stay in the hospital for a few days (1 to 3) after your surgery.
- A physical therapist will help you keep your shoulder muscles relaxed.
- Active movement of your shoulders will not be allowed until sufficient time has been given for healing your shoulder muscles.
- You will be given instructions in how to care for your shoulder at home. Make sure to follow them.

PAIN MANAGEMENT

Pain management is an essential part of your recovery. After surgery, you will feel some pain but, with physical therapy, you will be on the path to recovery soon. The pain gradually reduces as you recover your strength and start exercising your shoulder again. Keep your doctor informed in the event of any complications as you exercise your shoulder muscles. Pain relief medications include opioids, nonsteroidal anti-inflammatory drugs (NSAIDs), and local anesthetics that can help you manage your pain. The doctor may prescribe a combination of medicines and, over time, reduce your need for opioids. The use of opioids are critical and must be taken only under your doctor's approval. However, if the pain does not reduce after the surgery, make sure to inform your doctor.

REHABILITATION

A rehabilitation program is essential to the success of a shoulder replacement. Regular exercises and physical therapy are mandatory after surgery. Your physical therapist will demonstrate exercises to strengthen your shoulder and improve flexibility. The following guidelines will ensure a successful recovery from your surgery:

1. Follow the exercises demonstrated by the physical therapist two or three times a day.
2. Do not exert pressure on your arm when you get out of bed or up from a chair since this causes additional strain on your shoulder muscles.
3. Overuse of your shoulder may result in excess pain afterward. Try to limit your shoulder movements as much as possible.
4. Ask for assistance at home.
5. Limit your involvement in sports that involve excessive action, as this may cause unnecessary strain on your shoulders.
6. Ask for help when you want to lift something heavy.
7. Keep your arm in the position demonstrated by the physical therapist. Avoid extreme movements, such as moving your arms to one side or behind your body for the first weeks after surgery.

Shoulder replacement surgery has greatly improved the quality of life for thousands of patients, improving motion and flexibility. Following the rehabilitation program, you will make several trips to see your doctor and keep her or him informed of your progress.

References

1. "Shoulder Joint Replacement," American Academy of Orthopedic Surgeons (AAOS), December 2011.
2. "Shoulder Replacement," MedlinePlus, National Institutes of Health (NIH), April 5, 2018.
3. J. Martin, Laura. "Shoulder Replacement Surgery: What to Know," WebMD, December 21, 2017.
4. "Joint Replacement: Shoulder," The Cleveland Clinic Foundation, August 21, 2009.

Section 33.7 | **Spine Surgery**

This section includes text excerpted from "Low Back Pain Fact Sheet," National Institute of Neurological Disorders and Stroke (NINDS), August 13, 2019.

SURGERY FOR SPINE

When other therapies fail, surgery may be considered an option to relieve pain caused by serious musculoskeletal injuries or nerve compression. It may be months following surgery before the patient is fully healed, and she or he may suffer permanent loss of flexibility.

Surgical procedures are not always successful, and there is little evidence to show which procedures work best for their particular indications. Patients considering surgical approaches should be fully informed of all related risks. Surgical options include:

- **Vertebroplasty and kyphoplasty** are minimally invasive treatments to repair compression fractures of the vertebrae caused by osteoporosis. Vertebroplasty uses three-dimensional imaging to assist in guiding a fine needle through the skin into the vertebral body, the largest part of the vertebrae. A glue-like bone cement is then injected into the vertebral body space, which quickly hardens to stabilize and strengthen the bone and provide pain relief. In kyphoplasty, prior to injecting the bone cement, a special balloon is inserted and gently inflated to restore height to the vertebral structure and reduce spinal deformity.
- Spinal laminectomy (also known as "spinal decompression") is performed when spinal stenosis causes a narrowing of the spinal canal that causes pain, numbness, or weakness. During the procedure, the lamina or bony walls of the vertebrae, along with any bone spurs, are removed. The aim of the procedure is to open up the spinal column to remove pressure on the nerves.
- **Discectomy or microdiscectomy** may be recommended to remove a disc, in cases where it has herniated and presses on a nerve root or the

spinal cord, which may cause intense and enduring pain. Microdiscectomy is similar to a conventional discectomy; however, this procedure involves removing the herniated disc through a much smaller incision in the back and a more rapid recovery. Laminectomy and discectomy are frequently performed together and the combination is one of the more common ways to remove pressure on a nerve root from a herniated disc or bone spur.

- **Foraminotomy** is an operation that "cleans out" or enlarges the bony hole (foramen) where a nerve root exits the spinal canal. Bulging discs or joints thickened with age can cause narrowing of the space through which the spinal nerve exits and can press on the nerve, resulting in pain, numbness, and weakness in an arm or leg. Small pieces of bone over the nerve are removed through a small slit, allowing the surgeon to cut away the blockage and relieve pressure on the nerve.

- **Intradiscal electrothermal therapy (IDET)** is a treatment for discs that are cracked or bulging as a result of degenerative disc disease. The procedure involves inserting a catheter through a small incision at the site of the disc in the back. A special wire is passed through the catheter and an electrical current is applied to heat the disc, which helps strengthen the collagen fibers of the disc wall, reducing the bulging and the related irritation of the spinal nerve. IDET is of questionable benefit.

- **Nucleoplasty,** also called "plasma disc decompression" (PDD), is a type of laser surgery that uses radiofrequency energy to treat people with low back pain associated with mildly herniated discs. Under x-ray guidance, a needle is inserted into the disc. A plasma laser device is then inserted into the needle and the tip is heated to 40 to 70 degrees Celsius, creating a field that vaporizes the tissue in the disc, reducing its size and relieving pressure on the nerves. Several channels may be made depending on how tissue needs to be removed to decompress the disc and nerve root.

- **Radiofrequency denervation** is a procedure using electrical impulses to interrupt nerve conduction (including the conduction of pain signals). Using x-ray guidance, a needle is inserted into a target area of nerves and a local anesthetic is introduced as a way of confirming the involvement of the nerves in the person's back pain. Next, the region is heated, resulting in localized destruction of the target nerves. Pain relief associated with the technique is temporary and the evidence supporting this technique is limited.
- **Spinal fusion** is used to strengthen the spine and prevent painful movements in people with degenerative disc disease or spondylolisthesis (following laminectomy). The spinal disc between two or more vertebrae is removed and the adjacent vertebrae are "fused" by bone grafts and/or metal devices secured by screws. The fusion can be performed through the abdomen, a procedure known as an "anterior lumbar interbody fusion," or through the back, known as "posterior fusion." Spinal fusion may result in some loss of flexibility in the spine and requires a long recovery period to allow the bone grafts to grow and fuse the vertebrae together. Spinal fusion has been associated with an acceleration of disc degeneration at adjacent levels of the spine.
- **Artificial disc replacement** is considered an alternative to spinal fusion for the treatment of people with severely damaged discs. The procedure involves removal of the disc and its replacement by a synthetic disc that helps restore height and movement between the vertebrae.

Section 33.8 | **Carpal Tunnel Surgery**

This section includes text excerpted from "Carpal Tunnel Syndrome Fact Sheet," National Institute of Neurological Disorders and Stroke (NINDS), April 7, 2020.

SURGERY FOR CARPAL TUNNEL

Carpal tunnel release is one of the most common surgical procedures in the United States. Generally, surgery involves severing a ligament around the wrist to reduce pressure on the median nerve. Surgery is usually done under local or regional anesthesia (involving some sedation) and does not require an overnight hospital stay. Many people require surgery on both hands. While all carpal tunnel surgery involves cutting the ligament to relieve the pressure on the nerve, there are two different methods used by surgeons to accomplish this.

- **Open release surgery,** the traditional procedure used to correct carpal tunnel syndrome, consists of making an incision up to 2 inches in the wrist and then cutting the carpal ligament to enlarge the carpal tunnel. The procedure is generally done under local anesthesia on an outpatient basis, unless there are unusual medical conditions.

- **Endoscopic surgery** may allow somewhat faster functional recovery and less postoperative discomfort than traditional open release surgery, but it may also have a higher risk of complications and the need for additional surgery. The surgeon makes one or two incisions (about ½ inch each) in the wrist and palm, inserts a camera attached to a tube, observes the nerve, ligament, and tendons on a monitor, and cuts the carpal ligament (the tissue that holds joints together) with a small knife that is inserted through the tube.

The ligaments usually grow back together and allow more space than before. Although symptoms may be relieved immediately after surgery, full recovery from carpal tunnel surgery can take months.

Almost always there is a decrease in grip strength, which improves over time. Some individuals may develop infections, nerve damage, stiffness, and pain at the scar. Most people need to modify work activity for several weeks following surgery, and some people may need to adjust job duties or even change jobs after recovery from surgery.

Although recurrence of carpal tunnel syndrome following treatment is rare, fewer than half of individuals report their hand(s) feeling completely normal following surgery. Some residual numbness or weakness is common.

Section 33.9 | Surgery for Upper and Lower Limb Fractures

"Surgery for Upper and Lower Limb Fractures," © 2020 Omnigraphics. Reviewed April 2020.

Fractures occur due to various reasons and a bone fracture depends on the force that is exerted on that particular bone. If the force exerted is not too high, the bone just cracks but if the force is too high, such as in automobile crashes or a gunshot, the bones may break into pieces. Surgeries are, therefore, performed to fix these damaged bones.

There are a number of ways to treat people who suffer from fractures in their upper extremities such as hand, wrist, forearm, elbow, upper arm, and shoulder; and lower extremities such as hip, thigh, knee, lower leg, ankle, and foot.

Some common types of fractures are:

- **Stable fracture.** In this type of fracture, the broken bones are in line and they do not require realignment.
- **Open, compound fracture.** The broken bone fragments pierce through the skin or the force causes an open wound at the time of fracture.
- **Transverse fracture.** This is a complete fracture and has a horizontal fracture line.
- **Oblique fracture.** In this type of fracture, the fracture occurs diagonally.

- **Comminuted fracture.** In this type of fracture, the bone breaks into two or more fragments.

SURGICAL TREATMENTS FOR LIMB FRACTURES
Internal Fixators for Fractures

It is important to carefully stabilize and support the broken bone until it is strong enough to support mobility. Physicians used casts and splints to stabilize the broken bone from outside the body during earlier days but the emergence of the sterile surgical procedures has reduced the risk of infection allowing the doctors to internally fix and stabilize the fracture.

During a surgical treatment, the bone fragments are initially repositioned into their normal alignments and are then held together with special implants such as plates screws, nails, and wires. These implants are compatible with the body and can rarely cause an allergy and are durable and strong since they are made from stainless steel and titanium. These implants can also be made from cobalt and chrome if the joint is to be replaced rather than fixing it.

The following are the internal fixators used for the surgery:

Plates. Plates are like the internal splints that are attached to the bone with screws to hold the broken pieces of bone together. The plates may be left in place after complete healing or in certain cases they may be removed.

Screws. Screws are mostly used for internal fixation than any other type of implant. The screws used differ in size and design based on the type of fracture and how they will be used. For certain fractures, only screws are used to hold the bones in place, while they can also be used along with plates, or rods. Once the bone heals, the screws may be left in place or removed.

Nails or Rods. The best way to hold the bones in case of fractures of the long bones is by inserting a rod or nail through the hollow center of the bone that contains some bone marrow. Screws are fixed at each end of the rod to keep the fracture from shortening or rotating and to hold the rod in place till the fracture heals. This method is used to treat fractures in the femur and tibia and these rods can be left in the bone even after complete healing.

Wires or Pins. Wires are often used to fix the broken bones that are too small to be fixed with screws. In several cases, wires or pins are used in conjunction with other forms of internal fixation or they can be used alone to treat small bone fractures, such as fractures in the hand or foot. In some cases of fractures, the wires are permanently left in or they are removed after a certain amount of time.

External Fixators for Fractures

An external fixator is a stabilizing frame that is used to hold the broken bones in a proper position. An external fixator has metal pins or screws that are placed into the bone through small surgical cuts made on the skin and muscle. The pins and screws are attached to the bar outside the skin and these external fixators are different from casts and splints which rely completely on external support. In many cases, external fixation is considered to be a temporary treatment that is used to fix fractures. External fixators can be easily applied and are used when the patient has multiple injuries and is not ready for a longer surgery to fix the fracture. Until the patient is healthy enough to undergo the final surgery, good support and stability are provided by the external fixators.

References

1. "Different Types of Fractures," Premier Orthopaedics, July 20, 2015.
2. "Fractures (Broken Bones)," American Academy of Orthopaedic Surgeons (AAOS), February 1, 2001.
3. "Internal Fixation for Fractures," American Academy of Orthopaedic Surgeons (AAOS), April 22, 2019.

Chapter 34 | Gastrointestinal Surgery

Chapter Contents

Section 34.1 | Appendectomy

This section contains text excerpted from the following sources: Text beginning with the heading "Basics of Appendicitis" is excerpted from "Treatment for Appendicitis," National Institute of Diabetes and Digestive and Kidney Diseases (NIDDK), November 2014. Reviewed April 2020; Text beginning the heading "Appendicitis for Elderly People" is excerpted from "Recurrent Appendicitis," Agency for Healthcare Research and Quality (AHRQ), U.S. Department of Health and Human Services (HHS), October 2010. Reviewed April 2020.

BASICS OF APPENDICITIS
What Is Appendicitis?
Appendicitis is inflammation of your appendix.

How Common Is Appendicitis?
In the United States, appendicitis is the most common cause of acute abdominal pain requiring surgery. Over 5 percent of the population develops appendicitis at some point.

Who Is More Likely to Develop Appendicitis?
Appendicitis most commonly occurs in the teens and twenties but may occur at any age.

What Are the Complications of Appendicitis?
If appendicitis is not treated, it may lead to complications. The complications of a ruptured appendix are:
- Peritonitis, which can be a dangerous condition. Peritonitis happens if your appendix bursts and infection spreads in your abdomen. If you have peritonitis, you may be very ill and have:
  - Fever
  - Nausea
  - Severe tenderness in your abdomen
  - Vomiting
- An abscess of the appendix called an appendiceal abscess

TREATMENT FOR APPENDICITIS
How Do Doctors Treat Appendicitis?

Doctors typically treat appendicitis with surgery to remove the appendix. Surgeons perform the surgery in a hospital with general anesthesia. Your doctor will recommend surgery if you have continuous abdominal pain and fever, or signs of a burst appendix and infection. Prompt surgery decreases the chance that your appendix will burst.

Healthcare professionals call the surgery to remove the appendix an appendectomy. A surgeon performs the surgery using one of the following methods:

- **Laparoscopic surgery.** During laparoscopic surgery, surgeons use several smaller incisions and special surgical tools that they feed through the incisions to remove your appendix. Laparoscopic surgery leads to fewer complications, such as hospital-related infections, and has a shorter recovery time.
- **Laparotomy.** Surgeons use laparotomy to remove the appendix through a single incision in the lower right area of your abdomen.

After surgery, most patients completely recover from appendicitis and do not need to make changes to their diet, exercise, or lifestyle. Surgeons recommend that you limit physical activity for the first 10 to 14 days after a laparotomy and for the first 3 to 5 days after laparoscopic surgery.

What If the Surgeon Finds a Normal Appendix?

In some cases, a surgeon finds a normal appendix during surgery. In this case, many surgeons will remove it to eliminate the future possibility of appendicitis. Sometimes surgeons find a different problem, which they may correct during surgery.

Can Doctors Treat Appendicitis without Surgery?

Some cases of mild appendicitis may be cured with antibiotics alone. All patients suspected of having appendicitis are treated with antibiotics before surgery, and some patients may improve completely before surgery is performed.

How Do Doctors Treat Complications of a Burst Appendix?

Treating the complications of a burst appendix will depend on the type of complication. In most cases of peritonitis, a surgeon will remove your appendix immediately with surgery. The surgeon will use laparotomy to clean the inside of your abdomen to prevent infection and then remove your appendix. Without prompt treatment, peritonitis can cause death.

A surgeon may drain the pus from an appendiceal abscess during surgery or, more commonly, before surgery. To drain an abscess, the surgeon places a tube in the abscess through the abdominal wall. You leave the drainage tube in place for about 2 weeks while you take antibiotics to treat infection. When the infection and inflammation are under control, about 6 to 8 weeks later, surgeons operate to remove what remains of the burst appendix.

APPENDICITIS FOR ELDERLY PEOPLE

Appendicitis is one of the most common surgical diseases encountered, with approximately 250,000 appendectomies performed annually in the United States. Although appendectomy (either open or laparoscopic) is a relatively safe operation compared with other surgical procedures, appendicitis in the elderly can be a challenging problem, with substantially higher rates of missed and delayed diagnoses, perforation, and postoperative morbidity and mortality. For the general population, the mortality rate following appendectomy is less than 1 percent; however, in elderly patients, reported mortality rates range from 4 percent to 8 percent. Similarly, complication rates of 20 percent to 30 percent are reported for patients older than 65 years of age compared to 7 percent to 10 percent for those younger than 65 years of age. The higher rate of complications in the elderly may be due in part to the higher observed rates of perforation (50% to 70% in the elderly compared to approximately 20% in the general population).

445

MEDICAL ERROR IN THE TREATMENT OF APPENDICITIS FOR ELDERLY PEOPLE

The most common medical error encountered in the treatment of appendicitis is a missed or delayed diagnosis, especially in the elderly. In one study, a preoperative diagnosis of appendicitis was made in fewer than half of elderly patients and an incorrect admitting diagnosis was associated with an increased risk of perforation. The most common misdiagnoses were bowel obstruction in patients with perforated appendicitis and diverticulitis in those without perforations. Because both of these conditions are generally treated nonoperatively, such misdiagnoses can be associated with a significant delay in operative intervention and subsequent increased risk of perforation.

Overdiagnosis of appendicitis is also an issue. Although the use of computed tomography (CT) scanning has decreased this rate, a recent multi-institutional study suggests that the negative appendectomy rate (i.e., surgery is performed for presumed appendicitis, but the appendix proves to be normal) is still 6 percent. In such cases, the surgeon traditionally removes the normal-appearing appendix because 20 percent to 40 percent will have pathological abnormalities not visible to the surgeon's eye—primarily endo appendicitis or inflammation that is confined to the mucosa or inner wall of the appendix. In addition, if the operation was performed open, future physicians might be confused when a patient sporting a right lower quadrant "appendectomy" incision presents with true appendicitis in the future. However, such a "telltale" incision is not found following laparoscopic exploration, and many surgeons will choose to leave a normal-appearing appendix in place. In a study of more than 1500 such patients, only a tiny minority (0.2%) went on to develop clinical appendicitis requiring reoperation. Taken together, this suggests that a normal-appearing appendix seen on laparoscopic evaluation may safely be left in place.

Once in the operating room, there are several technical errors that can occur, primarily accidental injury to adjacent bowel or bleeding (either intraoperative or postoperative). If a laparoscopic approach is used, there is an additional risk of injury during trocar (the port used to access the abdomen) placement to the bowel (which can go unrecognized) or vasculature (which can be particularly harrowing if injury occurs in a major vessel, such as the aorta, vena cava, or iliac vessels) and the rare risk of air embolus.

RECURRENT OR RESIDUAL APPENDICITIS

"Recurrent" or "residual" appendicitis can occur when the appendix is not completely removed at the time of the first operation. Most often this is "stump" appendicitis, in which a portion of the distal appendix was removed, but the base of the appendix and some of the proximal appendix were inadvertently left behind. The appendix can vary in size and position relative to the ileocecum, making it challenging to identify the base of the appendix, especially in the setting of acute inflammation. A laparoscopic approach can magnify these issues given the limited visual field, two-dimensional image, and lack of tactile feedback for the surgeon.

Section 34.2 | Bowel Diversion Surgeries

This section includes text excerpted from "Ostomy Surgery of the Bowel," National Institute of Diabetes and Digestive and Kidney Diseases (NIDDK), August 2014. Reviewed April 2020.

WHAT IS OSTOMY SURGERY OF THE BOWEL?

Ostomy surgery of the bowel, also known as "bowel diversion," refers to surgical procedures that reroute the normal movement of intestinal contents out of the body when part of the bowel is diseased or removed. Creating an ostomy means bringing part of the intestine through the abdominal wall so that waste exits through the abdominal wall instead of passing through the anus.

Ostomy surgery of the bowel may be temporary or permanent, depending on the reason for the surgery. A surgeon specially trained in intestinal surgery performs the procedure in a hospital. During the surgery, the person receives general anesthesia.

Ostomy surgeries of the bowel include:
- Ileostomy
- Colostomy
- Ileoanal reservoir
- Continent ileostomy

WHY DOES A PERSON NEED OSTOMY SURGERY OF THE BOWEL?
A person may need ostomy surgery of the bowel if she or he has:
- Cancer of the colon or rectum
- An injury to the small or large intestine
- Inflammatory bowel disease—longlasting disorders, such as Crohn disease and ulcerative colitis, that cause irritation or sores in the GI tract
- Obstruction—a blockage in the bowel that prevents the flow of fluids or solids
- Diverticulitis—a condition that occurs when small pouches in the colon called "diverticula" become inflamed, or irritated and swollen, and infected

WHAT IS A STOMA?
During ostomy surgery of the bowel, a surgeon creates a stoma by bringing the end of the intestine through an opening in the abdomen and attaching it to the skin to create an opening outside the body. A stoma maybe three-fourths of an inch to a little less than two inches wide. The stoma is usually located in the lower part of the abdomen, just below the beltline. However, sometimes the stoma is located in the upper abdomen. The surgeon and a wound, ostomy, and continence (WOC) nurse or an enterostomal therapist will work together to select the best location for the stoma. A removable external collection pouch, called an "ostomy pouch" or "ostomy appliance," is attached to the stoma and worn outside the body to collect intestinal contents or stool. Intestinal contents or stool passes through the stoma instead of passing through the anus. The stoma has no muscle, so it cannot control the flow of stool, and the flow occurs whenever other digestive muscles contract. Ileostomy and colostomy are the two main

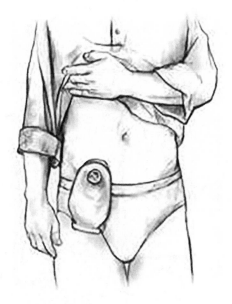

Figure 34.1. Ostomy Pouch

types of ostomy surgery of the bowel during which a surgeon creates a stoma.

WHAT IS AN ILEOSTOMY?

An ileostomy is a stoma created from a part of the ileum. For this surgery, the surgeon brings the ileum through the abdominal wall to make a stoma. An ileostomy may be permanent or temporary. An ileostomy is permanent when the surgeon removes or bypasses the entire colon, rectum, and anus. A surgeon may perform a temporary ileostomy for a damaged or an inflamed colon or rectum that only needs time to rest or heal from injury or surgery. After the colon or rectum heals, the surgeon repairs the opening in the abdominal wall and reconnects the ileum so stool will pass into the colon normally. An ileostomy is the most common temporary bowel diversion. A surgeon performs an ileostomy most often to treat inflammatory bowel disease or rectal cancer.

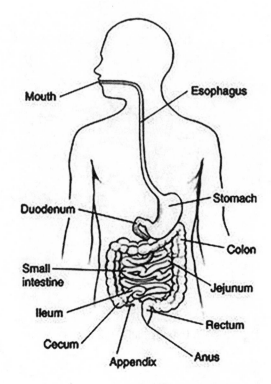

Figure 34.2. Ileostomy

WHAT IS A COLOSTOMY?

A colostomy is a stoma created from a part of the colon. For this surgery, the surgeon brings the colon through the abdominal wall and makes a stoma. A colostomy may be temporary or permanent. The colostomy is permanent when the surgeon removes or bypasses the lower end of the colon or rectum. A surgeon may perform a temporary colostomy for damaged or an inflamed lower part of the colon or rectum that only needs time to rest or heal from injury or surgery. Once the colon or rectum heals, the surgeon repairs the opening in the abdominal wall and reconnects the colon so stool will pass normally. A surgeon performs a colostomy most often to treat rectal cancer, diverticulitis, or fecal incontinence—the accidental loss of stool.

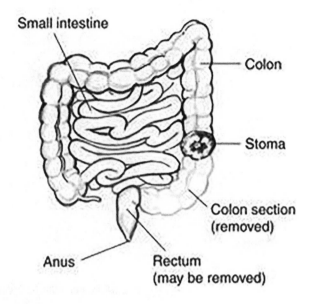

Small intestine

Colon

Stoma

Colon section
(removed)

Anus

Rectum
(may be removed)

Figure 34.3. Colostomy

WHAT IS AN ILEOANAL RESERVOIR?

An ileoanal reservoir is an internal pouch made from the ileum. This surgery is a common alternative to an ileostomy and does not have a permanent stoma. Also known as a "J-pouch" or "pelvic pouch," the ileoanal reservoir connects to the anus after a surgeon removes the colon and rectum. Stool collects in the ileoanal reservoir and then exits the body through the anus during a bowel movement. An ileoanal reservoir is an option after removal of the entire large intestine when the anus remains intact and disease-free. The surgeon often makes a temporary ileostomy before or at the time of making an ileoanal reservoir. Once the ileoanal reservoir heals from surgery, the surgeon reconnects the ileum to the ileoanal pouch and closes the temporary ileostomy. A person does not need a permanent external ostomy pouch for an ileoanal reservoir.

A surgeon creates an ileoanal reservoir most often to treat ulcerative colitis or familial adenomatous polyposis. Familial adenomatous polyposis is an inherited disease characterized by the presence of 100 or more polyps in the colon. The polyps may lead to

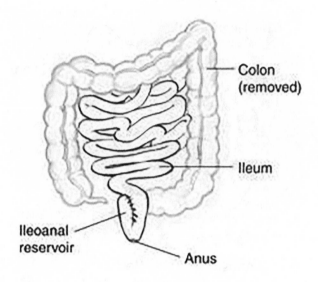

Figure 34.4. Ileoanal Reservoir

colorectal cancer if not treated. People with Crohn disease usually are not candidates for this procedure.

WHAT ARE THE COMPLICATIONS OF OSTOMY SURGERY OF THE BOWEL?

Complications of ostomy surgery of the bowel may include:
- Skin irritation
- Stoma problems
- Blockage
- Diarrhea
- Bleeding
- Electrolyte imbalance
- Infection
- Irritation of the internal pouch, or pouchitis
- Vitamin B_{12} deficiency
- Phantom rectum
- Short bowel syndrome
- Rectal discharge

Skin Irritation

Skin irritation is the most common complication for people with an ostomy. If the external ostomy pouch does not fit properly, stool or stool contents can leak out around the stoma and under the pouch. When irritated, a person's skin will become itchy, red, and uncomfortable. When changing the pouch, a person can use an ostomy powder on the skin around the stoma to treat skin irritation. If the skin irritation does not improve, the person should talk with a WOC nurse or an enterostomal therapist—who are specially trained in ostomy care and rehabilitation—or another healthcare provider about the symptoms. Skin irritation may occur around the stoma for people who have an ileostomy or a colostomy. People who have ileoanal reservoir surgery may have skin irritation around the anus. Sometimes, using a barrier ointment to protect the skin around the anus can help treat and prevent irritation.

Stoma Problems

Stoma problems include the following:

- **Hernia.** A stoma hernia, seen as a bulge in the skin around the stoma, is a weakening of the abdominal wall around the stoma site. As with all hernias, a stoma hernia continues to increase in size and may eventually need surgical repair when it becomes too large. Rarely, the intestine gets trapped or kinked within the hernia and becomes blocked. A blocked intestine that loses its blood supply requires emergency surgery.
- **Prolapse.** A stoma prolapse occurs when the bowel pushes itself through the stoma. A person may be able to push the bowel back through the stoma and keep it in place with a stoma shield. If not, the stoma prolapse may require special care and a larger ostomy pouch. A stoma prolapse that becomes blocked or loses its blood supply requires surgical repair.
- **Narrowing of the stoma.** Narrowing of the stoma makes it difficult for stool to pass through the stoma. A narrowed stoma may need surgical repair.

Blockage

Occasionally, an ileostomy or a colostomy does not function for a short time. If the stoma has not passed intestinal content or stool for four to six hours and the person is experiencing cramping or nausea, the ileum or colon may be blocked. Blockage may occur when foods that are hard to digest get stuck in the ileum or colon.

Abdominal adhesions in the ileum or colon may cause blockage as well. Abdominal adhesions are bands of fibrous tissue that form between abdominal tissues and organs, causing them to kink or narrow. Most blockages get better without additional surgery by not eating food and drinking only clear liquids to rest the bowel for a short time.

Diarrhea

Diarrhea is loose, watery stools. A person has diarrhea if she or he passes loose stools three or more times a day. Diarrhea occurs when intestinal contents pass through the small intestine too quickly for fluid and mineral absorption. When fluids and minerals, such as sodium and potassium are not absorbed, they leave the body. Diarrhea can lead to dehydration, malnutrition, and weight loss. Diarrhea is common, even normal, with an ileostomy or ileoanal reservoir. In most cases of diarrhea, the only treatment necessary is replacing lost fluids and electrolytes to prevent dehydration. Electrolytes are minerals in body fluids that are part of salts, including sodium, potassium, magnesium, and chloride. People should maintain good daily hydration by drinking plenty of water and liquids such as fruit juices, sports drinks, caffeine-free soft drinks, and broths. In some cases of diarrhea, a healthcare provider may recommend changes in diet and may prescribe medications to treat diarrhea.

Bleeding

As with any major surgery, ostomy surgery may cause internal bleeding. If too much blood is lost, the person may require a blood transfusion. Bleeding may also occur through the stoma or through the anus after surgery.

Electrolyte Imbalance

The main function of the large intestine is to absorb water, nutrients, and electrolytes from partially digested food that enters from the ileum. When a surgeon removes the large intestine, absorption of electrolytes does not occur to the same extent, making electrolyte imbalance more likely. Diarrhea, excessive sweating, and vomiting can increase the chance of developing electrolyte imbalance. Symptoms of electrolyte imbalance may include:

- Fatigue, or feeling tired
- Weakness
- Nausea
- Muscle problems such as spasms, weakness, uncontrolled twitching, and cramps
- Dizziness and confusion
- People with these symptoms require medical care and should contact a healthcare provider

People who have had their large intestine removed should talk with a healthcare provider or dietitian about diets that help maintain electrolyte balance.

Infection

The gastrointestinal (GI) tract is filled with bacteria that can leak out during ostomy surgery and infect areas inside the abdomen. Bacteria entering the body through the stoma or anus can also cause an infection. The person's skin around the stoma may also become infected with bacteria or skin fungus. Healthcare providers treat infections with antibiotics. Symptoms of infection may include:

- Fever
- Back pain
- Poor appetite
- Nausea and vomiting

Irritation of the Internal Pouch, or Pouchitis

Pouchitis is an irritation or inflammation of the lining of an ileoanal reservoir or a continent ileostomy pouch. A healthcare provider treats pouchitis with antibiotics. For severe or chronic pouchitis, a healthcare provider may prescribe immunosuppressive medications, such as corticosteroids. Symptoms of pouchitis include:

- Frequent bowel movements with diarrhea
- An urgent need to have a bowel movement
- A feeling of pressure in the pouch
- Abdominal pain
- Cramping or bleeding
- Dehydration
- Low-grade fever
- A general unwell feeling

Vitamin B$_{12}$ Deficiency

Ostomy surgery of the bowel may affect vitamin B$_{12}$ absorption from food and result in a gradual drop in vitamin B$_{12}$ levels in the body. Low levels of vitamin B$_{12}$ can affect the body's ability to use nutrients and may cause anemia. Anemia is a condition in which red blood cells are fewer or smaller than normal, which prevents the body's cells from getting enough oxygen. Healthcare providers treat vitamin B$_{12}$ deficiency with vitamin B$_{12}$ supplements.

Phantom Rectum

Phantom rectum is the feeling of needing to have a bowel movement even though the rectum is not present. Phantom rectum is relatively common. Symptoms are usually mild and often go away without treatment. However, for some people, phantom rectum may occur for years after a surgeon removes the rectum. Some people with phantom rectum may feel pain. Healthcare providers treat rectal pain with medications, such as pain relievers and sometimes antidepressants. To help control phantom rectum, a healthcare provider may recommend complementary therapies, such as guided imagery and other relaxation techniques.

Short Bowel Syndrome

Short bowel syndrome is a group of problems related to inadequate absorption of nutrients after removal of a part of the small intestine.

People with short bowel syndrome cannot absorb enough water, vitamins, and other nutrients from food to sustain life. Diarrhea is the main symptom of short bowel syndrome. Other symptoms may include:
- Cramping
- Bloating
- Heartburn
- Weakness and fatigue
- Vomiting
- Excessive gas
- Foul-smelling stool

Short bowel syndrome is uncommon and can occur with Crohn disease, trauma, or other conditions that lead to removal of a large amount of the small intestine.

A healthcare provider will recommend a treatment for short bowel syndrome based on a person's nutritional needs. Treatment may include nutritional support, medications, and surgery.

Rectal Discharge

People with an ileostomy or a colostomy whose lower colon, rectum, and anus are still present may experience a discharge of mucus from their rectum. Mucus is a clear fluid made by the GI tract that coats and protects the lining of the bowel. Mucus within the bypassed part of the colon may leak out of the rectum from time to time or gradually build up, forming a small, stool-like ball that passes out of the rectum. A person cannot control mucus production and rectal discharge. However, people who have rectal discharge can learn how to manage and cope with this problem.

Section 34.3 | **Colectomy**

WHAT IS A COLECTOMY?

A colectomy is the surgical removal of all or a part of the colon, or large intestine, from the digestive system. The esophagus, stomach, small intestine, and large intestine (colon) are part of the human digestive system. Digestion involves processing vitamins, minerals, carbohydrates, fats, proteins, and water from food and removing waste from the body. When a colectomy is performed, the severed portions of the colon may be reattached to facilitate bowel movement. Otherwise, a surgical procedure known as a "colostomy" becomes necessary. In this procedure, an opening known as a "stoma" is made to the outside body to excrete stool.

WHEN IS A COLECTOMY RECOMMENDED?

A colectomy is recommended for conditions like bowel obstruction, colon cancer, diverticulitis, inflammatory disease, such as Crohn disease and ulcerative colitis, infection, and bleeding.

WHAT IS THE SURGICAL PROCEDURE USED IN A COLECTOMY?

Surgeons use one of two methods to perform a colectomy:

Open surgery. The colon is accessed by making a long vertical incision on the abdomen and the surgeon operates on the infected/damaged part. This is termed an "open colectomy."

Laparoscopic surgery. The surgeon makes a few small incisions using specialized surgical tools. A video camera is then inserted into one of the incisions so that the surgeon can operate by looking at a screen. This is termed a "laparoscopic-assisted colectomy" and is the procedure of choice for certain types of cancerous conditions. There is less pain and blood loss, and recovery is usually faster than after open surgery.

WHAT ARE THE CATEGORIES OF COLECTOMY?

Depending on whether all or part of the colon is removed, a colectomy is categorized into the following types:

- **Total colectomy.** The entire colon is surgically removed.
- **Segmental resection.** Removal is confined to only the affected part of the colon.
- **Partial colectomy.** Part of the colon is removed. This is also known as a "subtotal colectomy."
- **Sigmoidectomy.** The lower section of the colon is removed in this procedure.
- **Hemicolectomy.** Only the right or left quadrants of the colon is removed.
- **Total proctocolectomy.** The entire colon and the rectum are removed and the small intestine is attached to the anus for excretion of stool.
- **Abdominal perineal resection.** This involves the removal of the sigmoid colon, rectum, and anus and replaced with a permanent colostomy.
- **Low anterior resection.** The top section of the rectum is removed.

HOW DO YOU PREPARE BEFORE SURGERY?

A few days before surgery you need to take care of a few things as listed below:

- Follow the diet advised by the surgeon.
- Stay hydrated with at least eight glasses of water daily.
- Cleanse your colon by following the instructions given by your surgeon. This could include laxatives, enemas, and special liquid preparations and diets.
- Take medicines as prescribed by your surgeon.
- Shower with an antibacterial soap the night before the procedure.
- Make arrangements for help at home and have someone drive you to the hospital.
- Wear comfortable clothing.

- Stop taking regular medication as instructed by your surgeon.

WHAT HAPPENS IN A COLECTOMY

During a laparoscopic colectomy, the surgeon makes an incision that is less than half an inch in the abdomen and inserts a tube-like instrument known as a "cannula" or "port" into the abdomen. Carbon dioxide (CO_2) gas is pumped into the abdomen through the cannula to create enough space to carry out the procedure. A laparoscope is then inserted through the cannula. The laparoscope is a device with a camera and light source on it. It illuminates the surgical site and relays images of it to a high definition monitor for the surgeon to view. Up to four ports are used to insert specialized surgical instruments for the surgeon to perform the surgery. One of the incisions is made slightly bigger and the portion of the colon targeted for removal is pulled out of the abdomen. Depending on the type of surgery, the ends of the intestines are then joined together and inserted back into the abdomen.

An open surgery happens more or less the same way, except that the surgeon uses handheld instruments through a large incision made in the abdomen.

If most of the colon is removed, reattachment may not be possible and an ileostomy or a colostomy may be required. A stoma, or opening, is made in the abdominal wall and the open end of the intestine is attached to it. This allows waste to exit from the stoma. The patient will need to wear an ostomy bag which collects the waste material. Depending on the patient, the stoma could be temporary or permanent. People are able to lead a healthy and active life even with a permanent stoma.

WHAT ARE THE COMPLICATIONS AND SIDE EFFECTS ASSOCIATED WITH A COLECTOMY?

A colectomy is a generally safe procedure. But as with any operation, there are risks. If you are concerned, discuss them with your healthcare provider. Some of the risks include:

- Bleeding

- Difficulty breathing
- Heart attack
- Injury to nearby organs during surgery
- Blood clots in the legs and lungs
- Obstruction caused by scar tissue after surgery
- Infection
- Tearing of sutures
- Anastomotic leaks in the colon because of failure of sutures
- Hematoma (accumulation of blood in the wound)

WHAT HAPPENS AFTER THE PROCEDURE

You may need to spend up to a week in the hospital after surgery to recover. You will be administered pain medication and put on a limited liquid diet. After a few days, solid food may be advised. Your surgeon, as well as other doctors (such as your oncologist or general practitioner), will schedule a series of follow-up appointments. Make sure you attend all of them. You will also be given instructions on specific things to watch out for in order to spot complications that may arise when you are at home. Make sure you remain alert to them. You will also be given information on how to take care of the stoma.

HOW SHOULD YOU TAKE CARE OF YOURSELF AT HOME AFTER SURGERY

Keep the following things in mind for a normal recovery and to identify complications at home:

- Watch for problems such as swelling, redness, bleeding, or discharge at the site of surgery. Intimate your healthcare provider immediately if you find something.
- If you experience pain, chills, or fever, contact your healthcare provider immediately.
- Do not lift heavy weights and do not engage in demanding activities at home for up to six weeks.
- Seek help at home for your daily activities until you can take care of yourself again.

- Follow a diet as per instructions from your healthcare provider.
- Do not expose the surgical site to water.
- Drink plenty of water to stay hydrated.
- Do not drive while on narcotic medication for pain.
- Follow instructions on showering, sexual activity, and taking care of your stoma.
- Use a thermometer to check for fever.
- Wear loose fitting clothes.
- Remain on medication as directed for pain, infection, and constipation. Call your healthcare provider if in doubt.
- Engage in deep breathing and relaxation techniques if you find yourself getting anxious.

WHAT IS THE OUTCOME OF A COLECTOMY?

The outcome of a colectomy depends on why exactly you needed the procedure. For cancerous conditions, if the diseased section has been removed entirely, the possibility of a good outcome is greater. For precancerous conditions, such as polyps and ulcerative colitis, the outcome is similar. Most people go on to lead a healthy and productive life postsurgery.

References

1. "Frequently Asked Questions about Colectomy (Colon Resection)," The University of Chicago Medical Center, n.d.
2. Tresca, Amber J. "Types of Colectomy Surgery," VeryWell, January 4, 2017.
3. "Surgical Procedures: Colectomy," Trustees of the University of Pennsylvania, September 19, 2016.
4. "Colectomy," EBSCO Publishing, n.d.
5. "Colectomy," The Regents of the University of California, n.d.
6. "Colectomy," The Johns Hopkins University, The Johns Hopkins Hospital, and Johns Hopkins Health System, n.d.

7. Mayo Clinic Staff, "Colectomy," Mayo Foundation for Medical Education and Research (MFMER), November 17, 2015.

Section 34.4 | Gastric, Colon, and Rectal Cancer Surgery

This section contains text excerpted from the following sources: Text beginning with the heading "About Colon Cancer" is excerpted from "Colon Cancer Treatment (PDQ®)—Patient Version," National Cancer Institute (NCI), January 31, 2020; Text beginning with the heading "About Rectal Cancer" is excerpted from "Rectal Cancer Treatment (PDQ®)—Patient Version," National Cancer Institute (NCI), January 31, 2020. Text beginning with the heading "About Gastric Cancer" is excerpted from "Gastric Cancer Treatment (PDQ®)—Patient Version," National Cancer Institute (NCI), April 10, 2020.

ABOUT COLON CANCER

Colon cancer is a disease in which cancer cells form in the tissues of the colon. The colon is part of the body's digestive system. The digestive system removes and processes nutrients (vitamins, minerals, carbohydrates, fats, proteins, and water) from foods and helps pass waste material out of the body. The digestive system is made up of the esophagus, stomach, and the small and large intestines. The colon (large bowel) is the first part of the large intestine and is about five feet long. Together, the rectum and anal canal make up the last part of the large intestine and are about six to eight inches long. The anal canal ends at the anus (the opening of the large intestine to the outside of the body).

COLON CANCER SURGERY

Surgery is the most common treatment for all stages of colon cancer. A doctor may remove the cancer using one of the following types of surgery:

- **Local excision.** If the cancer is found at a very early stage, the doctor may remove it without cutting through the abdominal wall. Instead, the doctor may put a tube with a cutting tool through the rectum into the colon and cut the cancer out. This is called a "local excision." If the cancer is found in a polyp (a

463

small bulging area of tissue), the operation is called a "polypectomy."

- **Resection of the colon with anastomosis.** If the cancer is larger, the doctor will perform a partial colectomy (removing the cancer and a small amount of healthy tissue around it). The doctor may then perform an anastomosis (sewing the healthy parts of the colon together). The doctor will also usually remove lymph near the colon and examine them under a microscope to see whether they contain cancer.
- **Resection of the colon with colostomy.** If the doctor is not able to sew the two ends of the colon back together, a stoma (an opening) is made on the outside of the body for waste to pass through. This procedure is called a "colostomy." A bag is placed around the stoma to collect the waste. Sometimes the colostomy is needed only until the lower colon has healed, and then it can be reversed. If the doctor needs to remove the entire lower colon, however, the colostomy may be permanent.

After the doctor removes all the cancer that can be seen at the time of the surgery, some patients may be given chemotherapy or radiation therapy after surgery to kill any cancer cells that are left. Treatment given after the surgery, to lower the risk that the cancer will come back, is known as "adjuvant therapy."

CRYOSURGERY

Cryosurgery is a treatment that uses an instrument to freeze and destroy abnormal tissue. This type of treatment is also called "cryotherapy."

ABOUT RECTAL CANCER

Rectal cancer is a disease in which malignant cells form in the tissues of the rectum. The rectum is part of the body's digestive system. The digestive system takes in nutrients (vitamins, minerals, carbohydrates, fats, proteins, and water) from foods and helps pass waste material out of the body. The digestive system is made up of the esophagus, stomach, and the small and large intestines. The colon is the first part of the large intestine and is about five feet long. Together, the rectum and anal canal make up the last part of the large intestine and are six to eight inches long. The anal canal ends at the anus (the opening of the large intestine to the outside of the body).

RECTAL CANCER SURGERY

Surgery is the most common treatment for all stages of rectal cancer. The cancer is removed using one of the following types of surgery:

- **Polypectomy.** If the cancer is found in a polyp (a small piece of bulging tissue), the polyp is often removed during a colonoscopy.
- **Local excision.** If the cancer is found on the inside surface of the rectum and has not spread into the wall of the rectum, the cancer and a small amount of surrounding healthy tissue is removed.
- **Resection.** If the cancer has spread into the wall of the rectum, the section of the rectum with cancer and nearby healthy tissue is removed. Sometimes the tissue between the rectum and the abdominal wall is also removed. The lymph nodes near the rectum are removed and checked under a microscope for signs of cancer.
- **Radiofrequency ablation.** The use of a special probe with tiny electrodes that kill cancer cells. Sometimes the probe is inserted directly through the skin and only local anesthesia is needed. In other cases, the probe is inserted through an incision in the abdomen. This is done in the hospital with general anesthesia.
- **Cryosurgery.** A treatment that uses an instrument to freeze and destroy abnormal tissue. This type of treatment is also called "cryotherapy."

- **Pelvic exenteration.** If the cancer has spread to other organs near the rectum, the lower colon, rectum, and bladder are removed. In women, the cervix, vagina, ovaries, and nearby lymph nodes may be removed. In men, the prostate may be removed. Artificial openings (stoma) are made for urine and stool to flow from the body to a collection bag.

After the cancer is removed, the surgeon will either: do an anastomosis (sew the healthy parts of the rectum together, sew the remaining rectum to the colon, or sew the colon to the anus); make a stoma (an opening) from the rectum to the outside of the body for waste to pass through. This procedure is done if the cancer is too close to the anus and is called a "colostomy." A bag is placed around the stoma to collect the waste. Sometimes the colostomy is needed only until the rectum has healed, and then it can be reversed. If the entire rectum is removed, however, the colostomy may be permanent.

ABOUT GASTRIC CANCER

Gastric cancer is a disease in which cancer cells form in the lining of the stomach. The stomach is a J-shaped organ in the upper abdomen. It is part of the digestive system, which processes nutrients (vitamins, minerals, carbohydrates, fats, proteins, and water) in foods that are eaten and helps pass waste material out of the body. Food moves from the throat to the stomach through a hollow, muscular tube called the "esophagus." After leaving the stomach, partly-digested food passes into the small intestine and then into the large intestine.

The wall of the stomach is made up of five layers of tissue. From the innermost layer to the outermost layer, the layers of the stomach wall are: mucosa, submucosa, muscle, subserosa (connective tissue), and serosa. Gastric cancer begins in the mucosa and spreads through the outer layers as it grows.

Stromal tumors of the stomach begin in supporting connective tissue and are treated differently from gastric cancer.

GASTRIC CANCER SURGERY

Surgery is a common treatment for all stages of gastric cancer. The following types of surgery may be used:

- **Subtotal gastrectomy.** Removal of the part of the stomach that contains cancer, nearby lymph nodes, and parts of other tissues and organs near the tumor. The spleen may be removed. The spleen is an organ that makes lymphocytes, stores red blood cells and lymphocytes, filters the blood, and destroys old blood cells. The spleen is on the left side of the abdomen near the stomach.

- **Total gastrectomy.** Removal of the entire stomach, nearby lymph nodes, and parts of the esophagus, small intestine, and other tissues near the tumor. The spleen may be removed. The esophagus is connected to the small intestine so the patient can continue to eat and swallow.

If the tumor is blocking the stomach, but the cancer cannot be completely removed by standard surgery, the following procedures may be used:

- **Endoluminal stent placement.** A procedure to insert a stent in order to keep a passage (such as arteries or the esophagus) open. For tumors blocking the passage into or out of the stomach, surgery may be done to place a stent from the esophagus to the stomach or from the stomach to the small intestine to allow the patient to eat normally.

- **Endoluminal laser therapy.** A procedure in which an endoscope with a laser attached is inserted into the body. A laser is an intense beam of light that can be used as a knife.

- **Gastrojejunostomy.** Surgery to remove the part of the stomach with cancer that is blocking the opening into the small intestine. The stomach is connected to the jejunum (a part of the small intestine) to allow food and medicine to pass from the stomach into the small intestine.

ENDOSCOPIC MUCOSAL RESECTION

Endoscopic mucosal resection is a procedure that uses an endoscope to remove early-stage cancer and precancerous growths from the lining of the digestive tract without surgery. An endoscope is a thin, tubelike instrument with a light and a lens for viewing. It may also include tools to remove growths from the lining of the digestive tract.

Section 34.5 | Gallbladder Removal Surgery (Cholecystectomy)

This section includes text excerpted from "Treatment for Gallstones," National Institute of Diabetes and Digestive and Kidney Diseases (NIDDK), November, 2017.

HOW DO HEALTHCARE PROFESSIONALS TREAT GALLSTONES?

If your gallstones are not causing symptoms, you probably do not need treatment. However, if you are having a gallbladder attack or other symptoms, contact your doctor. Although your symptoms may go away, they may appear again and you may need treatment. Your doctor may refer to you a gastroenterologist or surgeon for treatment.

The usual treatment for gallstones is surgery to remove the gallbladder. Doctors sometimes can use nonsurgical treatments to treat cholesterol stones, but pigment stones usually require surgery.

Surgery

Surgery to remove the gallbladder, called "cholecystectomy," is one of the most common operations performed on adults in the United States. The gallbladder is not an essential organ, which means you can live normally without a gallbladder.

A healthcare professional will usually give you general anesthesia for surgery. Once the surgeon removes your gallbladder, bile flows out of your liver through the hepatic duct and common bile duct and directly into the duodenum, instead of being stored in the gallbladder.

Surgeons perform two types of cholecystectomy:

- **Laparoscopic cholecystectomy.** Almost all surgeons perform cholecystectomies with laparoscopy. Surgeons perform many laparoscopic cholecystectomies on an outpatient basis, meaning you may be able to go home the same day. You will probably be able to return to normal physical activity in about a week.
- **Open cholecystectomy.** A surgeon performs an open cholecystectomy. when your gallbladder is severely inflamed, infected, or scarred from other operations. Your doctor may perform a cholecystectomy if problems occur during a laparoscopic cholecystectomy. After the surgery, you may need to stay in the hospital for up to a week. You will probably be able to return to normal physical activity after about a month.

WHAT HAPPENS AFTER GALLBLADDER REMOVAL

A small number of people have softer and more frequent stools after gallbladder removal, because bile now flows into your duodenum more often. Changes in bowel habits are usually temporary; however, discuss them with your doctor.

All surgeries come with a possible risk of complications; however, gallbladder surgery complications are very rare. The most common complication is injury to the bile ducts, which can cause infection. You may need one or more additional operations to repair the bile ducts.

Nonsurgical Treatments

Doctors use nonsurgical treatments for gallstones only in special situations, like if you have cholesterol stones and you have a serious medical condition that prevents surgery. Even with treatment, gallstones can return. Therefore, you may have to be regularly treated for gallstones for a very long time, or even for the rest of your life.

A doctor may use the following types of nonsurgical treatments to remove or break up cholesterol gallstones:

- **Endoscopic retrograde cholangiopancreatography (ERCP).** Sometimes doctors use ERCP to remove a gallstone that is stuck in the common bile duct.
- **Oral dissolution therapy.** Ursodiol (Actigall) and chenodiol (Chenix) are medicines that contain bile acids that can break up gallstones. These medicines work best to break up small cholesterol stones. You may need months or years of treatment to break up all stones.
- **Shock wave lithotripsy.** A doctor can use shock wave lithotripsy to blast gallstones into small pieces. Doctors use this procedure only rarely, and sometimes along with ursodiol.

Section 34.6 | Hemorrhoid Surgery

This section includes text excerpted from "Hemorrhoids," National Diabetes Education Program (NDEP), National Institute of Diabetes and Digestive and Kidney Diseases (NIDDK), October 2016, Reviewed April 2020.

WHAT ARE HEMORRHOIDS?

Hemorrhoids, also called "piles," are swollen and inflamed veins around your anus or in your lower rectum.

The two types of hemorrhoids are:

- External hemorrhoids, which form under the skin around the anus
- Internal hemorrhoids, which form in the lining of the anus and lower rectum

HOW COMMON ARE HEMORRHOIDS?

Hemorrhoids are common in both men and women and affect about 1 in 20 Americans. About half of adults older than 50 years of age have hemorrhoids.

WHO IS MORE LIKELY TO GET HEMORRHOIDS?

You are more likely to get hemorrhoids if you:
- Strain during bowel movements
- Sit on the toilet for long periods of time
- Have chronic constipation or diarrhea
- Eat foods that are low in fiber
- Are older than 50 years of age
- Are pregnant
- Often lift heavy objects

WHAT ARE THE COMPLICATIONS OF HEMORRHOIDS?

Complications of hemorrhoids can include the following:
- Blood clots in an external hemorrhoid
- Skin tags—extra skin left behind when a blood clot in an external hemorrhoid dissolves
- Infection of a sore on an external hemorrhoid
- Strangulated hemorrhoid—when the muscles around your anus cut off the blood supply to an internal hemorrhoid that has fallen through your anal opening
- Anemia

WHAT ARE THE SYMPTOMS OF HEMORRHOIDS?

The symptoms of hemorrhoids depend on the type you have.
  If you have external hemorrhoids, you may have:
- Anal itching
- One or more hard, tender lumps near your anus
- Anal ache or pain, especially when sitting

Too much straining, rubbing, or cleaning around your anus may make your symptoms worse. For many people, the symptoms of external hemorrhoids go away within a few days.
  If you have internal hemorrhoids, you may have:
- Bleeding from your rectum—bright red blood on stool, on toilet paper, or in the toilet bowl after a bowel movement
- A hemorrhoid that has fallen through your anal opening, called "prolapse"

Internal hemorrhoids that are not prolapsed most often are not painful. Prolapsed internal hemorrhoids may cause pain and discomfort.

Although hemorrhoids are the most common cause of anal symptoms, not every anal symptom is caused by a hemorrhoid. Some hemorrhoid symptoms are similar to those of other digestive tract problems. For example, bleeding from your rectum may be a sign of bowel diseases, such as Crohn disease, ulcerative colitis, or cancer of the colon or rectum.

HOW DO DOCTORS TREAT HEMORRHOIDS?
The outpatient center or hospital treatments include the following:
- **Hemorrhoidectomy.** A doctor, most often a surgeon, may perform a hemorrhoidectomy to remove large external hemorrhoids and prolapsing internal hemorrhoids that do not respond to other treatments. Your doctor will give you anesthesia for this treatment.
- **Hemorrhoid stapling.** A doctor, most often a surgeon, may use a special stapling tool to remove internal hemorrhoid tissue and pull a prolapsing internal hemorrhoid back into the anus. Your doctor will give you anesthesia for this treatment.

Sometimes complications of hemorrhoids also require treatment.

Section 34.7 | Hernia Surgery

This section includes text excerpted from "Hernia Surgical Mesh Implants," U.S. Food and Drug Administration (FDA), February 4, 2018.

WHAT IS A HERNIA?
A hernia occurs when an organ, intestine, or fatty tissue squeezes through a hole or a weak spot in the surrounding muscle or connective tissue. Hernias often occur at the abdominal wall. Sometimes a

hernia can be visible as an external bulge particularly when straining or bearing down.

TREATMENT FOR HERNIAS
Surgical

- **Laparoscopic**—The surgeon makes several small incisions in the abdomen that allow surgical tools into the openings to repair the hernia. Laparoscopic surgery can be performed with or without surgical mesh.
- **Open repair**—The surgeon makes an incision near the hernia and the weak muscle area is repaired. Open repair can be done with or without surgical mesh.
- **Open repair** that uses sutures without mesh is referred to as "primary closure." Primary closure is used to repair inguinal hernias in infants, small hernias, strangulated or infected hernias.

Hernias have a high rate of recurrence, and surgeons often use surgical mesh to strengthen the hernia repair and reduce the rate of recurrence. Since the 1980s, there has been an increase in mesh-based hernia repairs—by 2000, non-mesh repairs represented less than 10 percent of groin hernia repair techniques.

The use of surgical mesh may also improve patient outcomes through decreased operative time and minimized recovery time. However, recovery time depends on the type of hernia, the surgical approach, and the patient's condition both before and after surgery.

Information found in medical literature has consistently demonstrated a reduced hernia recurrence rate when surgical mesh is used to repair the hernia compared to hernia repair without surgical mesh. For example, inguinal hernia recurrence is higher with open repair using sutures (primary closure) than with mesh repair.

Despite reduced rates of recurrence, there are situations where the use of surgical mesh for hernia repair may not be recommended. Patients should talk to their surgeons about their specific circumstances and their best options and alternatives for hernia repair.

HERNIA REPAIR SURGERY COMPLICATIONS

Based on the U.S. Food and Drug Administration's (FDA) analysis of medical device adverse event reports and of peer-reviewed, scientific literature, the most common adverse events for all surgical repair of hernias—with or without mesh—are pain, infection, hernia recurrence, scar-like tissue that sticks tissues together (adhesion), blockage of the large or small intestine (obstruction), bleeding, abnormal connection between organs, vessels, or intestines (fistula), fluid buildup at the surgical site (seroma), and a hole in neighboring tissues or organs (perforation).

The most common adverse events following hernia repair with mesh are pain, infection, hernia recurrence, adhesion, and bowel obstruction. Some other potential adverse events that can occur following hernia repair with mesh are mesh migration and mesh shrinkage (contraction).

Many complications related to hernia repair with surgical mesh that have been reported to the FDA have been associated with recalled mesh products that are no longer on the market. Pain, infection, recurrence, adhesion, obstruction, and perforation are the most common complications associated with recalled mesh. In the FDA's analysis of medical adverse event reports to the FDA, recalled mesh products were the main cause of bowel perforation and obstruction complications.

If you are unsure about the specific mesh manufacturer and brand used in your surgery and have questions about your hernia repair, contact your surgeon or the facility where your surgery was performed to obtain the information from your medical record.

Section 34.8 | Inguinal Hernia

This section includes text excerpted from "Inguinal Hernia," National Diabetes Education Program (NDEP), National Institute of Diabetes and Digestive and Kidney Diseases (NIDDK), September 2019.

WHAT IS AN INGUINAL HERNIA?

An inguinal hernia is a bulging of the contents of the abdomen through a weak area in the lower abdominal wall. Inguinal hernias can occur at either of two passages through the lower abdominal wall, one on each side of the groin. These passages are called "inguinal canals." Inguinal hernias can also occur through two deeper passages in the groin known as the "femoral canals." Hernias through these passages are also known as "femoral hernias."

Inguinal hernias most often contain fat or part of the small intestine. In girls or women, inguinal hernias may contain part of the female reproductive system, such as an ovary. When an inguinal hernia occurs, part of the peritoneum—the lining of the abdominal cavity—bulges through the abdominal wall and forms a sac around the hernia.

Inguinal hernias may slide in and out of the abdominal wall. A doctor can often move an inguinal hernia back inside the abdominal wall with a gentle massage.

Inguinal hernias typically develop on one side of the groin and form on the right side more often than on the left. Some people who have an inguinal hernia on one side will have or will develop a hernia on the other side.

HOW DO DOCTORS TREAT INGUINAL HERNIAS?

Most people with inguinal hernias will need surgery to repair the hernia. Several different types of open and laparoscopic hernia surgeries are available. The type of surgery your doctor recommends may depend on factors, such as the size of the hernia and your age, health, and medical history.

Open Hernia Surgery

In open hernia surgery, a surgeon makes a cut in your groin to view and repair the hernia. After repairing the hernia, surgeons typically use stitches and a piece of mesh to close the abdominal wall. The mesh strengthens the weak area where the hernia occurred. In some cases, surgeons may use stitches alone to close and strengthen the weak area in the abdominal wall.

Patients most often receive local anesthesia and a sedative for open hernia surgery. In some cases, doctors may give patients general anesthesia or a spinal block to make the body numb from the waist down.

Laparoscopic Hernia Surgery

In laparoscopic hernia surgery, a surgeon makes several small cuts in your lower abdomen and inserts special tools to view and repair the hernia. The surgeon uses a piece of mesh to close and strengthen the abdominal wall.

Patients most often receive general anesthesia for laparoscopic hernia surgery. Recovery time after laparoscopic surgery may be shorter than after open hernia surgery.

Watchful Waiting

Research suggests that men with inguinal hernias that cause few or no symptoms may be able to safely delay surgery, an approach called "watchful waiting." Men who delay surgery should watch for symptoms and see a doctor regularly. About 70 percent of men who delay surgery will develop new or worsening symptoms and will need surgery within 5 years.

HOW DO DOCTORS TREAT THE COMPLICATIONS OF INGUINAL HERNIAS?

If an inguinal hernia causes complications, such as becoming stuck or strangulated, you will need emergency surgery to repair the hernia and treat the complications.

WHAT CAN YOU EXPECT AFTER SURGERY TO TREAT AN INGUINAL HERNIA?

You may have some pain or discomfort after hernia surgery. The pain is typically mild and goes away within two weeks after surgery.

Your doctor will recommend medicines to relieve pain. Talk with your doctor about when you can safely return to your usual activities after hernia surgery. Many people can go back to work and resume daily activities within three to five days after hernia surgery.

WHAT ARE THE RISKS OF HERNIA SURGERY?

Surgery to repair an inguinal hernia is quite safe. However, possible complications of hernia surgery include:

- Urinary retention
- Infection
- Swelling in the area you had surgery due to a buildup of blood, called a "hematoma," or a buildup of blood plasma, called a "seroma."
- Chronic or severe pain
- Return of the hernia, which may require another surgery

Serious complications, such as damage to blood vessels or organs, are rare.

Talk with your doctor about the risks of hernia surgery and symptoms you should watch for after surgery. For example, you should call your doctor right away if you have:

- Bleeding, drainage, or redness in the area where you had surgery
- Fever or chills
- Nausea or vomiting
- Pain or swelling in your abdomen
- Pain or swelling in your groin that gets worse
- Pain that is severe or does not get better when you take pain medicines
- Problems breathing
- Problems urinating

Chapter 35 | **Weight-Loss (Bariatric) Surgery**

Chapter Contents

Section 35.1 | **What Is Bariatric Surgery?**

This section contains text excerpted from the following sources: Text beginning with the heading "About Bariatric Surgery" is excerpted from "Definition and Facts for Bariatric Surgery," National Digestive Diseases Information Clearinghouse (NDDIC), National Institute of Diabetes and Digestive and Kidney Diseases (NIDDK), July 2016, Reviewed April 2020; Text beginning with the heading "Who Is a Good Adult Candidate for Bariatric Surgery?" is excerpted from "Potential Candidates for Bariatric Surgery," National Digestive Diseases Information Clearinghouse (NDDIC), National Institute of Diabetes and Digestive and Kidney Diseases (NIDDK), July 2016. Reviewed April 2020.

ABOUT BARIATRIC SURGERY

Bariatric surgery is an operation that helps you lose weight by making changes to your digestive system. Some types of bariatric surgeries make your stomach smaller, allowing you to eat and drink less at one time and making you feel full sooner. Other bariatric surgeries also change your small intestine—the part of your body that absorbs calories and nutrients from foods and beverages.

Bariatric surgery may be an option if you have severe obesity and have not been able to lose weight or keep from gaining back any weight you lost using other methods, such as lifestyle treatment or medications. Bariatric surgery also may be an option if you have serious health problems, such as type 2 diabetes or sleep apnea, related to obesity. Bariatric surgery can improve many of the medical conditions linked to obesity, especially type 2 diabetes.

DOES BARIATRIC SURGERY ALWAYS WORK?

Studies show that many people who have bariatric surgery lose about 15 to 30 percent of their starting weight on average, depending on the type of surgery they have. However, no method, including surgery, is sure to produce and maintain weight loss. Some people who have bariatric surgery may not lose as much as they hoped. Over time, some people regain a portion of the weight they lost. The amount of weight people regain may vary. Factors that affect weight regain may include a person's level of obesity and the type of surgery she or he had.

Bariatric surgery does not replace healthy habits, but may make it easier for you to consume fewer calories and be more physically active. Choosing healthy foods and beverages before and after the surgery may help you lose more weight and keep it off long term. Regular physical activity after surgery also helps keep the weight off. To improve your health, you must commit to a lifetime of healthy lifestyle habits and following the advice of your health-care providers.

HOW MUCH DOES BARIATRIC SURGERY COST?

On average, bariatric surgery costs between $15,000 and $25,000, depending on what type of surgery you have and whether you have surgery-related problems. Costs may be higher or lower based on where you live. The amount your medical insurance will pay varies by state and insurance provider.

Medicare and some Medicaid programs cover three common types of bariatric surgery—gastric bypass, gastric band, and gastric sleeve surgery—if you meet certain criteria and have a doctor's recommendation. Some insurance plans may require you to use approved surgeons and facilities. Some insurers also require you to show that you were unable to lose weight by completing a non-surgical weight-loss program or that you meet other requirements.

Your health insurance company or your regional Medicare or Medicaid office will have more information about bariatric surgery coverage, options, and requirements.

WHO IS A GOOD ADULT CANDIDATE FOR BARIATRIC SURGERY?

Bariatric surgery may be an option for adults who have:
- A body mass index (BMI) of 40 or more;
- A BMI of 35 or more with a serious health problem linked to obesity such as type 2 diabetes, heart disease, or sleep apnea; or
- A BMI of 30 or more with a serious health problem linked to obesity, for the gastric band only.

Having surgery to lose weight is a serious decision. If you are thinking about having bariatric surgery, you should know what is involved. Your answers to the following questions may help you decide if surgery is an option for you:

- Have you been unable to lose weight or keep it off using nonsurgical methods, such as lifestyle changes or drug treatment?
- Do you understand what the operation involves and its risks and benefits?
- Do you understand how your eating and physical activity patterns will need to change after you have surgery?
- Can you commit to following lifelong healthy eating and physical activity habits, medical follow-up, and the need to take extra vitamins and minerals?

WHO IS A GOOD TEEN CANDIDATE FOR BARIATRIC SURGERY?

Doctors sometimes use bariatric surgery to treat teens with severe obesity who also have obesity-related health problems. Bariatric surgery often improves health problems that could grow worse in adulthood if the teen remains obese.

Surgery may be an option for teens who have gone through puberty and reached their adult height, and have:

- A BMI of 35 or more with serious obesity-related health problems, such as type 2 diabetes or severe sleep apnea, or
- A BMI of 40 or more with less severe health problems, such as high blood pressure or high cholesterol.

Studies suggest that bariatric surgery is fairly safe for teens and can improve health problems, such as type 2 diabetes for at least 3 years after surgery. Teens who took part in a study that followed them for 3 years after surgery lost an average of 90 pounds and kept most of the weight off. They also reported improved quality of life-related to their weight. Researchers continue to study the long-term effects, which are unknown.

Like adults, teens who are thinking about weight-loss surgery should be prepared for the lifestyle changes they will need to make after the surgery. A surgical center that focuses on the unique needs of youth may help the teen patient prepare for and adjust to these changes. Parents and caregivers also should be prepared and ready to support their child.

Section 35.2 | Types of Bariatric Surgery

This section includes text excerpted from "Types of Bariatric Surgery," National Digestive Diseases Information Clearinghouse (NDDIC), National Institute of Diabetes and Digestive and Kidney Diseases (NIDDK), July 2016. Reviewed April 2020.

The type of surgery that may be best to help a person lose weight depends on a number of factors. You should discuss with your doctor what kind of surgery might be best for you or your teen.

WHAT IS THE DIFFERENCE BETWEEN OPEN AND LAPAROSCOPIC SURGERY?

In open bariatric surgery, surgeons make a single, large cut in the abdomen. More often, surgeons now use laparoscopic surgery, in which they make several small cuts and insert thin surgical tools through the cuts. Surgeons also insert a small scope attached to a camera that projects images onto a video monitor. Laparoscopic surgery has fewer risks than open surgery and may cause less pain and scarring than open surgery. Laparoscopic surgery also may lead to a faster recovery.

Open surgery may be a better option for certain people. If you have a high level of obesity, have had stomach surgery before, or have other complex medical problems, you may need open surgery.

WHAT ARE THE SURGICAL OPTIONS?

In the United States, surgeons use three types of operations most often:
- Laparoscopic adjustable gastric band
- Gastric sleeve surgery, also known as "sleeve gastrectomy"
- Gastric bypass

Surgeons use a fourth operation, biliopancreatic diversion with duodenal switch, less often.

Laparoscopic Adjustable Gastric Band

In this type of surgery, the surgeon places a ring with an inner inflatable band around the top of your stomach to create a small pouch. This makes you feel full after eating a small amount of food. The band has a circular balloon inside that is filled with salt solution. The surgeon can adjust the size of the opening from the pouch to the rest of your stomach by injecting or removing the solution through a small device called a "port" placed under your skin.

After surgery, you will need several follow-up visits to adjust the size of the band opening. If the band causes problems or is not helping you lose enough weight, the surgeon may remove it.

The U.S. Food and Drug Administration (FDA) has approved use of the gastric band for people with a BMI of 30 or more who also have at least one health problem linked to obesity, such as heart disease or diabetes.

Gastric Sleeve

In gastric sleeve surgery, also known as "vertical sleeve gastrectomy," a surgeon removes most of your stomach, leaving only a banana-shaped section that is closed with staples. Like gastric band surgery, this surgery reduces the amount of food that can fit in your stomach, making you feel full sooner. Taking out part of your stomach may also affect gut hormones or other factors, such as gut bacteria that may affect appetite and metabolism. This type of surgery cannot be reversed because some of the stomach is permanently removed.

Gastric Bypass

Gastric bypass surgery, also known as "Roux-en-Y gastric bypass," has two parts. First, the surgeon staples your stomach, creating a small pouch in the upper section. The staples make your stomach much smaller, so you eat less and feel full sooner.

Next, the surgeon cuts your small intestine and attaches the lower part of it directly to the small stomach pouch. Food then bypasses most of the stomach and the upper part of your small intestine so your body absorbs fewer calories. The surgeon connects the bypassed section farther down to the lower part of the small intestine. This bypassed section is still attached to the main part of your stomach, so digestive juices can move from your stomach

485

and the first part of your small intestine into the lower part of your small intestine. The bypass also changes gut hormones, gut bacteria, and other factors that may affect appetite and metabolism. Gastric bypass is difficult to reverse, although a surgeon may do it if medically necessary.

Duodenal Switch

This surgery, also called "biliopancreatic diversion" with duodenal switch, is more complex than the others. The duodenal switch involves two separate surgeries. The first is similar to gastric sleeve surgery. The second surgery redirects food to bypass most of your small intestine. The surgeon also reattaches the bypassed section to the last part of the small intestine, allowing digestive juices to mix with food.

This type of surgery allows you to lose more weight than the other three. However, this surgery is also the most likely to cause surgery-related problems and a shortage of vitamins, minerals, and protein in your body. For these reasons, surgeons do not perform this surgery as often.

WHAT SHOULD YOU EXPECT BEFORE SURGERY?

Before surgery, you will meet with several healthcare providers such as a dietitian, a psychiatrist or psychologist, an internist, and a bariatric surgeon.

- The doctor will ask about your medical history, do a thorough physical exam, and order blood tests. If you are a smoker, she or he will likely ask you to stop smoking at least 6 weeks before your surgery.
- The surgeon will tell you more about the surgery, including how to prepare for it and what type of follow-up you will need.
- The dietitian will explain what and how much you will be able to eat and drink after surgery and help you to prepare for how your life will change after surgery.
- The psychiatrist or psychologist may do an assessment to see if bariatric surgery is an option for you.

These healthcare providers also will advise you to become more active and adopt a healthy eating plan before and after surgery. In some cases, losing weight and bringing your blood sugar levels closer to normal before surgery may lower your chances of having surgery-related problems.

Some bariatric surgery programs have groups you can attend before and after surgery that can help answer questions about the surgery and offer support.

WHAT SHOULD YOU EXPECT AFTER SURGERY?

After surgery, you will need to rest and recover. Although the type of follow-up varies by type of surgery, you will need to take supplements that your doctor prescribes to make sure you are getting enough vitamins and minerals.

Walking and moving around the house may help you recover more quickly. Start slowly and follow your doctor's advice about the type of physical activity you can do safely. As you feel more comfortable, add more physical activity.

After surgery, most people move from a liquid diet to a soft diet such as cottage cheese, yogurt, or soup, and then to solid foods over several weeks. Your doctor, nurse, or dietitian will tell you which foods and beverages you may have and which ones you should avoid. You will need to eat small meals and chew your food well.

HOW MUCH WEIGHT CAN YOU EXPECT TO LOSE?

The amount of weight people lose after bariatric surgery depends on the individual and on the type of surgery she or he had. A study following people for 3 years after surgery found that those who had gastric band surgery lost an average of about 45 pounds. People who had gastric bypass lost an average of 90 pounds. Most people regained some weight over time, but weight regain was usually small compared to their initial weight loss.

Researchers know less about the long-term results of gastric sleeve surgery, but the amount of weight loss seems to be similar to or slightly less than gastric bypass.

Your weight loss could be different. Remember, reaching your goal depends not just on the surgery, but also on sticking with healthy lifestyle habits throughout your life.

WEIGHT-LOSS DEVICES

The FDA has approved several new weight-loss devices that do not permanently change your stomach or small intestine. These devices cause less weight loss than bariatric surgery, and some are only temporary. The devices may have risks, so talk with your doctor if you are thinking about any of these options. Researchers have not studied any of them over a long period of time and do not know the long-term risks and benefits.

- The electrical stimulation system uses a device implanted in your abdomen, by way of laparoscopic surgery, that blocks nerve activity between your stomach and brain. The device works on the vagus nerve, which helps signal the brain that the stomach feels full or empty.
- The gastric balloon system consists of one or two balloons placed in your stomach through a tube inserted through your mouth. Your doctor or nurse will give you a sedative before the procedure. Once the balloons are in your stomach, doctors inflate them with salt water so they take up space in your stomach and help you feel fuller. You will need to have the balloons removed after 6 months or a year.
- A new device uses a pump to drain part of the food in your stomach after a meal. The device includes a tube that goes from the inside of your stomach to a port on the outside of your abdomen. The port is a small valve that fits over the opening in your abdomen. About 20 to 30 minutes after eating, you attach tubing from the port to the pump and open the valve. The pump drains your stomach contents through a tube into the toilet, so that your body does not absorb about 30 percent of calories you ate. You can have the device removed at any time.

Section 35.3 | **Benefits and Side Effects of Bariatric Surgery**

This section contains text excerpted from the following sources: Text in this section begins with excerpts from "Understanding the Health Benefits and Risks of Bariatric Surgery," National Digestive Diseases Information Clearinghouse (NDDIC), National Institute of Diabetes and Digestive and Kidney Diseases (NIDDK), March 20, 2015, Reviewed April 2020; Text under the heading "What Are the Benefits of Bariatric Surgery?" is excerpted from "Bariatric Surgery Benefits," National Digestive Diseases Information Clearinghouse (NDDIC), National Institute of Diabetes and Digestive and Kidney Diseases (NIDDK), July 2016. Reviewed April 2020. Text under the heading "What Are the Side Effects of Bariatric Surgery?" is excerpted from "Bariatric Surgery Side Effects," National Digestive Diseases Information Clearinghouse (NDDIC), National Institute of Diabetes and Digestive and Kidney Diseases (NIDDK), July 2016. Reviewed April 2020.

Severe obesity is a chronic condition that, for many people, is difficult to treat with diet or exercise alone, and increases risks for type 2 diabetes, cardiovascular disease, fatty liver disease, and many other devastating health conditions. Bariatric surgical procedures, which restrict stomach size and/or alter the intestinal tract, have been increasingly performed to treat severe obesity when other interventions have not worked. Additionally, bariatric surgery is used in clinical practice for people who have milder levels of obesity along with type 2 diabetes or other serious obesity-related disease. These surgical procedures can have dramatic benefits—such as significant and sustained weight loss, improved control of blood glucose (sugar) levels, or even reversal of type 2 diabetes—especially when accompanied by exercise and a healthy diet. They also carry substantial risks, and researchers have been evaluating the benefits and risks of different procedures.

Despite the increasing popularity of bariatric surgery, crucial questions still remain, such as how best to select candidates for surgery, based on improved definition of specific benefits versus short- and long-term complications and survival rates, and the effects of different procedures on specific comorbidities in people with lesser degrees of obesity. While the surgical modifications of the stomach and intestines reduce food intake and the amount of nutrients—including calories absorbed, emerging evidence is revealing potential additional mechanisms for the effects on weight and metabolism. Researchers would thus like to determine precisely how certain types of bariatric surgical procedures work to help patients lose a considerable amount of weight, maintain weight loss, and improve obesity-related diseases. Finally, there is as yet unexplained heterogeneity in the outcomes of bariatric surgery, ranging from dramatic weight loss and improvement in comorbidities to subsets of patients who fail to lose weight, or who regain weight, and do not have a satisfactory outcome.

Scientists supported by the National Institute of Diabetes and Digestive and Kidney Diseases (NIDDK) and other organizations have been studying the risks and benefits of bariatric surgery, to help individuals with obesity and their doctors make more informed decisions. Additionally, research on the underlying mechanisms for the effects of bariatric surgical procedures could lead to the development of novel, nonsurgical treatments that confer the benefits without the risks of surgery.

BARIATRIC SURGICAL PROCEDURES

The first bariatric surgical procedure used for severe obesity dates back to 50 years and grew out of the results of operations for certain cancers or severe ulcers. Doctors became aware that their patients lost weight following surgeries that removed large portions of the stomach or small intestine. Some physicians began to use such operations to treat patients with severe obesity. Over time, these operations have been modified to improve patient safety and to incorporate technological advances in surgical procedure. There are several general problems involved in assessing the outcomes of bariatric surgery. Firstly, new surgical approaches and technologies evolve continuously, and are continuing to change at the present time. Secondly, the patient populations who receive bariatric surgery also continue to evolve and may be quite different in individual studies. Together, these issues often make direct comparisons of research studies difficult.

There are several different surgical procedures performed that work through restricting food intake, changing the way in which food is absorbed or metabolized, or both. Physicians performing restrictive operations, such as the laparoscopic adjustable gastric banding (LAGB) reduce the opening to the stomach or stomach size. Other procedures, such as the biliopancreatic diversion, with or without duodenal switch, restrict the amount of calories and nutrients the body absorbs. The most commonly performed procedure at this time, which has both a restrictive and malabsorptive component, is the Roux-en-Y Gastric Bypass (RYGB). RYGB connects the upper stomach to the lower part of the small intestine, so that food bypasses a large portion of the gastrointestinal tract in which digestion and nutrient absorption normally take place. Increasingly, surgeons are performing a sleeve gastrectomy (SG) procedure in which a portion of the stomach is removed, leaving a sleeve or tube through which food can pass. Over the past several decades, researchers have sought to understand the benefits and risks of different bariatric surgery procedures.

WHAT ARE THE BENEFITS OF BARIATRIC SURGERY?

Bariatric surgery can help you lose weight and improve many health problems related to obesity. These health problems include:

- Type 2 diabetes
- High blood pressure
- Unhealthy cholesterol levels
- Sleep apnea
- Urinary incontinence
- Body pain
- Knee and hip pain

You may be better able to move around and be physically active after surgery. You might also notice your mood improves and feel like your quality of life is better.

WHAT ARE THE SIDE EFFECTS OF BARIATRIC SURGERY?

Side effects may include:

- Bleeding
- Infection
- Leaking from the site where the sections of the stomach or small intestine, or both, are stapled or sewn together
- Diarrhea

- Blood clots in the legs that can move to the lungs and heart
- Rarely, surgery-related problems can lead to death

Other side effects may occur later. Your body may not absorb nutrients well, especially if you do not take your prescribed vitamins and minerals. Not getting enough nutrients can cause health problems, such as anemia and osteoporosis. Gallstones can occur after rapid weight loss. Some doctors prescribe medicine for about 6 months after surgery to help prevent gallstones. Gastric bands can erode into the stomach wall and need to be removed.

Other problems that could occur later include strictures and hernias. Strictures—narrowing of the new stomach or connection between the stomach and small intestine—make it hard to eat solid food and can cause nausea, vomiting, and trouble swallowing. Doctors treat strictures with special instruments to expand the narrowing. Two kinds of hernias may occur after bariatric surgery—at the incision site or in the abdomen. Doctors repair hernias with surgery.

Some research suggests that bariatric surgery, especially gastric bypass, may change the way your body absorbs and breaks down alcohol, and may lead to more alcohol-related problems after surgery.

Chapter 36 | Gynecologic and Obstetric Surgery

Chapter Contents

Section 36.1 | **Hysterectomy**

This section contains text excerpted from the following sources: Text in this section begins with excerpts from "Hysterectomy," Office on Women's Health (OWH), U.S. Department of Health and Human Services (HHS), December 4, 2014. Reviewed April 2020; Text under the heading "Ways to Perform a Hysterectomy" is excerpted from "Hysterectomy," *Eunice Kennedy Shriver* National Institute of Child Health and Human Development (NICHD), November 2, 2018.

A hysterectomy is a surgery to remove a woman's uterus (also known as the "womb"). The uterus is where a baby grows when a woman is pregnant. During the surgery the whole uterus is usually removed. Your doctor may also remove your fallopian tubes and ovaries. After a hysterectomy, you no longer have menstrual periods and cannot become pregnant.

WHAT ARE THE TYPES OF HYSTERECTOMY PROCEDURES?

Sometimes a hysterectomy may be medically necessary. But sometimes you can try medicines or other treatments first. Talk with your doctor about all of your treatment options. You may need a hysterectomy if you have one of the following:

- **Uterine fibroids.** Uterine fibroids are noncancerous growths in the uterine wall. In some women, they can cause pain and long-term heavy bleeding. Uterine fibroids tend to shrink after menopause, so you may choose to wait. Your doctor may also try other procedures, such as myomectomy or endometrial ablation, before a hysterectomy.
- **Heavy or unusual vaginal bleeding.** Changes in hormone levels, infection, cancer, or fibroids can cause heavy, prolonged bleeding. Hormonal birth control may help to lighten heavy bleeding, correct irregular bleeding, and relieve pain.
- **Uterine prolapse.** This is when the uterus slips from its usual place down into the vagina. This is more common in women who have had several vaginal births, but it can also happen after menopause or because of obesity. You can try Kegel exercises (squeezing the pelvic floor

muscles) to help restore tone to the muscle holding the uterus in place. Your doctor may also insert a pessary (rubber or plastic object) into your vagina to hold your uterus in place.

- **Endometriosis.** Endometriosis happens when the tissue that lines the uterus grows outside of the uterus on the ovaries. This can cause severe pain and bleeding between periods. Your doctor can prescribe medicine or do surgery to remove the scar tissue or growths without harming surrounding tissue.
- **Adenomyosis.** In this condition, the tissue that lines the uterus grows inside the walls of the uterus where it does not belong. The uterine walls thicken and cause severe pain and heavy bleeding. Hormonal birth control may help.
- **Cancer (or precancer) of the uterus, ovary, cervix, or endometrium.** Hysterectomy may be the best option if you have cancer in these organs.

WAYS TO PERFORM A HYSTERECTOMY

There are several ways to perform a hysterectomy:

Abdominal hysterectomy. The surgeon removes the uterus through a cut in the abdomen. This incision may be similar to what is done during a cesarean section. This type of hysterectomy requires a longer hospital stay and longer recovery time than others. Removal of the ovaries is not required for the treatment of fibroid symptoms. Similarly, some women may desire to preserve the cervix if there is no history of abnormal Pap smears.

Vaginal hysterectomy. Instead of making a cut into the abdomen, the surgeon removes the uterus through the vagina. This method is less invasive than an abdominal hysterectomy, so recovery time is usually shorter (three to four weeks). Vaginal hysterectomy may not be an option if your fibroids are very large.

Laparoscopic hysterectomy. Minimally invasive approaches include laparoscopic hysterectomy, laparoscopy-assisted vaginal hysterectomy, and robotic-assisted laparoscopic hysterectomy. Not all cases of uterine fibroids can be treated with such approaches,

496

but these methods may result in reduced postoperative recovery time.

Robotic hysterectomy. Robotic hysterectomy is becoming more common. The surgeon sits at a console near the patient and guides a robotic arm to perform laparoscopic surgery. Like laparoscopic myomectomies, this technique requires only small incisions in the uterus and abdomen. As a result, recovery can be shorter (three to four weeks) than with more invasive procedures. More research is needed to understand how these procedures work and to compare the outcomes with those of other established surgical treatments.

If you have not gone through menopause and are considering a hysterectomy for your fibroids, talk to your healthcare provider about keeping your ovaries. The ovaries make hormones that help maintain bone density and sexual health even if the uterus is removed. If your body can continue to make these hormones on its own, you might not need hormone replacement after the hysterectomy.

Having a hysterectomy means that you will no longer be able to get pregnant. This process cannot be reversed, so be certain about your choice before having the surgery.

Section 36.2 | Dilation and Curettage

WHAT IS DILATION AND CURETTAGE?

Dilation and curettage, also known as a "D&C" is a surgical procedure in which abnormal tissues are scraped from the lining (endometrium) of the uterus. It is an outpatient surgery and most women can return home the same day. In dilation and curettage, the cervix is dilated and a spoon-shaped instrument, called a "curette," is used to scrape and remove the abnormal tissue. A variation of this procedure is dilation and evacuation (D&E) in which the contents of the uterus are removed using suction force.

WHY IS DILATION AND CURETTAGE ADVISED?

Dilation and curettage serves diagnostic and therapeutic purposes. It is usually done for:

- Investigating abnormal or excessive uterine bleeding
- Removal of polyps (growths attached to the inner wall of the uterus)
- Removal of hyperplasia (abnormal growth in the lining of the uterus)
- Examination of potentially cancerous tissue
- Medical termination of pregnancy (up to 14 weeks of gestation) also called an "abortion"
- Abortion of abnormal fetus (having birth defects)
- Removal of placental and other tissues after miscarriage
- Removal of remnant placental tissue, postpartum
- Therapeutic abortion (termination of pregnancy that is dangerous to the mother)
- To determine the cause of infertility
- Other reasons as seen fit by a doctor

HOW DOES ONE PREPARE FOR DILATION AND CURETTAGE?

Make arrangements at home to take care of daily activities before you leave for the procedure. Ask someone to drive you home after surgery and arrange for a help when you are recovering. You will be informed as to when you need to stop eating before surgery in order to prevent vomiting during surgery. Inform the hospital about any allergies and medications that you are taking. You will not have to take regular medication on the day of surgery. You will be asked to avoid aspirin because it increases risk of bleeding. If you are allergic to local and general anesthetic agents—iodine, latex, or tape—volunteer this information in advance. If you are a smoker, you should quit at least eight weeks before surgery. Surgery leads to complications and healing time is increased in smokers. Follow instructions given to you by doctors and medical staff. Carry a sanitary napkin to wear when leaving for home.

HOW IS DILATION AND CURETTAGE PERFORMED?

The patient is given sedation for relaxation. The D&C is usually done under partial anesthesia, but in certain circumstances, at the request of the patient, she may be fully anesthetized. The patient also will be positioned with both legs harnessed onto stirrups. Prior to surgery, the cervix is dilated with a laminaria stick, which is a thick rod that is inserted in the cervix that absorbs fluid and dilates the cervix so that the uterus can be accessed. Medications are used to numb and soften the cervix to aid dilation. A speculum is then placed into the vagina and clamped into place. Once the cervix has dilated to one and a half inch, the surgeon uses a curette to scrape and clean the abnormal tissue from the uterus. Sometimes tissue samples are sent to the laboratory for analysis. The procedure results in cramps similar to menstrual cramps, which are usually controlled by pain medication.

WHAT ARE THE RISKS AND SIDE EFFECTS OF DILATION AND CURETTAGE?

- You may experience problems with anesthesia, such as nausea or vomiting
- Abdominal pain or cramping
- Infection or bleeding
- Perforation of the uterus or bowel and damage to the cervix
- Scar tissue may develop in the uterus
- Foul-smelling discharge
- Fever or chills
- Inability to get pregnant after surgery

Enquire with your medical practitioner about the risks applicable to you and other concerns prior to surgery.

WHAT HAPPENS AFTER THE PROCEDURE?

The type of recovery varies along with the kind of procedure applied in your case. You will need to recover from anesthesia and be kept under observation initially. Once your blood pressure, pulse, and breathing have returned to normal you will be taken to recovery and then discharged. Have another person drive you home in case you are discharged on the same day. Sufficient rest will be required if you were anesthetized. After surgery, you will experience spotting or slight vaginal bleeding for a few days. Wear a sanitary napkin. You will also experience cramping. You will be advised not to douche or use tampons and engage in sexual intercourse for a short period of time. Restrictions will be placed on intense physical activity, such as lifting heavy objects.

WHAT IS THE FOLLOW-UP REQUIRED AFTER DILATION AND CURETTAGE?

The endometrial lining will rebuild in a few days after surgery and regular menstrual periods will commence in due course of time. If you need pain medication, speak to your doctor. Aspirin could increase chances of bleeding and is not advised. Your cervix is under risk of bacterial infection until it is fully healed. Contact the clinic if you suffer from severe abdominal pain, fever, chills, or foul-smelling discharge.

References

1. "Dilation and Curettage (D and C)," The Johns Hopkins University, n.d.
2. "Dilation and Curettage (D and C)," University of Rochester Medical Center, n.d.
3. "Dilation and Curettage (D and C)," The Cleveland Clinic Foundation, n.d.
4. "Dilation and Curettage (D and C)," Memorial Sloan Kettering Cancer Center, April 3, 2017.
5. "Dilation and Curettage (D and C)," Oregon Right To Life, n.d.
6. "Dilation and Curettage (D and C)," Hallmark Health Medical Associates, n.d.
7. "Dilation and Curettage (D and C)," Novant Health Wound Care & Hyperbaric Medicine, n.d.

Section 36.3 | Cesarean Section (C-Section)

This section contains text excerpted from the following sources: Text beginning with the heading "What Is a C-Section?" is excerpted from "What Is a C-Section?" *Eunice Kennedy Shriver* National Institute of Child Health and Human Development (NICHD), September 1, 2017; Text beginning with the heading "What Is Vaginal Birth after Cesarean" is excerpted from "What Is Vaginal Birth after Cesarean," *Eunice Kennedy Shriver* National Institute of Child Health and Human Development (NICHD), September 1, 2017.

WHAT IS A C-SECTION?

A cesarean delivery, also called a "C-section" or "cesarean birth" is the surgical delivery of a baby through a surgical cut or incision in a woman's abdomen and uterus. After the baby is removed from the womb, the uterus and abdomen are closed with stitches that later dissolve.

According to the Centers for Disease Control and Prevention (CDC), in 2015, 32 percent of births were by cesarean delivery—the lowest rate since 2007. Between 1996 and 2008, the number of cesarean deliveries increased by 72 percent.

WHEN IS A CESAREAN DELIVERY NEEDED?

Cesarean delivery may be necessary in the following circumstances:

- **Labor is not progressing.** Contractions may not open the cervix enough for the baby to move into the vagina for delivery.
- **The infant's health is in danger.** The umbilical cord, which connects the fetus to the uterus, may become pinched, or the fetus may have an abnormal heart rate. In these cases, a cesarean delivery allows the baby to be delivered quickly to address and resolve the baby's health problems.
- **The baby is in the wrong position.** Most often when this occurs, the baby is breech, or in a breech presentation, meaning that the baby is coming out feet first instead of head first. The baby may also be in a transverse (sideways) or oblique (diagonal) position.
- **The pregnant woman is delivering two or more fetuses (multiple pregnancy).** A cesarean delivery may be needed if labor has started too early (preterm

labor), if the fetuses are not in good positions within the uterus for a natural delivery, or if there are other problems.

- **The baby is too large.** Larger infants are at risk for complications during delivery. These include shoulder dystocia when the infant's head is delivered through the vagina, but the shoulders are stuck. Women with gestational diabetes, especially if their blood sugar levels are not well controlled, are at increased risk for having large babies.
- **The placenta has problems.** Sometimes the placenta is not formed or working correctly, is in the wrong place in the uterus, or is implanted too deeply or firmly in the uterine wall. These issues can cause problems, such as preventing needed oxygen and nutrients from reaching the fetus or causing vaginal bleeding.
- **The mother has an infection,** such as HIV or herpes, that could be passed to the baby during vaginal birth. Cesarean delivery could help prevent transmission of the virus to the infant.
- **The mother has a specific medical condition.** A cesarean delivery enables the healthcare provider to better manage the mother's health issues.

Women who have a cesarean delivery may be given pain medication with an epidural block, a spinal block, or general anesthesia. An epidural block numbs the lower part of the body through an injection in the spine. A spinal block also numbs the lower part of the body, but through an injection directly into the spinal fluid. Women who receive general anesthesia, often used for emergency cesarean deliveries, will not be awake during the surgery.

WHAT ARE THE RISKS OF A CESAREAN DELIVERY?

Cesarean delivery is a type of surgery, so it has risks and possible complications for both mother and baby.

Possible risks from a cesarean delivery include:
- Infection

- Blood loss
- Blood clots in the legs, pelvic organs, or lungs
- Injury to surrounding structures, such as the bowel or bladder
- Reaction to medication or anesthesia used
- It is important to note that these risks also apply, to some degree, to vaginal birth.

A woman who has a cesarean delivery may also have to stay in the hospital longer than a woman who has had a vaginal delivery.

The more cesarean deliveries a woman has, the greater her risk of certain medical problems and problems with future pregnancies, such as uterine rupture and problems with the placenta.

CAN A CESAREAN DELIVERY BE REQUESTED?

Some women may want to have a cesarean birth even if vaginal delivery is an option. Women should discuss their options in detail with their healthcare provider before making a decision about a type of delivery. The decision should consider the impact of the delivery not only on the current pregnancy, but also on future pregnancies. The safest method of delivery for both the mother and the fetus is an uncomplicated vaginal delivery.

Regardless of the type of delivery, unless there is a medical necessity, delivery should not occur before 39 weeks of pregnancy called "full term."

WHAT IS VAGINAL BIRTH AFTER CESAREAN?

Vaginal birth after Cesarean (VBAC) refers to vaginal delivery of a baby after a previous pregnancy was delivered by cesarean delivery.

In the past, pregnant women who had one cesarean delivery would automatically have another. But research shows that, for many women who had prior cesarean deliveries attempting to give birth vaginally—called a "trial of labor after cesarean delivery" (TOLAC)—and VBAC might be safe options in certain situations.

In fact, *Eunice Kennedy Shriver* National Institute of Child Health and Human Development (NICHD) research shows that among appropriate candidates, about 75 percent of VBAC attempts are successful. A 2010 NIH Consensus Development Conference on VBAC evaluated available data and determined that VBAC was a reasonable option for many women.

The NICHD-supported researchers also developed a way to calculate a woman's chances of a successful VBAC. Access the calculator. Please note that this calculator only determines the likelihood of successful VBAC; it does not guarantee success.

Women should discuss VBAC and TOLAC with their healthcare providers early in pregnancy to learn whether these options are appropriate for them. Providers are encouraged to discuss plans for VBAC or refer women to a facility that can support VBAC when it is medically safe to consider.

When Is Vaginal Birth after Cesarean Appropriate?
The Vaginal Birth after Cesarean (VBAC) may be safe and appropriate for some women, including those:
- Whose prior cesarean incision was across the uterus toward its base (called a low-transverse incision)—the most common type of incision. Note that the incision on the uterus is different than the incision on the skin.
- With two previous low-transverse cesarean incisions
- Who are carrying twins
- With an unknown type of uterine incision

Benefits of VBAC include:
- No abdominal surgery
- A lower risk of hemorrhage and infection compared with a C-section
- Faster recovery
- Potential to avoid the risks of many cesarean deliveries such as hysterectomy, bowel and bladder injury, blood transfusion, infection, and abnormal placenta conditions
- Greater likelihood of being able to have more children in the future

If labor fails to progress or if there is another problem, a woman may need a C-section after trying TOLAC. Most risks associated with C-section after TOLAC are similar to those associated with choosing a repeat cesarean. They include:

- Uterine rupture
- Maternal hemorrhage and infection
- Blood clots
- Need for a hysterectomy

Section 36.4 | Episiotomy

"Episiotomy," © 2020 Omnigraphics. Reviewed April 2020.

An episiotomy is an incision made in the perineum (area between the vagina and anus) during childbirth. This incision is made to enlarge the vaginal opening before delivering a baby. In the past, an episiotomy was done to help prevent severe vaginal tears during childbirth but has become less common in recent years.

Recent research states that an episiotomy probably causes more problems than what it prevents. This procedure has an increased risk of infection and other complications. An episiotomy is done if:

- Baby's position is abnormal
- Baby is larger than normal
- Baby needs to be delivered early
- The woman is likely to experience a large vaginal tearing during delivery

TYPES OF EPISIOTOMY

The two most common types of episiotomy are:

- Midline Episiotomy
- Mediolateral Episiotomy

Midline Episiotomy

The surgical cut is made in the middle of the vaginal opening and goes straight down the anus.

The advantages include:
- Quick healing
- Easy repair
- Less likely to experience pain during sexual intercourse
- The blood loss is often less

The disadvantages include:
- High risk for tears that extend into or through the anal muscles
- Result in long-term problems, such as fecal incontinence or the inability to control bowel movements

Mediolateral Episiotomy

The surgical cut made in this procedure begins in the middle of the vaginal opening and extends down toward the buttocks at an angle of 45 degrees. There is a low risk of anal muscle tears, which is a major advantage of mediolateral episiotomy. However, there are also the disadvantages, which includes:
- The risk of increased blood loss
- Severe pain
- Difficult repair
- Discomfort during sexual intercourse

THE PROCEDURE

The midline and mediolateral episiotomies are common and easy to perform. The surgical cut for an episiotomy is made when the doctor is able to see three or four centimeters of your baby's head at the vaginal opening. The woman will be subjected to anesthesia before this procedure. The area will be cleaned with soap and then the doctor will insert two fingers into the vaginal opening to protect the baby's head before making a small incision. The incision made may be straight down or at a slight angle depending upon the type of the episiotomy being performed. After making an incision, the doctor will slightly pinch the tissue below the incision to prevent it from further tearing. Gentle pressure is given against the top of the baby's head to prevent it from coming out too quickly or abruptly.

After delivery, the vagina and perineum are cleaned and the doctor checks for any tearing in the vaginal walls using a special instrument called a "metal refractor." Once the doctor is sure that there are no further tears, the episiotomy will be cleansed and the incision site will be washed with sterile water or antibacterial soap solution. All the repairs are performed with suture or surgical thread that will be absorbed by the body and does not require removal. Thin sutures are used to close rectal lining and strong sutures are used to close anal sphincter. Once the rectal lining and anal sphincter are repaired, the doctor will close the remaining section of the incision.

COMPLICATIONS OF EPISIOTOMY

There are few risk factors associated with this procedure though it is necessary for some women. The possible complications include:

- Bleeding
- Infection
- Pain during sexual intercourse for few months after childbirth
- Hematoma
- Tear in the rectal tissue that can cause leakage of stool and gas
- Swelling

References

1. "Labor and Delivery: Types of Episiotomy," Healthline, January 27, 2016.
2. Stoppler, Melissa Conrad, "Episiotomy," MedicineNet, December 14, 2008.

Section 36.5 | Birth Control Sterilization

This section includes text excerpted from "Female Sterilization," Office of Population Affairs (OPA), U.S. Department of Health and Human Services (HHS), April 9, 2019.

WHAT IS FEMALE STERILIZATION?

Female sterilization permanently prevents women from becoming pregnant. There are two different procedures to achieve this goal: tubal ligation and tubal implants. They both work by blocking the fallopian tubes (tubes that lead from a woman's ovaries into the uterus or womb) so that sperm cannot meet with and fertilize an egg.

Because these methods cannot be undone, they are only recommended for women who are sure that they do not want to have any children in the future.

Tubal ligation. In this procedure—also known as "having your tubes tied"—the fallopian tubes are cut, sealed, clipped, or tied. With this method, very tiny cuts called "incisions" are made in the abdomen or belly. Tubal ligation prevents pregnancy immediately.

Tubal implant. A very small spring-like coil is placed into each fallopian tube. The coils cause scar tissue to form in the tubes, blocking the tubes. This method does not involve cuts or incisions. Instead, a healthcare provider uses a thin tube to thread the small coils through the vagina and uterus into the fallopian tubes, where the coils will remain.

With tubal implant, it may take up to three months for the scar tissue to fully block the tubes. So, it is important to use a back-up type of birth control (such as the birth control shot, birth control pills, the birth control ring, the birth control patch, or a condom) until your healthcare provider says it is no longer needed. After three months, your healthcare provider will do a confirmation test (an x-ray) to check that the coils are in the correct place and the scar tissue is blocking the fallopian tubes.

HOW EFFECTIVE IS IT?

In 100 women who have a sterilization procedure each year, less than one may become pregnant. Sterilization procedures are better at preventing pregnancy than condoms, the pill, the patch, the ring, or the shot.

HOW DO YOU GET IT?

Female sterilization is a relatively simple outpatient surgery done in a health center, doctor's office, or hospital. It can be performed under local or general anesthesia, depending on the method used to perform sterilization. You will go home the same day.

Some family planning centers offer sterilization procedures on site, but all family planning centers can refer you for the procedure.

Section 36.6 | Vasectomy

This section includes text excerpted from "Male Sterilization," Office of Population Affairs (OPA), U.S. Department of Health and Human Services (HHS), April 9, 2019.

WHAT IS MALE STERILIZATION OR VASECTOMY?

Male sterilization, or vasectomy, is a procedure performed on a man that will permanently keep him from being able to get a woman pregnant. This procedure keeps a man's sperm from going to his penis, ensuring that his ejaculate does not have any sperm in it that can fertilize an egg.

WHAT IS THE PROCEDURE LIKE?

Vasectomy is an outpatient procedure done under local anesthesia. After the local anesthesia is injected, the healthcare provider makes tiny cuts in the scrotum, the sac that holds the testes or "balls." The vas deferens—two tubes that carry sperm to the penis—are then cut, tied, or blocked.

Some men receive a no-scalpel vasectomy where, instead of cutting the skin of the scrotum, very tiny holes are made. The tubes that carry sperm are pulled through the holes and tied off and cut. A no-scalpel vasectomy does not require stitches.

After a vasectomy, a man will still produce semen (the fluid that comes out of his penis when he has sex). A man will need to return to his healthcare provider about three months after the vasectomy for testing to ensure there are no sperm in his semen. It takes about three months to completely clear the sperm out of the man's reproductive system. A man should use another type of birth control (like a condom) until his healthcare provider tells him there are no longer any sperm in his semen.

HOW EFFECTIVE IS IT?

In 100 women each year whose partner has had a vasectomy, less than one may become pregnant.

Section 36.7 | Uterine Fibroid Surgery

This section includes text excerpted from "Uterine Fibroids," Office on Women's Health (OWH), U.S. Department of Health and Human Services (HHS), April 1, 2019.

WHAT ARE FIBROIDS?

Fibroids are muscular tumors that grow in the wall of the uterus. Another medical term for fibroids is "leiomyoma" or just "myoma." Fibroids are almost always benign (not cancerous). Fibroids can grow as a single tumor, or there can be many of them in the uterus. They can be as small as an apple seed or as big as a grapefruit. In unusual cases they can become very large.

SURGICAL METHODS FOR TREATING FIBROIDS

If you have fibroids with moderate or severe symptoms, surgery may be the best way to treat them. Here are the options:

- **Myomectomy**—Surgery to remove fibroids without taking out the healthy tissue of the uterus. It is best for women who wish to have children after treatment for their fibroids or who wish to keep their uterus for other reasons. You can become pregnant after myomectomy.

But if your fibroids were imbedded deeply in the uterus, you might need a cesarean section to deliver. Myomectomy can be performed in many ways. It can be major surgery (involving cutting into the abdomen) or performed with laparoscopy or hysteroscopy. The type of surgery that can be done depends on the type, size, and location of the fibroids. After myomectomy new fibroids can grow and cause trouble later. All of the possible risks of surgery are true for myomectomy. The risks depend on how extensive the surgery is.

- **Hysterectomy**—Surgery to remove the uterus. This surgery is the only sure way to cure uterine fibroids. Fibroids are the most common reason that hysterectomy is performed. This surgery is used when a woman's fibroids are large, if she has heavy bleeding, is either near or past menopause, or does not want children. If the fibroids are large, a woman may need a hysterectomy that involves cutting into the abdomen to remove the uterus. If the fibroids are smaller, the doctor may be able to reach the uterus through the vagina, instead of making a cut in the abdomen. In some cases hysterectomy can be performed through the laparoscope. Removal of the ovaries and the cervix at the time of hysterectomy is usually optional. Women whose ovaries are not removed at the time of hysterectomy do not go into menopause. Hysterectomy is a major surgery. Although hysterectomy is usually quite safe, it does carry a significant risk of complications. Recovery from hysterectomy usually takes several weeks.
- **Endometrial ablation**—The lining of the uterus is removed or destroyed to control very heavy bleeding. This can be done with laser, wire loops, boiling water, electric current, microwaves, freezing, and other methods. This procedure usually is considered minor surgery. It can be done on an outpatient basis or even in a doctor's office. Complications can occur, but are

uncommon with most of the methods. Most people recover quickly. About half of women who have this procedure have no more menstrual bleeding. About three in 10 women have much lighter bleeding. But, a woman cannot have children after this surgery.

- **Myolysis**—A needle is inserted into the fibroids, usually guided by laparoscopy, and electric current or freezing is used to destroy the fibroids.
- **Uterine fibroid embolization (UFE), or uterine artery embolization (UAE)**—A thin tube is thread into the blood vessels that supply blood to the fibroid. Then, tiny plastic or gel particles are injected into the blood vessels. This blocks the blood supply to the fibroid, causing it to shrink. UFE can be an outpatient or inpatient procedure. Complications, including early menopause, are uncommon but can occur. Studies suggest fibroids are not likely to grow back after UFE, but more long-term research is needed. Not all fibroids can be treated with UFE. The best candidates for UFE are women who:
  - Have fibroids that are causing heavy bleeding
  - Have fibroids that are causing pain or pressing on the bladder or rectum
  - Do not want to have a hysterectomy
  - Do not want to have children in the future

Chapter 37 | **Organ and Tissue Transplantation**

Chapter Contents

Section 37.1 | How Organ Allocation and Transplant Process Works

This section includes text excerpted from "How Organ Allocation Works," Health Resources and Services Administration (HRSA), September 23, 2014. Reviewed April 2020.

THE FIRST STEP

Before an organ is allocated, all transplant candidates on the waiting list who are incompatible with the donor because of blood type, height, weight, and other medical factors are automatically screened from any potential matches. Then, the computer application determines the order in which the other candidates will receive offers, according to national policies.

GEOGRAPHY PLAYS A PART

There are 58 local donation service areas and 11 regions that are used for U.S. organ allocation. Hearts and lungs have less time to be transplanted, so use a radius from the donor hospital instead of regions when allocating those organs.

THE RIGHT-SIZED ORGAN

Proper organ size is critical to a successful transplant, which means that children often respond better to child-sized organs. Although pediatric candidates have their own unique scoring system, children essentially are first in line for other children's organs.

FACTORS IN ORGAN ALLOCATION

Blood type and other medical factors weigh into the allocation of every donated organ, but, other factors are unique to each organ-type.

Kidney
- Waiting time
- Donor/recipient immune system incompatibility
- Pediatric status

515

- Prior living donor
- How far from donor hospital
- Survival benefit

Heart
- Medical need
- How far from donor hospital

Lung
- Survival benefit
- Medical urgency
- Waiting time
- Distance from donor hospital

Liver
- Medical need
- Distance from donor hospital

PRESERVING ORGANS
Donated organs require special methods of preservation to keep them viable between the time of procurement and transplantation.

Transplant data show that more and more people receive transplants every year and that many people with transplants are living longer after receiving their organ(s) than ever before.

Common Maximum Organ Preservation Times
- Heart, lung: 4 to 6 hours
- Liver: 8 to 12 hours
- Pancreas: 12 to 18 hours
- Kidney: 24 to 36 hours

TRANSPLANT PROCESS
Waiting Times
Waiting times vary widely for many reasons. The shortage of organs causes most patients to wait for a transplant. The amount of time a

patient waits does not show how well a transplant center or Organ Procurement Organization (OPO) is doing its job. Each patient's situation is different. Some patients are more ill than others when they are put on the transplant waiting list. Some patients get sick more quickly than other patients, or respond differently to treatments. Patients may have medical conditions that make it harder to find a good match for them.

How long a patient waits depends on many factors. These can include:

- Blood type (some are rarer than others)
- Tissue type
- Height and weight of transplant candidate
- Size of donated organ
- Medical urgency
- Time on the waiting list
- The distance between the donor's hospital and the potential donor organ
- How many donors are there in the local area over a period of time
- The transplant center's criteria for accepting organ offers

Depending on the kind of organ needed, some factors are more important than others.

Patient Notification

Potential recipients often contact the OPTN to ask if they are on the national patient waiting list. Unfortunately, the OPTN cannot provide this information. A patient's presence and status on the waiting list should be discussed with the patient's transplant team.

- The transplant program must notify patients in writing within ten business days of registration that the patient has been placed on the national transplant waiting list (including the date the patient was listed), or
- The transplant program must notify the patient in writing ten days after completion of the evaluation that the patient will not be placed on the patient waiting list.

- Once listed, if the patient is removed from the waiting list for any reason other than transplantation or death, the transplant program must notify the patient in writing within ten business days that the patient has been removed from the list.

This policy is intended to improve communication between transplant centers and their patients and to help patients better understand the listing and transplant process.

Options to Consider

As an informed participant, it is important that transplant candidates know their treatment options. Some patients choose to list at hospitals in different parts of the country, change hospitals, and transfer their waiting time to a different center or receive a transplant from a living donor.

Multiple listing. Sometimes patients choose to register for a transplant at more than one hospital. When a patient lists at a transplant hospital, they are generally considered for organs from a donor in that local area first. If a patient is put on the list at more than one transplant hospital, they will be considered for donor organs that become available in more than one local area.

National transplant policy allows a patient to register for a transplant at more than one transplant hospital. However, each hospital may have its own rules for allowing its patients to be on the list at another hospital. Patients should ask each hospital whether it allows its patients to list at more than one transplant hospital. Being listed in more than one area does not guarantee an organ will become available faster than for patients registered at only one transplant hospital. Generally, each transplant center will require the patient to go through a separate evaluation, even if the patient is already listed at another hospital.

Transferring waiting time. Patients may switch to a different transplant hospital and transfer their waiting time to that hospital. Waiting time from the original center is added to the time collected at the new hospital.

The transplant teams at the first hospital and the new hospital will be responsible for coordinating the exchange of information and notifying UNOS of the transfer of waiting time. Patients should ask each hospital if transferred waiting time will be accepted.

Variability among transplant centers. Hospitals can vary widely in the number of transplants they perform and the characteristics of the donor and recipient pool. Organ procurement organizations can vary widely in the number and types of donors they receive each year.

Living donation. In addition to deceased organ donation, patients may also receive organs from living donors. In 2007, more than 6,300 living donor transplants were performed. With more than 100,000 people currently waiting for a transplant in the United States, the need for donor organs is far greater than the supply. Living donation offers an alternative for individuals awaiting transplantation.

Section 37.2 | Kidney Transplant

This section includes text excerpted from "Kidney Transplant," National Institute of Diabetes and Digestive and Kidney Diseases (NIDDK), January 2018.

Some people with kidney failure may be able to have a kidney transplant. During transplant surgery, a healthy kidney from a donor is placed into your body. The new, donated kidney does the work that your two kidneys used to do.

The donated kidney can come from someone you do not know who has recently died (deceased donor), or from a living person—a relative, spouse, or friend. Due to the shortage of kidneys, patients on the waiting list for a deceased donor kidney may wait many years.

A kidney transplant is a treatment for kidney failure; it is not a cure. You will need to take medicines every day to make sure your immune system does not reject the new kidney. You will also need to see your healthcare provider regularly.

A working transplanted kidney does a better job of filtering wastes and keeping you healthy than dialysis. However, a kidney transplant is not for everyone. Your doctor may tell you that you are not healthy enough for transplant surgery.

WHAT IS THE PROCESS FOR GETTING A KIDNEY TRANSPLANT?

If you want a kidney transplant, the process includes these steps:

- Tell your doctor or nurse you want to have a kidney transplant.
- Your doctor will refer you to a transplant center for tests to see if you are healthy enough to receive a transplant. Living donors need to be tested to make sure they are healthy enough to donate a kidney.
- If you do not have a living donor, you will be placed on a waiting list to receive a kidney. You will have monthly blood tests while you wait for a kidney.
- You must go to the hospital to have your transplant as soon as you learn a kidney is available. If you have a living donor, you can schedule the transplant in advance.

Talk with Your Doctor

The first step is to talk with your doctor to find out whether you are a candidate for a transplant. If you are on dialysis, your dialysis team will also be part of the process. If you and your doctor think a kidney transplant is right for you, your doctor will refer you to a transplant center.

Get Tested at a Transplant Center

At the transplant center, you will meet members of your transplant team. You will have tests to make sure you are a good candidate for transplant.

Tests will include blood tests and tests to check your heart and other organs—to make sure you are healthy enough for surgery. Some conditions or illnesses could make a transplant less likely to succeed, such as cancer that is not in remission, or current substance abuse.

You will also have tests to check your mental and emotional health. The transplant team must be sure you are prepared to care for a transplanted kidney. You will need to be able to understand and follow a schedule for taking the medicines you need after surgery.

In a process called "cross-matching," the transplant team tests the donor's blood against your blood to help predict whether your body's immune system will accept or reject the new kidney.

If a family member or friend wants to donate a kidney and is a good match, that person will need a health exam to make sure she or he is healthy enough to be a donor. If you have a living donor, you do not need to be on a waiting list for a kidney and can schedule the surgery when it is best for you, your donor, and your surgeon.

Testing and evaluation at the transplant center may take several visits over weeks to months.

Get on the Waiting List

If your tests show you can have a transplant, your transplant center will add your name to the waiting list. Wait times can range from a few months to years. Most transplant centers give preference to people who have been on the waiting list the longest. Other factors such as your age, where you live, and your blood type, may make your wait longer or shorter.

A transplant center can place you on the waiting list for a donor's kidney if your kidney function is 20 or less—even if you are not on dialysis. While you wait for a kidney transplant, you may need to start dialysis.

Have Monthly Blood Tests

While you wait for a kidney, you will need monthly blood tests. The center must have a recent sample of your blood to match with any kidney that becomes available.

Have Your Kidney Transplant

During kidney transplant surgery, a surgeon places a healthy kidney into your body. You will receive general anesthesia before the

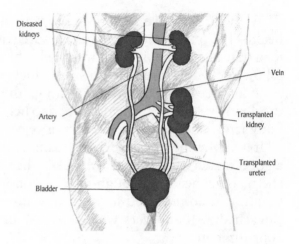

Diseased
kidneys

Vein

Artery

Transplanted
kidney

Transplanted
ureter

Bladder

Figure 37.1. Kidney Transplant Surgery

Your surgeon connects the transplanted kidney to your blood vessels and your bladder. Your blood flows through an artery into the transplanted kidney, and a vein takes filtered blood out. Your urine flows through a transplanted ureter to your bladder.

surgery. The surgery usually takes three or four hours. Unless your damaged kidneys cause infections or high blood pressure or are cancerous, they can stay in your body. Surgeons usually transplant a kidney into the lower abdomen near the groin.

If you are on a waiting list for a donor kidney, you must go to the hospital to have your transplant surgery as soon as you learn that a kidney is available.

If a family member or friend is donating the kidney, you will schedule the surgery in advance. Your surgical team will operate on you and your donor at the same time, usually in side-by-side rooms. One surgeon will remove the kidney from the donor, while another prepares you to receive the donated kidney.

WHO WILL BE IN YOUR TRANSPLANT TEAM?

A successful transplant involves working closely with your transplant team. Members of the team include:

- You—you are an important part of your transplant team.

- Your family members—this may include your spouse, parents, children, or any other family member you would like to involve.
- Transplant surgeon—the doctor who places the kidney in your body.
- Nephrologist—a doctor who specializes in kidney health and may work closely with a nurse practitioner or a physician's assistant.
- Transplant coordinator—a specially trained nurse who will be your point of contact, arrange your appointments, and teach you what to do before and after the transplant.
- Pharmacist—a person who tells you about all your medicines, fills your prescriptions, and helps you avoid unsafe medicine combinations and side effects.
- Social worker—a person trained to help you solve problems in your daily life and coordinate care needs after your transplant.
- Dietitian—an expert in food and nutrition who teaches you about the foods you should eat and avoid, and how to plan healthy meals.

Your transplant team will be able to provide the support and encouragement you need throughout the transplant process.

HOW WILL YOU FEEL AFTER YOUR TRANSPLANT?

Many people feel much better right after having transplant surgery. For some people, it takes a few days for the new kidney to start working. You probably will need to stay in the hospital for several days to recover from surgery—longer if you have any problems after the transplant. You will have regular follow-up visits with your nephrologist after leaving the hospital.

If you have a living donor, the donor will probably also stay in the hospital for several days. However, a new technique for removing a kidney for donation that uses a smaller cut may make it possible for the donor to leave the hospital in two to three days.

Before you leave the hospital, you need to learn how to stay healthy and take care of your donor kidney. You will have to take one or more antirejection medicines—also called "immunosuppressants." Without medicine, your immune system may treat your donor kidney as foreign, or not your own, and attack your new kidney. Antirejection medicines may have side effects.

You may also need to take other medicines—for example, antibiotics to protect against infections. Your transplant team will teach you what each medicine is for and when to take each one. Be sure you understand the instructions for taking your medicines before you leave the hospital.

HOW DO YOU KNOW YOUR NEW KIDNEY IS WORKING?

Blood tests help you know your donor's kidney is working. Before you leave the hospital, you will schedule an appointment at the transplant center to test your blood. The tests show how well your kidneys are removing wastes from your blood.

At first, you will need regular checkups and blood tests at the transplant center or from your doctor. As time goes on, you will have fewer checkups.

Your blood tests may show that your kidney is not removing wastes from your blood as well as it should. You also may have other symptoms that your body is rejecting your donor's kidney. If you have these problems, your transplant surgeon or nephrologist may order a kidney biopsy.

WHAT ARE THE POSSIBLE PROBLEMS AFTER A KIDNEY TRANSPLANT?

The donated kidney may start working right away or may take up to a few weeks to make urine. If the new kidney does not start working right away, you will need dialysis treatments to filter wastes and extra salt and fluid from your body until it starts working.

Other problems following kidney transplant are similar to other pelvic surgeries and may include:

- Bleeding
- Infection, especially a bladder infection

- Hernia
- Pain or numbness along the inner thigh that usually goes away without treatment

Transplant rejection is rare right after surgery and can take days or weeks to occur. Rejection is less common when the new kidney is from a living donor than when it is from a deceased donor.

WHAT ARE THE SYMPTOMS OF TRANSPLANT REJECTION?

Transplant rejection often begins before you feel any changes. The routine blood tests that you have at the transplant center will reveal early signs of rejection. You may develop high blood pressure or notice swelling because your kidney is not getting rid of extra salt and fluid in your body.

Your healthcare provider will treat early signs of rejection by adjusting your medicines to help keep your body from rejecting your new kidney.

Transplant rejection is becoming less common. However, your body may still reject the donor kidney, even if you do everything you should. If that happens, you may need to go on dialysis and go back on the waiting list for another kidney. Some people are able to get a second kidney transplant.

Seek Medical Care Right Away

When you are taking antirejection medicines, you are at a greater risk for infection. Antirejection medicines can dull symptoms of problems, such as infection. Call your transplant center right away if you are not feeling well or have:

- A fever of more than 100 degrees
- Drainage from your surgical scar
- Burning when you pass urine
- A cold or cough that would not go away

WHAT ARE THE SIDE EFFECTS OF ANTIREJECTION MEDICINES?

Some antirejection medicines may change your appearance. Your face may get fuller, you may gain weight, or you may develop acne or facial hair. Not all people have these side effects.

Antirejection medicines weaken your immune system, which can lead to infections. In some people over long periods of time, a weakened immune system can increase their risk of developing cancer. Some antirejection medicines cause cataracts, diabetes, extra stomach acid, high blood pressure, and bone disease.

When used over time, these medicines may also cause liver or kidney damage in some people. Your transplant team will order regular tests to monitor the levels of antirejection medicines in your blood and to measure your liver and kidney function.

WHAT SHOULD YOU EAT OR AVOID EATING WITH A KIDNEY TRANSPLANT?

You have more choices about what to eat after you receive a kidney transplant than you would if you were on dialysis. However, you will need to work with a dietitian to develop an eating plan that can change in response to your medicines, test results, weight, and blood pressure.

HOW DO YOU PAY FOR YOUR TRANSPLANT?

The federal government health insurance program, will pay for transplant and care for three years after the transplant. Medicare will also pay for your donor's surgery and her or his care.

Paying for Medicines

Medicare and private insurance may help pay for your medicines. Additionally, drug companies give discounts to people who can show that they cannot afford to pay for their prescriptions. Talk with your transplant social worker to find out what resources may be available to help you pay for your transplant.

Section 37.3 | The Liver Transplant Process

This section includes text excerpted from "Definition and Facts of Liver Transplant," National Institute of Diabetes and Digestive and Kidney Diseases (NIDDK), March 2017.

FACTS ABOUT LIVER TRANSPLANT
What Is a Liver Transplant?

A liver transplant is surgery to remove your diseased or injured liver and replace it with a healthy liver from another person, called a "donor." If your liver stops working properly, called "liver failure," a liver transplant can save your life.

How Common Are Liver Transplants?

In 2015, about 7,100 liver transplants were performed in the United States. Of these, almost 600 were performed in patients 17 years of age and younger.

When Do People Need a Liver Transplant?

People need a liver transplant when their liver fails due to disease or injury.

For adults in the United States, the most common reasons for needing a liver transplant in 2016 were:
- Alcoholic liver disease
- Cancers that start in the liver combined with cirrhosis
- Fatty liver disease (nonalcoholic steatohepatitis)
- Cirrhosis caused by chronic hepatitis C

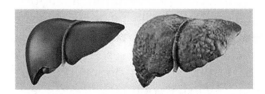

Figure 37.2. Healthy and Diseased Liver

A liver transplant removes your diseased or injured liver (right) and replaces it with a healthy liver (left).

Biliary atresia is the most common reason children need a liver transplant.

Doctors may consider a liver transplant to treat rare disorders, such as urea cycle disorders and familial hypercholesterolemia.

People may also need a liver transplant due to acute liver failure. Acute liver failure is an uncommon condition most often caused by taking too much acetaminophen. Other causes of acute liver failure include:

- Bad reactions to prescription medicines, illegal drugs, and herbal medicines
- Viral hepatitis
- Toxins
- Blockage of the blood vessels to the liver
- Autoimmune diseases
- Genetic disorders

What Are the Types of Liver Transplant?
DECEASED DONOR TRANSPLANTS

Most livers for transplants come from people who have just died, called "deceased donors." During a deceased donor transplant, surgeons remove your diseased or injured liver and replace it with the deceased donor's liver. Adults typically receive the entire liver from a deceased donor. However, surgeons may split a deceased donor's liver into two parts. The larger part may go to an adult, and the smaller part may go to a smaller adult or child.

LIVING DONOR TRANSPLANTS

Sometimes a healthy living person will donate part of her or his liver, most often to a family member who is recommended for a liver transplant. This type of donor is called a "living donor." During a living donor transplant, surgeons remove a part of the living donor's healthy liver. Surgeons remove your diseased or injured liver and replace it with the part from the living donor. The living donor's liver grows back to normal size soon after the surgery. The part of the liver that you receive also grows to normal size. Living donor transplants are less common than deceased donor transplants.

What Are the Survival Rates after a Liver Transplant?

For patients receiving liver transplants from deceased donors, the survival rates are:

- 86 percent at 1 year
- 78 percent at 3 years
- 72 percent at 5 years

The 20-year survival rate is about 53 percent.

Your chances of a successful liver transplant and long-term survival depend on your personal situation.

TRANSPLANT PROCESS

The liver transplant process has many steps, including talking with your doctor, visiting a transplant center, and getting evaluated.

Talk with Your Doctor about a Liver Transplant

The first step is to talk with your doctor to find out whether you are a candidate for a transplant. Doctors consider liver transplants only after they have ruled out all other treatment options. However, a liver transplant is not for everyone. Your doctor may tell you that you are not healthy enough for surgery. You may have a medical condition that would make a transplant unlikely to succeed. If you and your doctor think a liver transplant is right for you, your doctor will refer you to a transplant center.

Visit a Transplant Center

During your first visit to a transplant center, health professionals will provide information about:

- The evaluation and approval process
- Placement on the national waiting list
- Reasons for being removed from the national waiting list
- The waiting period
- How people are selected for liver transplants
- Surgery and recovery

- The long-term demands of living with a liver transplant, such as taking medicines for the rest of your life

Get Evaluated for a Liver Transplant

You will go through a series of evaluations at the transplant center, where you will meet members of your transplant team. You may need to visit the transplant center several times over the course of a few weeks or even months.

YOUR TRANSPLANT TEAM

Your transplant team has many members. The team will include all or some of the following people:
- **Transplant coordinator**—a specially trained nurse who will be your point of contact, arrange appointments, and provide information and education before and after your transplant.
- **Transplant surgeons**—specially trained doctors who perform the surgery and provide care before and after your transplant.
- **Hepatologist**—a doctor who specializes in liver disease and may provide care before and after your surgery.
- **Insurance case manager**—a person who will help you with your insurance coverage.
- **Financial coordinator**—a person who helps with financial matters.
- **Social worker**—a person who can help solve problems in your daily life and coordinate care needs after your transplant.
- **Psychiatrist**—a doctor who determines whether you are mentally and emotionally healthy and prepared for caring for a new liver.
- **Dietitian**—an expert in food and nutrition. A dietitian can teach you about the foods you should eat and how to plan healthy meals before and after your transplant.

Your team will ask you about your medical history and perform medical tests. These tests may include:

- A physical exam
- Blood and urine tests
- Tests that provide pictures of organs inside your body, called "imaging tests"
- Tests to see how well your heart, lungs, and kidneys are working

The team will use the results of these tests to tell them:

- How likely you are to survive transplant surgery
- What other diseases and conditions you have
- The cause and severity of your liver disease

Your team will find out if you are healthy enough for surgery. Some medical conditions or illnesses can make a liver transplant less likely to succeed. You may not be able to have a transplant if you have:

- A severe infection
- Alcohol or drug abuse problems
- Cancer outside the liver
- Serious heart or lung disease

Also, the transplant team will:

- Find out whether you or your caregivers are able to understand and follow your doctor's instructions for care after your transplant. They need to be sure you are mentally prepared for caring for a new liver.
- Find out whether you have a good support system of family members or friends to help care for you before and after the transplant
- Review your medical insurance and other financial resources. Many financial assistance programs are available to people receiving a liver transplant and their families to help with the cost of the surgery, medicines, and care.

Get Approved for a Liver Transplant

The transplant center's selection committee will review the results of your evaluation. Each transplant center has its own guidelines about who can get a liver transplant. Transplant centers often post their guidelines on their websites. The centers also follow national guidelines.

Keep in mind that you may choose not to have a transplant even though you have been approved.

Get Placed on the National Waiting List

If you are approved for a transplant and do not have a living donor, the transplant center will submit your name to be placed on the national waiting list for a liver from a deceased donor. If you have a living donor, the transplant center will not place you on the national waiting list.

The Organ Procurement and Transplantation Network (OPTN) has a computer network linking all regional organ-gathering organizations—known as "organ procurement organizations"—and transplant centers. The United Network for Organ Sharing (UNOS), a nonprofit organization, runs the OPTN under a contract with the federal government. When UNOS officially adds you to the national waiting list, UNOS will notify you and your transplant center.

UNOS policies let you register with more than one transplant center to increase your chances of receiving a liver. Each transplant center may require a separate medical evaluation.

WAIT FOR A MATCH

The waiting period for a deceased donor transplant can range from less than 30 days to more than five years. How long you will wait depends on how badly you need a new liver. Other factors—such your age, where you live, your blood type and body size, your overall health, and the availability of a matching liver—may make your wait time longer or shorter. The UNOS computer matches a deceased donor's liver based on your blood type and body size.

UNOS policies rank people with the most urgent need for a new liver to prevent death at the top of the national waiting list.

When a matching liver from a deceased donor is found, your transplant team coordinator will call you right away, tell you what you need to do before going to the hospital, and ask you to come to the hospital right away.

Confirm Living Donor Match If You Choose This Type of Liver Transplant

If a family member, spouse, or friend wants to be a living donor, the transplant team will determine whether you and the person have blood types that work together and a similar body size. The transplant team will:

- Ask the potential donor about her or his medical history
- Perform medical tests to make sure the person is in good general health, with no major medical or mental illnesses

The potential donor must be able to understand and follow instructions before and after surgery, be between 18 and 60 years of age, and have an emotional tie to the person receiving the liver transplant.

The OPTN and UNOS provide detailed information on the organ transplant process.

LIVER TRANSPLANT SURGERY
How Do You Prepare for Liver Transplant Surgery?

How you prepare for liver transplant surgery depends on the type of liver transplant you are having.

- **Deceased donor transplant.** If you are on the national waiting list for a deceased donor liver, your transplant team coordinator will call you as soon as a matching liver is found. You must go to the hospital right away. Your transplant team coordinator will tell you what you need to do before going to the hospital.

- **Living donor transplant.** If you are receiving a liver from a living donor, you will schedule your surgery four to six weeks in advance. Your transplant team coordinator will tell you and the donor what you need to do before going to the hospital for the operations.

How Do Doctors Perform Liver Transplant Surgery?

Doctors perform liver transplant surgery by removing your diseased or injured liver and replacing it with the donor's liver. Liver transplant surgery can take up to 12 hours or longer. During the surgery, the surgical team will:
- Give you general anesthesia
- Put intravenous (IV) and other types of lines into your body so you receive medicines and fluids
- Monitor your heart and blood pressure

If you are getting a liver from a deceased donor, your surgery will start when the donor liver arrives at the transplant center. If you are getting a liver from a living donor, the surgical team will operate on you and your donor at the same time.

What Are the Possible Problems of Liver Transplant Surgery?

Possible problems of liver transplant surgery should be discussed with your surgeon. Some possible problems include:
- Bleeding
- Blood clots in your liver's blood vessels
- Damage to the bile ducts
- Failure of the donated liver
- Infection
- Rejection of the donated liver

What Happens after Liver Transplant Surgery

After your surgery, you will stay in an intensive care unit (ICU). Specially trained doctors and nurses will watch you closely while you are in the ICU. You will begin taking medicines called "immunosuppressants" to prevent problems with your new liver. The doctors and nurses will perform:

- Blood tests often to make sure your new liver is working properly
- Medical tests to make sure your heart, lungs, and kidneys are also working properly

When your doctors feel you are ready, you will move from the ICU to a regular room in the hospital.

Your transplant team will teach you how to take care of yourself before you get home. Transplant team members will give you information on follow-up medical care, the things you need to do to care for your new liver, and possible problems you may have with your new liver.

After a living donor's surgery, the donor will stay in a recovery room for a few hours and spend her or his first night in an ICU. Specially trained doctors and nurses will watch the donor closely in the ICU. The day after surgery, the donor will usually move to a hospital room. The doctors and nurses will encourage the donor to get out of bed and sit in a chair the day after surgery and to walk short distances as soon as she or he is able.

When Can You Go Home after Liver Transplant Surgery?

You can likely go home about 2 weeks after your transplant surgery. A living donor can typically go home about one week after surgery.

When Can You Go Back to Your Normal Activities?

Your doctor will let you know when you can go back to your normal activities. You can likely return to your normal activities after a few months. Most people are able to return to work, be physically active, and have a normal sex life. You will continue to have regular medical checkups to make sure that your liver is working properly and you have no other health problems. Doctors often recommend that women wait at least a year after their transplant before getting pregnant.

Although recovery times vary, most living donors can often return to their normal activities one month after surgery and can return to work within four to six weeks.

LIVING WITH A LIVER TRANSPLANT
What Is Organ Rejection?

Organ rejection occurs when your immune system sees your transplanted liver as "foreign" and tries to destroy it. You have the highest chance of organ rejection in the first three to six months after your transplant.

What Are the Signs and Symptoms of Organ Rejection?

Abnormal liver blood test results may be the first sign of organ rejection. Rejection does not always cause symptoms you may notice. When symptoms of rejection are present, they may include:

- Feeling tired
- Pain or tenderness in your abdomen
- Fever
- Yellowing of the skin and the whites of your eyes
- Dark-colored urine
- Light-colored stools

You should talk with your doctor right away if you have symptoms of organ rejection. Your doctor will often perform a liver biopsy to see if your body is rejecting the new liver.

How Can You Prevent Organ Rejection?

To help keep your body from rejecting the new liver, you will need to take medicines called "immunosuppressants." These medicines prevent and treat organ rejection by reducing your immune system's response to your new liver. You may have to take two or more immunosuppressants. You will need to take these medicines for the rest of your life.

Rejection can occur any time the immunosuppressive medicines fail to control your immune system's response to your new liver. If your transplanted liver fails as a result of rejection, your transplant team will decide whether another transplant is possible.

What Are the Side Effects of Immunosuppressants?

Immunosuppressants can have many serious side effects. You can get infections more easily because these medicines weaken your immune system. Other possible side effects include:

- Brittle bones
- Diabetes
- High blood pressure
- High levels of cholesterol and triglycerides in the blood
- Kidney damage
- Weight gain

Long-term use of these medicines can increase your chance of developing cancers of the skin and other areas of your body.

Prescription medicines, over-the-counter (OTC) medicines, vitamins, and dietary supplements can affect how well immunosuppressants work. Tell your doctor if you are prescribed any new medicines. Talk with your doctor before using OTC medicines, vitamins, dietary supplement, or any complementary or alternative medicines or medical practices.

How Do You Help Care for Your New Liver?

Do the following to help take care of your new liver:

- Take medicines exactly as your doctor tells you to take them.
- Talk with your doctor before taking any other medicines, including prescription and OTC medicines, vitamins, and dietary supplements.
- Keep all medical appointments and scheduled blood draws.
- Stay away from people who are sick.
- Tell your doctor when you are sick.
- Learn to recognize the symptoms of rejection.
- Have cancer screenings as recommended by your doctor.
- Keep up-to-date with vaccinations; however, "live" vaccines should not be used.

- Talk to your doctor, both before and after your liver transplant, about the use of contraceptives and the risks and outcomes of pregnancy.

Learn how to recognize the symptoms of infection. Symptoms of infection may include:
- Fever
- Chills
- A stuffy nose
- Sore throat
- Cough
- Diarrhea
- Vomiting

Talk with your doctor right away if you have symptoms of infection.

Make healthy choices and protect yourself.
- Eat healthy foods, exercise, and do not smoke cigarettes.
- Do not drink alcoholic beverages or use alcohol in cooking if you have a history of alcohol use disorder.
- Protect yourself from soil exposure by wearing shoes, socks, long-sleeve shirts, and long pants.
- Avoid pets such as rodents, reptiles, and birds.
- Protect yourself against organisms that can transmit diseases, such as ticks and mosquitoes, by:
  - Using insect repellent
  - Wearing shoes, socks, long-sleeve shirts, and long pants
  - Not going outdoors at times when organisms are most likely to be active, such as at dawn and dusk
- If you are planning on traveling, especially to developing countries, talk with your transplant team at least two months before leaving to determine the best ways to reduce travel-related risks.

What Should You Eat after Your Liver Transplant?

You should eat a healthy, well-balanced diet after your liver transplant to help you recover and keep you healthy. A dietitian or nutritionist can help you create a healthy eating plan that meets your nutrition and diet needs.

What Should You Avoid Eating after Your Liver Transplant?

Grapefruit and grapefruit juice can affect how well some immunosuppressants work. To help prevent problems with some of these medicines, avoid eating grapefruit and drinking grapefruit juice.

If you have a history of alcohol use disorder, do not drink alcoholic beverages or use alcohol in cooking.

You should avoid consuming the following:

- Water from lakes and rivers
- Unpasteurized milk products
- Raw or undercooked:
  - Eggs
  - Meats, particularly pork and poultry
  - Fish and other seafood

Your dietitian or nutritionist may recommend that you limit your intake of:

- Salt
- Cholesterol
- Fat
- Sugar

Section 37.4 | **Pancreas and Islet Transplantation**

This section contains text excerpted from the following sources: Text in this section begins with excerpts from "Pancreas," Organ Procurement and Transplantation Network (OPTN), Health Resources and Services Administration (HRSA), February 2001. Reviewed April 2020; Text beginning with the heading "What Are Islets?" is excerpted from "Pancreatic Islet Transplantation," National Institute of Diabetes and Digestive and Kidney Diseases (NIDDK), October 2018.

A pancreas transplant may involve either the whole pancreas or a pancreas segment. Whole organ transplants are far more common, but a segmental transplant is possible. Segmental transplants are done if a living donor is involved. Many pancreas transplants also involve transplantation of the duodenum.

The kidney is frequently transplanted with the pancreas in the United States, many people suffering from pancreas failure also have renal failure. In most cases, a kidney-pancreas transplant is performed from a deceased donor. But, there have been several transplants performed using a living donor, with one kidney and a pancreas segment being donated.

REASONS FOR PANCREAS TRANSPLANTS
Pancreas Diagnosis
- Retransplant/graft failure
- Diabetes mellitus—Type I
- Diabetes mellitus—Type II
- Diabetes secondary to chronic pancreatitis without pancreatectomy
- Diabetes secondary to cystic fibrosis without pancreatectomy
- Pancreatic cancer
- Bile duct cancer
- Other cancers
- Pancreatectomy prior to pancreas transplant

WHAT ARE ISLETS?
Pancreatic islets, also called "islets of Langerhans," are groups of cells in your pancreas. The pancreas is an organ that makes

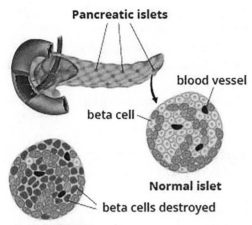

Pancreatic islets

blood vessel

beta cell

Normal islet

beta cells destroyed

Type 1 diabetes

Figure 37.3. Pancreatic Islets Compressor

Pancreatic islets contain beta cells that produce the hormone insulin.

hormones to help your body break down and use food. Islets contain several types of cells, including beta cells that make the hormone insulin. Insulin helps your body use glucose for energy and helps control your blood glucose levels, also called "blood sugar."

WHAT IS PANCREATIC ISLET TRANSPLANTATION AND HOW CAN IT TREAT TYPE 1 DIABETES?

In people with type 1 diabetes, the body's immune system attacks and destroys the beta cells. People with type 1 diabetes must take insulin because their bodies no longer make this hormone.

Pancreatic islet transplantation is an experimental treatment for type 1 diabetes. Because this is an experimental procedure, islet transplantation may only be performed as part of a U.S. Food and Drug Administration (FDA)-allowed clinical trial.

In the type of islet transplantation used to treat type 1 diabetes, also called "islet allotransplantation," doctors take islets with healthy beta cells from the pancreas of a deceased organ donor. Doctors then inject the healthy islet cells taken from the donor into a vein that carries blood to the liver of a person with type 1 diabetes. A person receiving a transplant is called a "recipient." These islets begin to make and release insulin in the recipient's body. More than one injection of transplanted islet cells is often needed to stop using insulin.

Researchers hope that islet transplantation will help people with type 1 diabetes:

- Improve their blood glucose levels
- Lower or remove the need for insulin injections
- Better recognize symptoms of low blood glucose, also called "hypoglycemia"
- Prevent severe hypoglycemia, which is when a person's blood glucose level becomes so low that she or he needs help from another person to treat the hypoglycemia

A whole pancreas transplant is another procedure that can give a person with type 1 diabetes healthy beta cells. However, a pancreas transplant is a major surgery that carries a greater risk of complications than an islet transplant.

WHO ARE CANDIDATES FOR ISLET TRANSPLANTATION?

Not all people with type 1 diabetes are good candidates for islet transplantation. Certain people with type 1 diabetes who have blood glucose levels that are difficult to manage, experience severe hypoglycemia, and have hypoglycemia unawareness—a dangerous condition in which a person cannot feel or recognize the symptoms of hypoglycemia—may be candidates.

Doctors consider people for islet transplantation if the possible benefits such as being better able to reach blood glucose targets without problems, such as hypoglycemia—outweigh the risks, such as the possible side effects of immunosuppressants. Immunosuppressants are medicines that recipients must take to prevent their immune system from attacking and destroying the transplanted islets.

People who have type 1 diabetes and have had, or are planning to have, a kidney transplant to treat kidney failure may be candidates for islet transplantation. Islet transplantation may be performed at the same time as or after a kidney transplant. Kidney transplant recipients will already be taking immunosuppressants to prevent rejection of the transplanted kidney. Therefore, the islet transplant does not add much more risk.

HOW DO DOCTORS PERFORM ISLET TRANSPLANTATION?

Special enzymes are used to remove islets from the pancreas of a deceased donor. The islets are purified and counted in a lab. On average, about 400,000 islets are transplanted in each procedure.

The transplant recipient will most often receive a local anesthetic and a sedative—medicine to help them relax—for the procedure. In some cases, the recipient may receive general anesthesia.

The islet transplant infusion procedure involves inserting a thin, flexible tube called a "catheter" through a small cut in the recipient's upper abdomen. A radiologist uses x-rays and ultrasound to guide the catheter into the portal vein of the liver. The islets are slowly infused through the catheter and into the liver by gravity. Alternatively, a minimally invasive open procedure can be used to directly visualize a vein near the liver to insert the catheter.

Over the next two weeks, new blood vessels form and connect the islets with the blood vessels of the recipient. The beta cells in the islets begin to make and release insulin into the bloodstream immediately after transplant.

WHAT ARE THE BENEFITS OF ISLET TRANSPLANTATION?

Recipients may see the following benefits:
- Improved blood glucose levels
- Less need or no need for insulin injections to manage diabetes
- Fewer or no episodes of severe hypoglycemia
- Improved awareness of hypoglycemia, which helps prevent episodes of severe hypoglycemia

Research also suggests that islet transplantation may prevent or slow the development of diabetes complications such as heart disease, kidney disease, and nerve or eye damage.

HOW SUCCESSFUL IS ISLET TRANSPLANTATION?

A Phase 3 clinical trial conducted by the National Institutes of Health (NIH)-sponsored Clinical Islet Transplantation Consortium looked at outcomes associated with islet transplantation. Phase 3 trials test new treatments in large groups of people to confirm that treatments are effective and monitor side effects. Participants in this NIH-sponsored study included people with type 1 diabetes with problems managing their blood glucose levels, such as severe hypoglycemia and hypoglycemia unawareness.

The study found that, 1 year after islet transplantation, nearly 9 in 10 transplant recipients had an A1C level below 7 percent and did not have episodes of severe hypoglycemia. The A1C goal for many people with diabetes is below 7 percent. About half of the recipients did not need to take any insulin. Two years after islet transplantation, about 7 in 10 recipients had an A1C level of less than 7 percent and did not have episodes of severe hypoglycemia, and about 4 in 10 did not need insulin.

Ongoing research from this study also found that islet transplant recipients experienced significant improvements in their diabetes-related quality of life and reported better overall health status after the transplant. Even transplant recipients who still needed to take insulin to manage their diabetes experienced these improvements.

WHAT ARE THE RISKS OF ISLET TRANSPLANTATION?

Risks of islet transplantation include:

- Bleeding, blood clots, and pain after the procedure
- The chance that the transplanted islets may not work well or may stop working
- Side effects of antirejection medicines, also called "immunosuppressants," which are described below
- Development of antibodies against the donor cells that may make it more difficult to find an appropriate organ donor if another transplant is needed in the future

Immunosuppressants

After an islet transplant, recipients will take medicines, called "immunosuppressants," for as long as the transplanted islets are working. These medicines help prevent the body from rejecting the transplanted islets. Rejection occurs when the body's immune system sees the islets as "foreign" and tries to destroy them. If the recipient stops taking immunosuppressants, the recipient's body will reject the transplanted islets, and the islets will stop working.

Immunosuppressants can have many serious side effects. Possible side effects include:

- A higher chance of getting infections
- A higher chance of getting cancer
- Digestive side effects such as vomiting, nausea, or diarrhea
- Headaches, tremors, or confusion
- High blood pressure
- High blood glucose levels
- High levels of cholesterol and triglycerides in the blood
- Kidney damage

HOW COMMON IS ISLET TRANSPLANTATION?

Islet transplantation is not a common treatment for type 1 diabetes. In the United States, islet transplantation is considered an experimental treatment. Islet transplants are only performed at hospitals that have permission from the FDA to conduct clinical research—medical research that involves people—on this procedure.

The Collaborative Islet Transplantation Registry (CITR) has reported that, between 1999 and 2015, 1,086 people worldwide received islet transplants for type 1 diabetes. The CITR collects information on islet transplants performed at research centers in North America, Europe, Australia, and Asia. The National Institute of Diabetes and Digestive and Kidney Diseases (NIDDK) established and supports the CITR. The JDRF, formerly known as the "Juvenile Diabetes Research Foundation," also helped establish CITR.

WHY IS ISLET TRANSPLANTATION NOT USED MORE OFTEN TO TREAT TYPE 1 DIABETES?

Islet transplantation is not often used to treat type 1 diabetes for several reasons:

Islet Transplantation Is Considered an Experimental Procedure

In the United States, islet transplantation is considered an experimental procedure. Until islet transplantation is approved as a treatment for type 1 diabetes, the procedure can only be performed for research purposes through clinical trials. Health insurance plans generally do not cover the cost of experimental procedures.

Information from the NIH-supported Phase 3 clinical trial is being shared with the FDA to provide evidence to consider whether islet transplantation can be approved as a treatment for some people with type 1 diabetes.

You can view a filtered list of clinical studies on islet transplantation that are federally funded, open, and recruiting at www.ClinicalTrials.gov. You can expand or narrow the list to include clinical studies from industry, universities, and individuals; however, the NIH does not review these studies and cannot ensure they are safe. Always talk with your healthcare provider before you participate in a clinical study.

Islet Transplant Recipients Must Take Immunosuppressants

Islet transplant recipients must take long-term immunosuppressants, and these medicines may cause serious side effects. Researchers are looking for ways to prevent islet rejection without long-term immunosuppressants. In one approach, called "encapsulation," islets are coated with a material that protects them from being attacked by the recipient's immune system.

Donor Islets Are in Short Supply

Only a small number of donor pancreases are available for islet transplantation each year. According to the Organ Procurement and Transplantation Network (OPTN), 1,315 pancreases were recovered from deceased donors in 2017. Many donated pancreases are not suitable for islet isolation. Also, some donor islets may be damaged or destroyed during the transplant process.

Researchers are studying different ways to overcome the short supply of donor islets. For example, scientists are studying ways to transplant islets from pigs or create new human islets from stem cells.

IS ISLET TRANSPLANTATION USED TO TREAT ANY OTHER CONDITIONS?

Doctors may perform a different type of islet transplantation, called "islet auto-transplantation," in people who have their whole pancreas removed to treat severe and chronic pancreatitis. People with type 1 diabetes cannot receive islet auto-transplantation.

In islet auto-transplantation, doctors remove a patient's pancreas, remove the islets from the pancreas, and transplant the islets into the patient's liver. The goal is to give the body enough healthy islets that make insulin. Patients do not need to take immunosuppressants after islet auto-transplantation because they receive islets from their own bodies. Islet auto-transplantation is not considered experimental.

Section 37.5 | Vascularized Composite Allograft Transplantation

This section includes text excerpted from "10 Things to Know about VCA Organ Transplants," Organdonor. gov, Health Resources and Services Administration (HRSA), August 21, 2018.

WHAT IS A VASCULARIZED COMPOSITE ALLOGRAFT ORGAN TRANSPLANT?

VCA stands for "vascularized composite allograft" organs. VCA transplants involve multiple tissue types including skin, bone, nerves, and blood vessels (vascular means vessels) which are transplanted onto a patient.

WHAT ARE SOME TYPES OF VASCULARIZED COMPOSITE ALLOGRAFT TRANSPLANTS?

The VCA transplants that you probably hear about most often are hand, arm, and face transplants. But, they can also include the larynx, genitalia, the abdominal wall, and other body parts.

WHY A TRANSPLANT SERVES BETTER THAN ARTIFICIAL LIMBS OR RECONSTRUCTIVE SURGERY?

The VCA transplants can restore abilities and independence in ways that artificial limbs and surgery cannot. These transplants can completely transform lives.

HOW COMMON ARE THESE TRANSPLANTS?

As of 2017, about 85 hand and arm transplants and 20 full or partial face transplants had been performed around the world. The first VCA transplants were performed about 20 years ago, but it is still a relatively new, developing surgery.

HOW DOES A HAND OR ARM TRANSPLANT WORK?

The surgery is very complicated. Bones have to be connected to the arm; arteries, and veins must be reattached; and tendons and nerves need to be repaired. The medical and surgical team can include dozens of professionals and take up to 16 hours to perform.

HOW DOES A FACE TRANSPLANT WORK?

These transplants also take teams of doctors and many hours to perform—how long depends on the recipient's injury or illness. For example, if the mouth and jaw need to be replaced, then teeth, bone, tongue, chin, and skin might need to be transplanted, increasing the complexity of the process.

WILL A FACE RECIPIENT "LOOK LIKE" THE DONOR?

The answer is yes and no. Yes, skin characteristics such as moles, freckles, and scars will transfer to the recipient. However, since the recipient's underlying bone structure is apt to be different from the donor's, any resemblance will likely be minimal.

HOW DOES VASCULARIZED COMPOSITE ALLOGRAFT ORGAN MATCHING HAPPEN?

Criteria for matching donors and recipients in a traditional transplant also apply for VCA, such as compatible blood and tissue types. VCA also requires matching other features such as skin tone, body size, hair color, and sometimes gender.

ARE THERE SOME RISKS WITH THIS SURGERY?

Yes, there is a risk of rejection, just as any organ transplant can be rejected. Patients will be on medication for the rest of their lives. Rehabilitation can be a full-time job for years. And anytime a person undergoes a surgical procedure there can be complications.

WHEN YOU SIGN UP AS AN ORGAN DONOR, ARE YOU AGREEING TO DONATE YOUR HANDS AND FACE?

No, you are not authorizing a VCA donation when you sign up as an organ, eye, and tissue donor. Your family makes the decision about VCA donation after your death, so make sure your wishes are known.

Section 37.6 | Heart Transplantation and Artificial Heart

This section contains text excerpted from the following sources: Text under the heading "About Heart Transplant" is excerpted from "Heart Transplant," National Heart, Lung, and Blood Institute (NHLBI), July 25, 2011, Reviewed April 2020; Text beginning with the heading "About Total Artificial Heart" is excerpted from "Total Artificial Heart," National Heart, Lung, and Blood Institute (NHLBI), February 11, 2018.

ABOUT HEART TRANSPLANT

Most heart transplants are done on patients who have end-stage heart failure—a condition in which your heart is severely damaged or weakened—and on people who have failed other treatment options. End-stage heart failure may be caused by conditions such as coronary heart disease, viral infections, or hereditary conditions. In rare instances, heart transplant may be performed at the same time as lung transplant in patients who have severe heart and lung disease.

You may be eligible for heart transplant surgery if you have severe heart disease that does not respond to other treatments. If you are otherwise healthy enough for surgery, you will be placed on the National Organ Procurement and Transplantation Network's (OPTN) waiting list. This national network handles the organ-sharing process for the United States. If a match is found, you will need to have your heart transplant surgery right away.

Heart transplant surgery will be done in a hospital. You will have general anesthesia and will not be awake during the surgery. You will receive medicine through an intravenous (IV) line in your arm. A breathing tube connected to a ventilator will help you breathe. A surgeon will open your chest, connect your heart's arteries and veins to a heart-lung bypass machine, and remove your diseased heart. The body's arteries and veins will be taken off the bypass machine and reconnected to the healthy donor heart. The heart transplant is complete after the surgeon closes your chest.

After the surgery, you will recover in the hospital's intensive care unit (ICU) and stay in the hospital for up to three weeks. During your recovery, you may start a cardiac rehabilitation program. Before leaving the hospital, you will learn how to keep track of your overall health; monitor your weight, blood pressure, pulse, and temperature; and learn the signs of heart transplant rejection and infection. For the first three months after leaving the hospital, you will return often for tests to check for infection or rejection of your new heart, to test your heart function, and to make sure that you are recovering well.

Practicing good hygiene, obtaining routine vaccines, and making healthy lifestyle choices are very important after a heart transplant to reduce your risk of infection. Regular dental care is also important. Your doctor or dentist may prescribe antibiotics before any dental work to prevent infection. Following your doctor's advice will help you recover and stay as healthy as possible.

Heart transplant has some serious risks. Primary graft dysfunction happens when the donor heart fails and cannot function. This is the most frequent cause of death for the first month after transplant. Your immune system also may reject your new heart. Rejection is most likely to occur within six months after the transplant. You will need to take medicines for the rest of your life to suppress your immune system and help prevent your body from rejecting your new heart. These medicines weaken your immune system and increase your chance for infection. Their long-term use also can increase your risk for cancer, cause diabetes and osteoporosis, and damage your kidneys. Cardiac allograft vasculopathy is a common and serious complication of heart transplant. Cardiac allograft vasculopathy is an aggressive form of atherosclerosis that over months or a few years can quickly block the heart's arteries and cause the donor heart to fail. Over time, your new heart may fail due to the same reasons that caused your original heart to fail. Some patients who have a heart transplant that fails may be eligible for another transplant.

Despite these risks, heart transplant has a good success rate that has improved over many decades of research. Recent survival rates are about 85 percent at one year after surgery, with survival rates decreasing by about three to four percent each additional year after surgery because of serious complications. Mechanical circulatory support, possibly from left ventricular assist devices, may be an alternative to heart transplant. But, more research is needed to determine long-term survival rates for these new devices.

ABOUT TOTAL ARTIFICIAL HEART

A total artificial heart (TAH) is a pump that is surgically installed to provide circulation and replace heart ventricles that are diseased or damaged. The ventricles pump blood out of the heart to the lungs and other parts of the body. Machines outside the body control the implanted pumps, helping blood flow to and from the heart.

A doctor may recommend a TAH if you have heart failure caused by ventricles that no longer pump blood well enough, and you need long-term support. TAH surgery may be an alternative treatment in certain patients who are unable to receive a heart transplant.

As with any surgery, TAH surgery can lead to serious complications, such as blood clots or infection. You may have to stay in the hospital to prevent or manage these complications. In some cases, people with a TAH can leave the hospital to wait for a heart transplant.

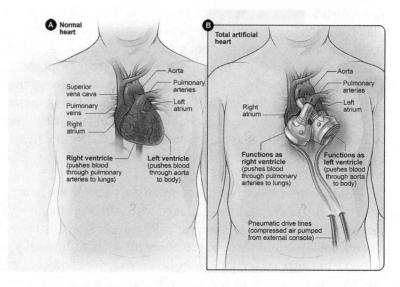

Figure 37.4. Normal Heart and a Total Artificial Heart Device

Figure A shows the normal structure and location of the heart. Figure B shows a total artificial heart, including the tubes that exit the body and connect to a machine that powers and controls the total artificial heart.

HOW DOES IT WORK?

The TAH replaces the lower chambers of the heart, known as "ventricles." Tubes connect the TAH to a power source that is outside the body. The TAH then pumps blood through the heart's major artery to the lungs and the rest of the body.

The TAH has four mechanical valves that work like the heart's own valves to control blood flow. These valves connect the TAH to your heart's upper chambers, known as the "atrium," and to the major arteries, the pulmonary artery, and the aorta. Once the TAH is connected, it duplicates the action of a normal heart, providing mechanical circulatory support and restoring normal blood flow through the body. The TAH is powered and controlled by a bedside console for patients in the hospital. After they leave the hospital, people with a TAH use a portable control device that fits in a shoulder bag or backpack and weighs about 14 pounds. It can be recharged at home or in a car.

BEFORE SURGERY

If you are not already in the hospital, you will likely spend at least a week in the hospital to prepare for the TAH surgery. You will continue to take any heart medicines your doctor gave you. During this time, you will learn about the TAH that you are getting and how to live with it.

You and your loved ones will meet with your surgeons, your cardiologist, and other doctors and nurses who specialize in the heart. The members of your healthcare team will provide you with the information that you need before surgery, including steps you need to take at home to prepare. You can ask to see what the device looks like and how it will be attached inside your body.

Your doctors will make sure that your body is strong enough for the surgery. You may need to get extra nutrition through a feeding tube.

You may have the following tests before your surgery:

- **Blood tests.** Doctors use these tests to determine your blood type for any blood you may need during surgery and to check how well your liver and kidneys are working. The tests will also show your blood cell levels, as well as important chemicals in your blood.
- **Chest computed tomography (CT) scan.** This test takes pictures of the inside of your chest. Doctors use these pictures to make sure that the TAH, which is large, will fit in your chest.
- **Chest MRI.** This test creates detailed pictures of the organs in your chest, including your heart, lungs, and blood vessels.
- **Chest x-ray.** This test also takes pictures of the inside of your chest. Doctors use these pictures to check your lungs, your heart, and your major arteries.
- **Electrocardiogram.** Doctors use this test to monitor your heart's rhythm. It can show how well your ventricles are working before surgery.
- **Echocardiogram.** This test uses sound waves to create moving pictures of your heart. It shows the movement of the blood through your heart and major blood

vessels to see, for example, whether there are any blockages.
- **Pulmonary function tests.** These tests measure how well your lungs work to help determine your risk for needing a ventilator for a long time after the surgery.

DURING SURGERY

The surgery to connect the TAH is complex and can last from five to nine hours. Learn about the team that performs the surgery and the steps involved in connecting a TAH to your body.

Surgical Team

As many as 15 people might be in the operating room during the surgery, including:
- Surgeons, who do the operation
- Surgical nurses, who assist the surgeons
- Anesthesiologists, who give you medicine that makes you sleep during the surgery
- Perfusionists, who oversee the heart-lung bypass machine that keeps blood flowing through your body while the TAH is placed in your chest
- Engineers, who assemble the TAH and make sure that it is working well

Connecting the TAH Device

An anesthesiologist will give you medicine to make you sleep before the surgery. During the surgery, the anesthesiologist will check your heart rate, blood pressure, oxygen levels, and breathing.

A breathing tube is placed in your windpipe through your mouth. This tube is connected to a ventilator machine that will support your breathing during the surgery.

Medicines are used to stop your heart. This allows the surgeons to operate on your heart while it is not moving. A heart-lung bypass machine keeps oxygen-rich blood moving through your body during the surgery.

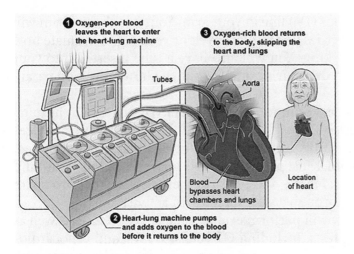

Figure 37.5. Heart-Lung Bypass Machine

The image shows how a heart-lung bypass machine works during surgery.

To perform the surgery, your surgeons will cut into your chest bone to get to your heart. Your surgeons will open your ribcage, remove your heart's ventricles, and attach the TAH to the upper chambers of your heart and to the aorta and the pulmonary artery. When everything is attached, the heart-lung bypass machine will be switched off and the surgical team will activate the TAH so it starts pumping. If the TAH is working properly and you are not bleeding abnormally, the surgeon will close your chest again. In some cases, it will remain partially closed for a few days. The medical team will fully close the chest once additional tests confirm that everything is working as it should.

AFTER SURGERY
Recovery from Surgery

Your hospital stay after surgery could last a month or more. Recovery time after TAH surgery will depend a lot on your health before the surgery.

Right after surgery, you will be moved to the hospital's intensive care unit. You may still need a ventilator to help you breathe. For a while, you may receive fluids and nutrition through a feeding tube or an intravenous (IV) line in your arm. Your healthcare team will monitor another IV line in your neck or your leg to evaluate how the TAH is working. You will also have a tube inserted into your urinary tract to drain urine and to evaluate how your kidneys are working.

After a few days or more, you will be moved to a regular hospital room. Nurses who have experience with TAHs and similar devices will take care of you. The nurses will help you sit, get out of bed, and walk around. Most patients are able to get up and move around after two weeks. Nurses and physical therapists will help you gain your strength through a slow increase in activity.

Medical staff will perform exams, such as blood tests as well as chest imaging tests, including CT scans, x-rays, and echocardiograms (ECG or EKG). Since most of the heart has been removed, electrocardiograms, heart monitors, and procedures, such as cardiopulmonary resuscitation will no longer be useful.

Once you become stronger, your healthcare team will remove your feeding, IV, and urine tubes. You will be able to begin eating regular food, go to the bathroom on your own, and take a shower. You will also learn how to care for your TAH at home.

During your recovery time in the hospital, you may enjoy visits from family or friends. These visitors can help you with various activities. They can also learn how to care for the TAH so that they can help you when you go home.

Possible Surgery-Related Complications
As with any surgery, there are possible surgery-related complications such as blood clots, bleeding, or infection after getting a TAH.

BLOOD CLOTS
Blood may clot more easily as a result of the contact with the human-made parts of the TAH. Blood clots can block blood vessels that deliver oxygen to important organs in your body and can cause severe complications, such as stroke; a type of venous thromboembolism known as "pulmonary embolism;" or death. For this reason, you need to take anticlotting medicine as long as you have a TAH.

BLEEDING

The surgery to connect a TAH to your heart is very complex. Bleeding can occur in your chest during and after the surgery. Anticlotting medicine also raises your risk of bleeding, because it thins your blood. Balancing the anticlotting medicine with the risk of bleeding can be hard. Be sure to take your medicine exactly as your doctor prescribes.

INFECTION

After surgery, you will be at risk for infection, so your doctor may prescribe medicine to reduce this risk. Your healthcare team will watch you closely for fever or other signs of infection. Other complications may develop.

OTHER COMPLICATIONS

The medical team will also watch you closely for the possibility of other complications including:

- High blood pressure
- Liver failure
- Kidney failure
- Anemia, which may require a blood transfusion

During the TAH surgery, there is a risk of dying. There is also a risk that your body may respond poorly to the medicine used to put you to sleep during the surgery.

Section 37.7 | Lung Transplantation

This section includes text excerpted from "Lung Transplant," National Heart, Lung, and Blood Institute (NHLBI), January 23, 2019.

Lung transplants are used to improve the quality of life (QOL) and extend the lifespan for people who have severe or advanced chronic lung conditions. In rare instances, a lung transplant may be performed at the same time as a heart transplant in patients who have severe heart and lung disease.

You may be eligible for lung transplant surgery if you have severe lung disease that does not respond to other treatments. If you are otherwise healthy enough for surgery, you will be placed on the National Organ Procurement and Transplantation Network's (OPTN) waiting list. This network handles the nation's organ-sharing process. If a match is found, you will need to have your lung transplant surgery right away.

This surgery will be performed in a hospital. You will have general anesthesia and will not be awake for the surgery. Tubes will help you breathe, give you medicine, and help with other bodily functions. A surgeon will open your chest, cut the main airway and blood vessels, and remove your diseased lung. The surgeon will connect the healthy donor lung, reconnect the blood vessels, and close your chest.

After the surgery, you will recover in the hospital's intensive care unit (ICU) before moving to a hospital room for one to three weeks. Your doctor may recommend pulmonary rehabilitation after your lung transplant surgery to help you regain and improve your breathing. Pulmonary rehabilitation may include exercise training, education, and counseling. Pulmonary function tests will help doctors monitor your breathing and recovery. After leaving the hospital, you will visit your doctor often to check for infection or rejection of your new lung, to test your lung function, and to make sure that you are recovering well.

The first year after lung transplant surgery is when you are most at risk for possibly life-threatening complications, such as rejection and infection. To help prevent rejection, you will need to take medicines for the rest of your life that suppress your immune system and help prevent your body from rejecting your new lungs. These important medicines weaken your immune system and increase your chance for infections, and over time they can increase your risk for cancer, diabetes, osteoporosis, and kidney damage. Practicing good hygiene, obtaining routine vaccines, and adopting healthy lifestyle choices, such as heart-healthy eating and not smoking are very important. Getting emotional support and following your doctor's advice will help you recover and stay as healthy as possible.

Chapter 38 | Urological Surgery

Chapter Contents

Section 38.1 | Circumcision

This section contains text excerpted from the following sources: Text in this section begins with excerpts from "Circumcision," Office on Women's Health (OWH), U.S. Department of Health and Human Services (HHS), January 30, 2019; Text under the heading "Circumcisions Performed in U.S. Community Hospitals" is excerpted from "Circumcisions Performed in U.S. Community Hospitals, 2009," Agency for Healthcare Research and Quality (AHRQ), U.S. Department of Health and Human Services (HHS), February 13, 2012. Reviewed April 2020; Text under the heading "Benefits and Risks" is excerpted from "South African National Guidelines for Medical Male Circumcision," U.S. Agency for International Development (USAID), 2016. Reviewed April 2020.

If you have a baby boy, you likely will be asked whether you want him to be circumcised. Circumcision is the removal of the foreskin, which is the skin that covers the tip of the penis. It is a good idea to think about this before going into labor because it is often offered before a new baby leaves the hospital.

The American Academy of Pediatrics (AAP) does not recommend routine circumcision because the medical benefits do not outweigh the risks. But, parents also need to consider their religious, cultural, and personal preferences when making the choice to circumcise their son.

There are medical benefits and risks to circumcision. Possible benefits include:

- **A lower risk of urinary tract infections (UTIs).** Keep in mind that UTIs affect only 1 percent or less of men who are not circumcised.
- **A lower risk of penile cancer.** Keep in mind that penile cancer is very rare in both men who are or are not circumcised.
- **A possible lower risk of sexually transmitted infections (STIs).** Keep in mind that practicing safe sex, including using a condom, is the best protection against STIs.

The risks of circumcision include:

- **Pain.** If you decide to have your baby circumcised, you can ask that a numbing medicine be put on your baby's penis to lessen the pain.
- **A low risk of bleeding or infection**

These risks are higher when circumcision is performed on older babies, boys, and men. Talk to your doctor if you have concerns about the risks or possible benefits.

CIRCUMCISIONS PERFORMED IN U.S. COMMUNITY HOSPITALS

Circumcision is the most commonly performed surgical procedure in newborns. Although circumcisions may be performed for cultural or religious reasons, there has been debate over the ethics and medical necessity for this procedure. As recently reported by the Centers for Disease Control and Prevention (CDC), the percent of male newborn circumcisions declined over the past decade.

In 1999, the American Academy of Pediatrics (AAP) issued a policy position stating that the evidence of medical benefits from circumcisions was not compelling enough to warrant routine newborn circumcision. In recent years however, evidence has been accumulating on the potential health benefits associated with circumcisions, including reductions in infant urinary tract infections and rates of penile cancer. In heterosexual men, circumcision has been linked to decreased acquisition and transmission of sexually transmitted infections such as syphilis, human immunodeficiency virus (HIV), and herpes simplex virus types. Since 2005, three randomized controlled studies have been published indicating benefits from circumcision in reducing HIV acquisition in heterosexual males in Africa. These findings have renewed the debate over AAP's current position that there is insufficient evidence to issue recommendations for routine neonatal circumcisions.

This statistical brief presents data from the Healthcare Cost and Utilization Project (HCUP) on hospitalizations involving circumcision procedures in male newborns, updating previously published information from 2005. It provides details on characteristics of infants receiving circumcisions, complementing recently published data on trends in circumcision in the United States and also on circumcision rates in hospitals across regions of the country by median income, by patient residence, and by payer. Findings by payer are of particular interest because it was recently reported that circumcision rates were 24 percent higher in hospitals located in

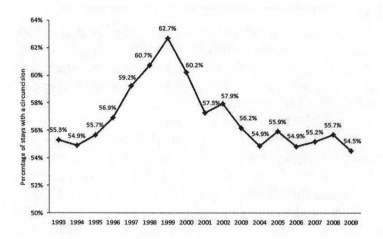

Figure 38.1. Percentage of circumcisions per 1,000 male newborns, 1993–2009 *(Source: AHRQ, Center for Delivery, Organization, and Markets, Healthcare Cost and Utilization Project, Nationwide Inpatient Sample, 1993–2009)*

Percentage of circumcisions per 1,000 male newborns, 1993–2009. Trend line chart; percentage of stays with a circumcision in 1993, 55.53 percent; in 1994, 54.9 percent; in 1995, 55.7 percent; in 1996, 56.9 percent; in 1997, 59.2 percent; in 1998, 60.7 percent; in 1999, 62.7 percent; in 2000, 60.2 percent; in 2001, 57.3 percent; in 2002, 57.9 percent; in 2003, 56.2 percent; in 2004, 54.9 percent; in 2005, 55.9 percent; in 2006, 54.9 percent; in 2007, 55.2 percent; in 2008, 55.7 percent; in 2009, 54.5 percent. Source: AHRQ, Center for Delivery, Organization, and Markets. Healthcare Cost and Utilization Project, Nationwide Inpatient Sample, 1993–2009.

states where Medicaid pays for circumcisions than in states where Medicaid does not pay for the procedure.

All differences between estimates noted are statistically significant at the 0.05 level or better.

Between 1993 and 1999, the rate of male newborn circumcisions performed in the hospital increased by 13 percent, from 55.3 to 62.7 percent of male newborn hospital stays (figure 37.1). However, between 1999 and 2004, the rate of male newborn circumcisions decreased by 12 percent, from 62.7 to 54.9 percent of male newborn hospital stays. This coincides with the American Academy of Pediatrics (AAP) policy statement on circumcision published in 1999. From 2004 to 2009, the rate of male newborn circumcisions remained relatively stable in the range of 55 to 56 percent of male newborns in the hospital.

BENEFITS AND RISKS

The necessity for male circumcision is a subject of heated debate in many countries. In some settings male circumcision is widely performed for religious or cultural reasons, while in others it is performed mainly for medical reasons. Every potential client or parent has to get full information about the benefits and risks of circumcision to make an informed decision.

Voluntary male medical circumcision (VMMC) services add value by connecting men to healthcare and offering them, at a minimum, a package of services including education on safer sex, access to condoms and HIV testing and counselling services, with links to HIV care and treatment.

The decision of a male to be circumcised, or the decision of a parent to have her or his son circumcised, should not only be based on culture, religion, or personal preference, but should also be informed by information provided by a healthcare worker.

Benefits

If male circumcision is being done for reasons other than the treatment of a medical problem, health benefits are primarily preventive, and may only be accrued long after the procedure. Male circumcision may reduce the risk of getting some infections and related complications, but does not guarantee complete protection. Some of these conditions are common, while others are less so, and the degree of risk for the person is likely to depend on his behaviour and where he lives. Medical male circumcision offers excellent value for money in high HIV prevalence settings. It saves costs by averting new HIV infections and reducing the number of people needing HIV treatment and care.

Benefits of male circumcision (the strength of the evidence varies by disease):

- It is easier to keep the penis clean
- It reduces the risk of urinary tract infections in childhood
- It prevents balanitis and posthitis
- It prevents the potential development of scar tissue on the foreskin, which may lead to phimosis and paraphimosis

- It reduces the risk of some STIs, especially ulcerative diseases like chancroid and syphilis
- It reduces the risk of getting infected with HIV
- It reduces the risk of penile cancer
- It reduces the risk of cancer of the cervix in female sex partners
- It reduces the risk of prostate cancer

Risks

As with any surgical procedure, there are risks associated with male circumcision. While the benefits of male circumcision may be wide-ranging and long-term, any problems generally occur during or soon after the procedure.

Risks of male circumcision include:
- Pain
- Bleeding
- Haematoma
- Infection at the site of the circumcision
- Increased sensitivity of the glans penis for the first few months after the procedure
- Irritation of the glans
- Meatitis
- Injury to the penis
- Adverse reaction to the anaesthetic used during the male circumcision

These complications are rare when the circumcision is done by well trained, adequately equipped, experienced healthcare personnel, and are usually easily and rapidly resolved. Data from controlled trials show that fewer than 1 in 50 circumcisions result in complications.

Section 38.2 | **Prostate Cancer Surgery**

This section includes text excerpted from "Prostate Cancer Treatment (PDQ®)—Patient Version," National Cancer Institute (NCI), June 12, 2019.

GENERAL INFORMATION ABOUT PROSTATE CANCER

- Prostate cancer is a disease in which malignant (cancer) cells form in the tissues of the prostate.
- Signs of prostate cancer include a weak flow of urine or frequent urination.
- Tests that examine the prostate and blood are used to detect (find) and diagnose prostate cancer.
- A biopsy is done to diagnose prostate cancer and find out the grade of the cancer (Gleason score).
- Certain factors affect prognosis (chance of recovery) and treatment options.

TREATMENT OPTIONS OVERVIEW
Surgery

Patients in good health whose tumor is in the prostate gland only may be treated with surgery to remove the tumor. The following types of surgery are used:

- **Radical prostatectomy.** A surgical procedure to remove the prostate, surrounding tissue, and seminal vesicles. There are two types of radical prostatectomy:
- **Retropubic prostatectomy.** A surgical procedure to remove the prostate through an incision (cut) in the abdominal wall. Removal of nearby lymph nodes may be done at the same time.
- **Perineal prostatectomy.** A surgical procedure to remove the prostate through an incision (cut) made in the perineum (area between the scrotum and anus). Nearby lymph nodes may also be removed through a separate incision in the abdomen.
- **Pelvic lymphadenectomy.** A surgical procedure to remove the lymph nodes in the pelvis. A pathologist views the tissue under a microscope to look for cancer

cells. If the lymph nodes contain cancer, the doctor will not remove the prostate and may recommend other treatment.

- **Transurethral resection of the prostate (TURP).** A surgical procedure to remove tissue from the prostate using a resectoscope (a thin, lighted tube with a cutting tool) inserted through the urethra. This procedure is done to treat benign prostatic hypertrophy and it is sometimes done to relieve symptoms caused by a tumor before other cancer treatment is given. TURP may also be done in men whose tumor is in the prostate only and who cannot have a radical prostatectomy.

In some cases, nerve-sparing surgery can be done. This type of surgery may save the nerves that control erection. However, men with large tumors or tumors that are very close to the nerves may not be able to have this surgery.

Possible problems after prostate cancer surgery include the following:

- Impotence
- Leakage of urine from the bladder or stool from the rectum
- Shortening of the penis (1 to 2 centimeters). The exact reason for this is not known.
- Inguinal hernia (bulging of fat or part of the small intestine through weak muscles into the groin). Inguinal hernia may occur more often in men treated with radical prostatectomy than in men who have some other types of prostate surgery, radiation therapy, or prostate biopsy alone. It is most likely to occur within the first 2 years after radical prostatectomy.

Cryosurgery

Cryosurgery is a treatment that uses an instrument to freeze and destroy prostate cancer cells. Ultrasound is used to find the area that will be treated. This type of treatment is also called "cryotherapy."

Cryosurgery can cause impotence and leakage of urine from the bladder or stool from the rectum.

Section 38.3 | Urinary Incontinence Surgery

This section contains text excerpted from the following sources: Text beginning with the heading "What Is Stress Urinary Incontinence?" is excerpted from "Stress Urinary Incontinence (SUI)," U.S. Food and Drug Administration (FDA), April 16, 2019; Text under the heading "Surgery for Bladder Problems" is excerpted from "Treatments for Bladder Control Problems (Urinary Incontinence)," National Institute of Diabetes and Digestive and Kidney Diseases (NIDDK), June 1, 2018.

WHAT IS STRESS URINARY INCONTINENCE?

Stress urinary incontinence (SUI) is a leakage of urine during moments of physical activity that increases abdominal pressure, such as coughing, sneezing, laughing, or exercise. SUI is the most common type of urinary incontinence in women.

Stress urinary incontinence can happen when pelvic tissues and muscles, which support the bladder and urethra, become weak and allow the bladder "neck" (where the bladder and urethra intersect) to descend during bursts of physical activity. This descent can prevent the urethra from working properly to control the flow of urine. SUI can also occur when the sphincter muscle that controls the urethra weakens. The weakened sphincter muscle is not able to stop the flow of urine under normal circumstances and when there is an increase in abdominal pressure. Weakness may occur from pregnancy, childbirth, aging, or prior pelvic surgery. Other risk factors for SUI include chronic coughing or straining, obesity, and smoking.

It is important for you to consult with your healthcare provider for proper diagnosis of SUI.

WHAT QUESTIONS SHOULD YOU ASK YOUR SURGEON IF YOU ARE CONSIDERING SURGERY TO TREAT STRESS URINARY INCONTINENCE?

Ask your surgeon about all SUI treatment options, including nonsurgical options and surgical options that do and do not use

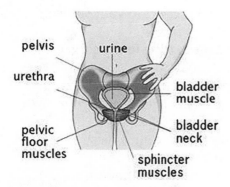

Figure 38.2. Bladder Control System
(Source: National Kidney and Urologic Diseases Information Clearinghouse (NKUDIC))

mesh slings. It is important for you to understand why your surgeon may be recommending a particular treatment option to treat your SUI.

Any surgery for SUI may put you at risk for complications, including additional surgery. One complication that may occur when mesh slings are used is vaginal mesh erosion, which could require additional surgery to resolve.

If mesh erosion occurs through the vaginal tissue, it is possible that men may experience penile irritation and/or pain during sexual intercourse.

Ask your surgeon the following questions before you decide to have SUI surgery:

- What surgical or nonsurgical treatment options are available and what do you recommend to treat my SUI?
- Have you had specialized training in the surgical treatment of SUI, and if so, what type of training have you had with this particular product and/or procedure?
- What can I expect after surgery and what is the recovery time?
- If I also have pelvic organ prolapse, will that change how you treat my SUI?
- What if the surgery does not correct my problem?

- Which side effects should you report to your surgeon after the surgery?
- Are you planning to use a mesh sling in my surgery? If so:
  - How often have you performed this surgery using this particular product? What results have your other patients had with this product?
  - What are the pros and cons of using a mesh sling in my particular case? How likely is it that my repair could be successfully performed without using a mesh sling?
  - Are recovery times different for mesh sling surgery compared to nonmesh surgery?
  - Will my partner be able to feel the mesh sling during sexual intercourse?
  - If I have a complication related to the mesh sling, how likely is it that the complication can be resolved? Will you treat it or will I be referred to a specialist experienced with mesh sling complications?
  - Is there patient information that comes with the product, and can I have a copy?

What Should You Do after Your Surgery to Treat Stress Urinary Incontinence?

Continue with annual checkups and follow-up care, notifying your healthcare provider if complications develop, such as persistent vaginal bleeding or discharge, pelvic or groin pain, or pain during sexual intercourse. There is no need to take additional action if you are satisfied with your surgery and are not having complications or symptoms.

- If you have complications or other symptoms:
  - Discuss complications and treatment options with your healthcare provider. Only your healthcare provider can give you personalized medical advice.
  - Consider getting a second opinion from a surgeon who specializes in female pelvic reconstruction if

you are not satisfied with the discussion with your healthcare provider.

- Let your healthcare provider know you have a mesh sling, especially if you plan to have another surgery, plan to become pregnant or have other medical procedures.
- If you have had SUI surgery, but do not know whether your surgeon used a mesh sling, ask your healthcare provider.
- Talk to your healthcare provider about any additional questions you may have.
- Submit a voluntary report about any problems experienced with surgical mesh slings through Medwatch, the FDA Safety Information and Adverse Event Reporting program.

SURGERY FOR BLADDER PROBLEMS

If you have overflow incontinence caused by a blockage or a narrowed urethra, a doctor can treat it with surgery to remove the blockage.

For women. A weak bladder neck or poorly supported urethra can cause stress incontinence and may be treated with some type of surgery. In sling surgery, a surgeon works through the vagina to insert a strip of material—usually mesh—in the tissue between the vagina and urethra. Mesh is a screenlike material that doctors can implant in your body to support the bladder or urethra or repair a hernia. A doctor performs the operation in a hospital or surgery center. You will receive general, spinal, or local anesthesia. Most women can leave the hospital the same day, though some may need to stay overnight. Full recovery takes 2 to 3 weeks.

Although sling surgeries with surgical mesh, sometimes called "mid-urethral slings," can be successful and safe, serious complications can occur in some women. Your doctor can explain the risks and benefits of surgery for stress incontinence and what kind of results you can expect. She or he can help you decide whether surgery is right for you.

For men. Stress incontinence in men is sometimes treated with surgery. Surgery includes the artificial urinary sphincter (AUS) and the male sling procedures. A doctor performs the operations in a hospital. You will receive general or spinal anesthesia. Most men can leave the hospital the same day, though some may need to stay overnight. Your doctor can explain the risks and benefits of surgery for urinary incontinence (UI) and what kind of results you can expect.

Minimally invasive surgeries are available for men with an enlarged prostate.

Section 38.4 | Urinary Diversion

This section includes text excerpted from "Urinary Diversion," National Institute of Diabetes and Digestive and Kidney Diseases (NIDDK), September 2013. Reviewed April 2020.

WHAT IS TEMPORARY URINARY DIVERSION?

Temporary urinary diversion reroutes the flow of urine for several days or weeks. Temporary urinary diversions drain urine until the cause of blockage is treated or after urinary tract surgery. This type of urinary diversion includes a nephrostomy and urinary catheterization.

WHAT IS A NEPHROSTOMY?

A nephrostomy involves a small tube inserted through the skin directly into a kidney. The nephrostomy tube drains urine from the kidney into an external drainage pouch. Nephrostomy tubes are often used for less than a week after a percutaneous nephrolithotomy—a surgical procedure to break up and remove a kidney stone.

This treatment is often used when a kidney stone is quite large or in a location that does not permit effective use of other treatments. For this procedure, a surgeon makes a tiny incision in the back and creates a tunnel into one of the kidneys. As the kidney heals after surgery, the nephrostomy provides an alternative route for urine drainage until normal urinary flow resumes. A person may also need a nephrostomy if narrowing, blockage, or inflammation of the ureters keeps urine from draining properly. Under

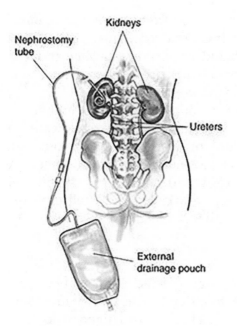

Kidneys

Nephrostomy
tube

Ureters

External
drainage pouch

Figure 38.3. Nephrostomy Tube Pouch

these circumstances, the nephrostomy may stay in place for several weeks until the problem is resolved.

WHAT IS PERMANENT URINARY DIVERSION?

Permanent urinary diversion requires surgery to reroute urine flow to an external pouch through an opening in the wall of the abdomen, called a "stoma," or to a surgically created internal reservoir. Stomas range from three-fourths of an inch to 3 inches wide. Surgeons perform permanent urinary diversion when a patient has a damaged bladder or no longer has a bladder. Advanced bladder cancer ranks as the most common reason for bladder removals. Bladder damage may result from nerve damage, birth defects, or chronic-or long lasting-inflammation. Nerve damage severe enough to require permanent urinary diversion generally occurs from multiple sclerosis, among other disease, spinal cord injuries, and damage caused by pelvic trauma or radiation injury. The most common birth defect requiring bladder surgery is spina bifida.

Chronic bladder inflammation can result from severe cases of interstitial cystitis (IC) or chronic urinary retention. Interstitial cystitis is a condition that causes the bladder to become swollen and irritated, leading to decreased bladder capacity. Urinary retention is the inability to empty the bladder completely.

The two permanent types of urinary diversion include urostomy and continent urinary diversion. A urostomy, also called a "noncontinent urinary diversion," requires an external pouch—a disposable plastic bag that sticks to the skin of the abdomen. A continent urinary diversion involves the creation of an internal reservoir with a segment of bowel—also called the "small and large intestines"—that stores urine until it can be drained.

CUTANEOUS URETEROSTOMY

In cutaneous ureterostomy, the surgeon detaches one or both ureters and attaches them directly to a stoma. This type of urostomy is not as common as an ileal conduit because of a higher complication rate and the need for follow-up surgery. A surgeon performs cutaneous ureterostomy when the bowel cannot be used to create a stoma because of certain diseases and conditions or exposure to high doses of radiation.

WHAT SPECIAL CARE IS NEEDED
AFTER URINARY DIVERSION SURGERY?

After urinary diversion surgery, a wound, ostomy, and continence (WOC) nurse or an enterostomal therapist helps patients learn how to take care of their permanent urinary diversions. WOC nurses and enterostomal therapists specialize in ostomy care and rehabilitation. Patients should ask how to care for their stomas and pouches.

CARING FOR A CONTINENT CUTANEOUS RESERVOIR

For a continent cutaneous reservoir, patients learn how to insert a catheter through the stoma or urethra to drain the internal reservoir. Patients can drain the reservoir by inserting the catheter while standing in front of the toilet or sitting on the toilet. During the first few weeks after urinary diversion surgery, patients need to drain the

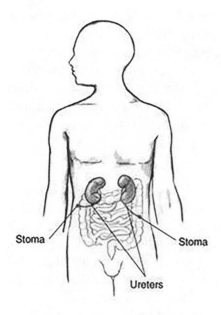

Stoma

Stoma

Ureters

Figure 38.4. Cutaneous Ureterostomy

internal reservoir every couple of hours. Over time, the reservoir capacity will increase and patients will be able to go four to six hours between reservoir drainings. Patients should wash their hands with soap and water each time they use a catheter. Before and after catheterization, patients should clean the stoma and skin around it with a wet towelette or washcloth and completely dry the stoma and skin.

The reservoir is made from part of the bowel, so it may produce mucus that normally lines the digestive tract. To clear this mucus, patients may need to irrigate, or flush out, the reservoir using a syringe with sterile water or normal saline. Patients should talk with a WOC nurse, an enterostomal therapist, or a urologist—a doctor who specializes in the urinary tract—about how often they should irrigate the reservoir.

ACTIVITIES

To help the stoma heal, patients need to restrict their activities, including driving and heavy lifting, during the first two to three weeks after urinary diversion surgery. Once the stoma has healed, patients should be able to do most of the activities they enjoyed before urinary diversion surgery, even swimming and other water sports. The only exceptions may be contact sports, such as football or karate. Patients whose jobs include strenuous physical activities should talk with their healthcare providers and employers about making adjustments to their job responsibilities.

RELATIONSHIPS

Patients may worry that people will have negative reactions to their urinary diversion. Most people will never know patients are wearing a pouch or have a continent urinary diversion. Friends and relatives are likely to be aware of the patient's health problems. However, only a spouse, intimate partner, or primary caretaker needs to know the details of the urinary diversion. Patients can choose how much they share about their condition.

Urinary diversion surgery may reduce sexual function, especially when the bladder has been removed because of cancer. Patients who have good sexual function may resume sexual activities after urinary diversion surgery as soon as their healthcare providers say it is safe. Patients should talk with their healthcare providers about any concerns they have about maintaining a satisfying sexual relationship. Healthcare providers can give information about ways to protect the stoma during sexual activity. Patients may want to ask about specially designed apparel to enhance intimacy for people with urostomies. Communicating with a sexual partner is essential. Patients should share their concerns and wishes and listen carefully to their partner's concerns.

Chapter 39 | Amputation

Chapter Contents

This section includes text excerpted from "VA/DoD Clinical Practice Guideline for the Management of Upper Extremity Amputation Rehabilitation," U.S. Department of Veterans Affairs (VA), 2014. Reviewed April 2020.

DECISION FOR AMPUTATION

The informed consent process is essential to any surgical intervention and is required by law. The discussion prior to surgery is usually the first contact between the patient and the surgeon who will conduct the operation. This discussion is the opportunity to form a trusting relationship and open communication to address any patient's fears, wishes, and concerns. The surgeon must make the patient aware of the risks and benefits of each viable treatment option. The patient should be encouraged to ask questions and to express her or his own personal desires, verbalize a good understanding of the options, and agree to a treatment plan before undertaking upper extremity amputation. Special consideration must be given in cases where the patient is unable to consent to surgery. The decision regarding amputation should be based upon accepted surgical and medical standards of care. The surgeon should be familiar with the multiple approaches available for the various levels of amputation, muscle balancing strategies, and wound closure techniques. Emerging and advanced surgical techniques may be performed in a specialized setting under the care of experienced surgeons. Combined with sophisticated medical and rehabilitation care, amputation surgeries can also serve as a refined reconstructive procedure to prepare the residual limb not only for motor function, but also for sensory feedback and cosmesis.

The presence of severe trauma, critical extremity ischemia and/ or overwhelming infection generally requires that amputation surgery be performed urgently. An urgent amputation may also be required when vessel occlusion and subsequent extremity tissue necrosis results from using vasoconstrictor agents to treat infections (sepsis). In trauma cases in which the immediate threat to life is not serious, a period of conservative management may be observed to monitor the evolution of the patient's condition. In certain cases this period may allow for restoration of collateral circulation in the extremity and help to avoid amputation or minimize the segment to be removed. Emergency repair of torn blood vessels by the vascular surgeon can make extremities viable and even help to avoid amputation. Healthcare providers should be aware that extensive reconstructive surgery to preserve an extremity may result in a painful, nonfunctional, and less efficient and effective limb than an amputated limb with a prosthesis. Conversely, the opposite of this statement can also be true. An upper limb with very minimal function can sometimes be more useful than an amputation with a prosthesis. Therefore, careful consideration should be made with respect to the decision about limb salvage versus amputation.

When considering amputation as a treatment for cancer, the care team should involve the Orthopedic Oncology or General Surgery Oncology teams (if available) to add more subject matter expertise in the patient and care team decision-making process. Elective, or delayed, amputations may be considered in situations when the affected extremity is considered nonfunctional secondary to the loss of compensated vascular, neurologic, or musculoskeletal function resulting in significant decline in patient health, quality of life (QOL), and patient wellbeing. It is in the best interest of the patient and care team that the patient undergoes a comprehensive mental health assessment to ensure that patient is of sound decision-making capacity and has been determined to be able to make a well-informed decision regarding elective or delayed amputation. With any amputation surgery, thought should be given to the surgical technique that will result in the highest level of functional ability, including consideration of available prosthesis treatment options. This can be best accomplished through early consultations and collaboration with other members of the care team with subject matter expertise (prosthetist, physiatrist, etc.) that will provide the best opportunity for the patient to achieve the maximal level of postsurgical function and outcome.

PRIMARY GOAL OF AMPUTATION

Although the primary goal of amputation is removal of the diseased, damaged, or dysfunctional portion of the limb, the surgery must also result in a residual limb that is optimized for motion, motion control, and proprioceptive feedback to achieve the most successful outcomes. In general, maximum preservation of length is desirable in the upper limb amputation. With increasing length and preservation of joints, the patient becomes more capable of positioning the residual limb and/or prosthetic device in space, allowing optimal functional result and leading to improved outcomes. There may be instances when preserving maximal limb length in an amputation would actually hinder functional outcomes with a prosthesis, thereby limiting functional independence. These should be thoroughly discussed with the surgeon and care team. In a traumatic amputation, the scope of injury will often determine the level of amputation, while in cases of vascular disease, the level of amputation is often dictated by the amount of blood flow and tissue viability. However, it is important for the surgeon to understand the requirements and capabilities of available prostheses for each amputation level, allotransplantation and/or other evolving treatments, and direct opportunities for limb length preservation when available.

SURGICAL LEVELS AND CONSIDERATIONS
Generally accepted surgical considerations and levels:
- Do not perform "guillotine" style amputation.
- Complete the amputation within the zone of injury to maximize length.
- Preserve at least 5cm of humerus length to preserve a transhumeral amputation level.
- Preserve at least 5cm of ulnar length to preserve a transradial amputation.
- Special consideration must be taken in cases of disarticulation at the elbow or wrist level, partial hand amputation, and with other complex or unusual cases.
- Perform myodesis for all primary function muscles. Myoplasty and myofascial closure may be utilized to secure secondary muscles and to contour muscles for final amputation closure.
- Skin grafts and dermal substitutes may be used to allow amputation closure, if a primary fasciocutaneous closure is not available.

Section 39.2 | Lower Limb Amputation

This section contains text excerpted from the following sources: Text under the heading "Description of Lower Limb Amputation" is excerpted from "VA/DoD Clinical Practice Guideline for Rehabilitation of Individuals with Lower Limb Amputation," U.S. Department of Veterans Affairs (VA), 2017; Text beginning with the heading "The Appropriate Level of Surgery" is excerpted from "VA/DoD Clinical Practice Guideline for Rehabilitation of Lower Limb Amputation," U.S. Department of Veterans Affairs (VA), 2007. Reviewed April 2020.

DESCRIPTION OF LOWER LIMB AMPUTATION
Dysvascular Amputation

In civilian and elderly U.S. Department of Veterans Affairs (VA) populations, the most common cause of lower limb amputation (LLA) is dysvascular complications from diabetes, arteriosclerosis, smoking, or a combination of these. In these patients, amputation may occur when medical or revascularization options do not exist or have failed, when significant tissue loss has occurred, or when infectious complications can only be managed by surgical interventions. In diabetic patients, protective and prophylactic foot care and early detection of any deformity or skin breakdown may prevent the development of ulcers and reduce the risk of amputation. Smoking cessation and control of cardiovascular risk factors, including glycemic control in diabetics, are additional approaches to the prevention of LLA. Due to the systemic nature of arteriosclerosis and diabetes, patients with these conditions are at high risk for further complications to their amputated residual limb and/or amputation of the contralateral limb. In addition, they are at higher risk for other health problems such as cardiovascular disease, cerebrovascular accident, renal disease, peripheral neuropathy, etc. While this focuses on rehabilitation of patients with LLA, preservation of the residual and contralateral limb, as well as the patients' general health, wellness, and functional independence remain integral parts of ongoing care.

Traumatic Amputation

Trauma is another major cause of LLA, though not as common as dysvascular amputations. Traumatic amputation may occur from a variety of causes, including motor vehicle and industrial accidents, electrical, chemical and thermal burns, and injuries associated with power tool or heavy machinery use. Of particular concern to military and Veteran populations are amputations associated with combat-related injuries, such as those occurring from explosions, penetrating, or crush injuries. These injuries are also typically complicated by a multitude of other comorbid conditions (e.g., traumatic brain injury, post-traumatic stress, other soft tissue injuries).

Other Causes of Amputation

Other less prevalent causes of amputation include malignant musculoskeletal tumors, infection, iatrogenic complications of vascular access procedures for other medical problems, and congenital limb development deficiency. The goal in treating musculoskeletal tumors with the lowest risk of recurrence is to remove the tumor and salvage the limb, while for tumors with high risk of local recurrence or metastasis, amputation is often indicated. Treatment of infection may require amputation when the initial treatment leads to vessel occlusion and extremity necrosis. Chronic or recurring infection after total knee arthroplasty may also lead to transfemoral amputation. Congenital limb deficiencies account for a small percentage of lower limb loss. Depending on the location of the deficiency, definitive amputation is performed at a time that considers skeletal growth, while also supporting physical, behavioral, and psychological development.

Limb Salvage and Delayed Amputation

For severe limb injury, patients and surgeons are often faced with the decision between amputation versus limb reconstruction and salvage. While limb salvage may initially be the therapeutic option of choice, complications such as infection, chronic pain, or persistent dysfunction may result in delayed amputation. In some cases, the decision to attempt limb salvage may result in increased complication rates, increased pain, and more procedures than if a primary amputation had been performed. To mitigate these risks, several scoring systems have been developed to assist with the decision to amputate or salvage the limb. Unfortunately, these systems may not accurately predict functional recovery and, therefore, should be used in combination with other criteria, including patient preferences. Unsuccessful attempts at limb salvage may result in increased morbidity and mortality. One study showed that there were a greater number of hospitalization days (49.8 days versus 24.3 days) and more operative procedures (6.7 procedures versus 1.6 procedures) for individuals who underwent delayed versus primary amputation surgery. Additionally, a retrospective cohort study of 324 service members with combat-related amputations secondary to injuries sustained in Afghanistan or Iraq demonstrated better functional outcomes compared to those with limb salvage.

THE APPROPRIATE LEVEL OF SURGERY

Once the patient is optimized for surgery, the surgeon must determine the level of amputation. The level of amputation will affect the patient's rehabilitation, functional outcome, and long-term quality of life. Several factors are incorporated in this decision that include the patient and family perspective, input from other members of the rehabilitation team, and principles of amputation surgery.

THE APPROPRIATE LEVEL OF AMPUTATION PRIOR TO SURGERY

1. The choice of amputation level should take into consideration the risks and benefits. The factors in the risk–benefit assessment include the patient's goals and priorities, the patient's general condition and risk of additional surgeries, the potential for healing of the limb, and the predicted probable functional outcome.
2. Optimal residual limb length:
   - Transtibial
     - Optimum—length that allows space for the prosthetic foot and sufficient muscle padding over the residual limb—typically mid tibia.
     - Minimum—junction of middle third and proximal third of tibia just below the flair of the tibial plateau to allow sufficient tibia for weight-bearing.

Amputation

- Transfemoral
  - Optimum—length that allows space for an uncompromised knee system—typically just above the condylar flair
  - Minimum—junction of middle third and proximal third (below the level of the lesser trochanter) to allow sufficient femur length/lever arm to operate the prosthesis

If there is uncertainty of the optimal length of the residual limb, preoperative consultation with an experienced physiatrist or prosthetist should be considered.

The potential for wound healing should be determined. The following may be considered:

- Laboratory studies:
  - C-reactive protein to check for infection
  - Hemoglobin to check for treatable anemia to ensure an appropriate oxygenation level necessary for wound healing
  - Absolute lymphocyte count to check for immune deficiency and/or infection
  - Serum albumin/prealbumin level to check for malnutrition and diminished ability to heal the wound
- Imaging studies:
  - Anteroposterior and lateral radiography of the involved extremity
  - CT scanning and MRI as necessary
  - Doppler ultrasonography to measure arterial pressure
- Additional tests:
  - Ischemic index (II) is the ratio of Doppler pressure at the level being tested to the brachial systolic pressure—a II of 0.5 or greater at the surgical level is necessary to support healing.
  - Assess preoperative amputation TcPO2 levels—preoperative levels greater than 20mmHg are associated with successful healing after amputation.

Determining the optimum amputation level involves balancing the patient's goals and expectations, the risks associated with additional surgery, the functional and cardiovascular consequences of more proximal amputations, the surgeons' clinical experience, and the physiological potential for the residual limb to heal. Other factors that might be considered include cosmesis, mobility goals, and specialized vocational or recreational priorities. The ultimate functional desires and expectations of the patient need to be included in the decision-making process. Whether the patient wishes to return to high-level athletics versus nonambulatory status may significantly influence the ultimate level of ambulation, and may lead a surgeon to preserve a longer limb with a lower chance of healing. Conversely, if the patient's underlying medical condition makes any surgical intervention potentially life-threatening, the surgeon may elect to perform the amputation at a more proximal level with a greater chance of healing.

Due to the patient's underlying comorbid cardiovascular disease, this increased energy expenditure may result in the patient having a lower level of function, and possibly not being able to ambulate at all. In fact, the level of amputation is more predictive for mobility than other factors including age, sex, diabetes, emergency admission, indication for amputation, and previous vascular surgery. The decision regarding the level of amputation must also consider the reason for the amputation (e.g., disease process, trauma), the vascular supply to the skin flaps, and the requirements of limb fitting procedures and techniques available at the time.

Additionally, the physiological potential for the amputated wound to heal is a significant factor which must be balanced into the decision-making. Many noninvasive tests have been advocated. Amputation should preserve as much of the limb as possible, because the longer the lever arm, the more control a patient will have over a prosthesis. If possible, the knee should be salvaged to decrease the energy consumption required for ambulating. In transtibial amputations, the increased energy expenditure in walking is 25 to 40 percent above normal, and in transfemoral amputations, it is 68 to 100 percent above normal; hence, patients with transtibial amputations usually have better mobility than those with transfemoral amputations. The site of an injury largely determines the decision regarding the level of section. In addition to preserving length, it is important to ensure that the residual limb be covered with skin that has normal sensation and is free of scar tissue as much as possible and that the end of the residual limb is adequately covered with muscles.

Section 39.3 | Postamputation Pain and Other Complications

This section includes text excerpted from "Amputation System of Care Traumatic Amputation," U.S. Department of Veterans Affairs (VA), May 7, 2014. Reviewed April 2020.

AMPUTATION SPECIFIC CONSIDERATIONS
Residual Limb Care

Following amputation, the residual limb undergoes a number of changes over time which can potentially result in secondary complications and result in a limited ability to wear a prosthesis for functional activities.

These changes and secondary complications include:
- Soft tissue and muscle atrophy
- Skin irritation and breakdown
- Joint contracture
- Infection (soft tissue and bone)
- Proximal Osteoarthritis/musculoskeletal complications
- Heterotopic Ossification
- Osteopenia and Osteoporosis

Pain Management

Pain following amputation can generally be classified as residual limb pain or phantom limb pain. Residual limb pain typically improves following amputation surgery, but can be persistent and associated with prosthetic use. Phantom limb pain (pain perceived in the part of the body that is missing) can be chronic and severe enough to interfere with prosthetic use and functional abilities.

OTHER TRAUMATIC INJURY CONSIDERATIONS

Amputations related to combat and other trauma are commonly associated with moderate to severe injury severity scores, and multiple comorbid injuries that require long-term management and care. These associated injuries have the potential to impact Veterans' medical and rehabilitation outcomes such as functional independence, satisfaction, and quality of life. Frequently associated injuries include:

- Traumatic brain injury (TBI)
- Fractures and other musculoskeletal injuries
- Soft tissue injuries and burns
- Peripheral nerve injuries
- Abdominal injuries
- Hearing loss and tinnitus
- Vision impairment or loss
- Genitourinary injuries (common with dismounted blast explosions)
- Mental-health conditions such as PTSD, depression, and adjustment disorder

SECONDARY COMPLICATIONS

Amputation of one or more limbs has a longitudinal impact on many areas outside of the residual limb itself. The two areas most commonly affected are the musculoskeletal and the cardiovascular systems. Many of the considerations in these areas gradually progress or worsen over time, whereas other conditions may be more intermittent. These conditions highlight the importance of comprehensive prevention strategies including proper nutrition, exercise, tobacco cessation, and wellness counseling for individuals with amputations. Wellness promotion and preventive measures should be part of one's lifestyle. Medical monitoring and education should be routine in amputation clinics and rehabilitation services.

Musculoskeletal Considerations

Longitudinal considerations for musculoskeletal conditions include:

- Osteoarthritis in the nonamputated extremity
- Overuse syndromes
- Delayed amputation after initial limb salvage
- General musculoskeletal pain and low back pain

Weight Gain/Obesity

Decreased activity levels and metabolic changes can result in weight gain and obesity. This weight gain can lead to a vicious cycle where weight gain makes prosthetic fitting and use more difficult, thus resulting in even greater declines in activity.

Cardiovascular Disease

The aging amputee population has significantly worse cardiovascular and metabolic issues that appear to be directly related to their traumatic amputation, and not accounted for by obesity, sedentary lifestyle, or tobacco use. Persons with traumatic amputations have been identified as having increased hypertension, ischemic heart disease, and diabetes mellitus. Lower extremity amputees should be monitored for aortic aneurysms; occurring at a reported rate of 6 percent versus 1 percent in the nonamputee population.

Chapter 40 | **Plastic Surgery Procedures**

Chapter Contents

Section 40.1 | Plastic Surgery: An Overview

"Plastic Surgery: An Overview," © 2020 Omnigraphics. Reviewed April 2020.

Plastic surgery is a surgical specialty that deals with both the improvement in a person's appearance (aesthetic or cosmetic surgery) and the reconstruction of facial or body tissue defects caused due to illness, trauma, or birth disorders. The term "plastic" does not refer to an artificiality that the field is unfairly known for. The word originated from the ancient Greek word "plastikos," which means to mold or give form.

HISTORY OF PLASTIC SURGERY

The field of plastic surgery roots back to ancient Egypt and has developed over many thousands of years. The otolaryngologist (head and neck surgeon) Sir Harold Gillies, who was from New Zealand but practiced in London, is considered as the father of modern plastic surgery. He is known for the development of several techniques used in modern plastic surgery, which was developed by him when he set out to help World War I soldiers who suffered injuries that disfigured their faces. His first patient who underwent plastic surgery was Walter Yeo, who received a flap surgery (tissue transfer) in 1917.

In order to practice plastic surgery today, an individual must possess an undergraduate degree with premed units, be a Doctor of Medicine and Osteopathic Medicine, along with extensive training in the field.

Plastic surgery is growing in popularity each year among both women and men, with almost 18 million surgical procedures taking place in the United States each year. Americans spent more than $6.5 billion on cosmetic surgery in 2017.

BRANCHES OF PLASTIC SURGERY

Plastic surgery restores and improves function, along with the appearance. It can involve surgery on any part of the body, other than the central nervous system, including:

- Skin (including removal of scars, burns, skin cancer, birthmarks, and tattoo removal)
- Maxillofacial (the facial skeleton)
- Congenital anomalies (such as cleft palate, deformed ears, and cleft lip)

FORMS OF PLASTIC SURGERY
Microsurgery

Microsurgery requires the use of an operating microscope to perform the surgical intervention in extremely small nerves and blood vessels, around one millimeter in diameter. It is used for performing free tissue transfer. This reconstructive surgery involves the culling of donor tissues to be transferred to another part of the body that requires reconstruction. Microsurgery is also used to reconstruct a mandible (the lower jaw) as a part of oral cancer treatment or management, traumatic tissue loss in most parts of the body, and the absence of congenital tissue. It is also used in reconstructing surgery after the resection (removal) of the breasts as a part of breast cancer treatment or management.

Hand Surgery

Hand surgery is another branch of plastic surgery that involves the reattachment or reconstruction of limbs and soft tissues in the hand.

Craniofacial Surgery

Craniofacial surgery is a subspecialty of plastic surgery that usually involves procedures performed on the skull, head, face, jaws, neck, and other associated structures. Craniofacial surgeons work on soft tissues, muscles, teeth, nerves, blood vessels, bones, and skin. Craniofacial surgery can involve the improvement or restoration of form and function for disfiguring ailments such as rare clefts in the craniofacial structures (cleft palate and cleft lip), facial fractures, Treacher Collins syndrome, Crouzon's syndrome, hemifacial microsomia, and Apert Syndrome.

Reconstructive Surgery

Reconstructive surgery is one of the most popular forms of plastic surgery, as it aims to perform a surgical intervention on various parts of the body, aside from the craniofacial area, to restore appearance and function. Reconstructive surgery is usually recommended for severe trauma and injuries; or after the management or treatment of certain types of cancer.

Burn Treatments

Restoration of the function and appearance of body parts affected or damaged by severe burns is the primary aim of burn treatments in the field of plastic surgery. It includes skin grafts, free flap procedure, tissue expansion, and microsurgery to restore the function of blood vessels and nerves.

Cosmetic Surgery

Cosmetic surgery is the most well-known branch of plastic surgery that is considered completely optional, while the other branches of the field are concerned with necessary treatments for damage caused by injuries, illnesses, or accidents. It is performed with the aim of improving the appearance of a patient or removing the visible signs of aging. It is also the most lucrative, with millions of people around the world having procedures done to enhance or preserve their looks. Popular cosmetic procedures include eyelid surgery, rhinoplasty, abdominoplasty, breast augmentation, facelifts, and liposuction. Other procedures include penile surgery, breast reduction, breast lift, butt implants, butt lift, chemical peels for scar removal and other unsightly marks, filler injections, and resurfacing or rejuvenation of the skin through laser treatments.

COMPLICATIONS OF PLASTIC SURGERY
Hematoma

Hematoma is a pocket of blood similar to a large, painful bruise that occurs in one percent of breast augmentation procedures. It is also the most common complication after a facelift, occurring in an average of one percent of patients, more commonly in males than females. Treatment includes additional operations to drain the blood if the accumulation of blood is large or growing rapidly.

Seroma

Seroma is an accumulation of serum, or sterile body fluid under the surface of the skin, leading to swelling and sometimes pain. This can happen after most surgeries, and it is the most common complication after a tummy tuck surgery, occurring in 15 to 30 percent of patients. Since seromas can become infected, they are often drained using a needle, although there is a chance of recurrence.

Blood Loss

Some blood loss is expected as with any surgery. However, uncontrolled blood loss results in a drop in blood pressure, along with fatal outcomes. Blood loss can happen while on the operating table, as well as internally postsurgery.

Infection

Postoperative care usually includes steps to reduce the risk of infection. However, it remains a common complication of plastic surgery. Infections are known to occur in 1.1 to 2.5 percent of people who undergo breast augmentation. In some cases, infections can be severe and internal, and might require intravenous (IV) antibiotics. A skin infection, known as "cellulitis," may also occur after surgery.

Nerve Damage

Nerve damage is a potential complication in many types of surgical procedures. Signs of nerve damage include numbness and tingling that are common after a plastic surgery. Nerve damage is often temporary; but, in some cases, it can end up being permanent. Most women undergo a change in sensitivity after breast augmentation surgery, and 15 percent experienced a lasting change in nipple sensation.

Deep Vein Thrombosis and Pulmonary Embolism

Deep vein thrombosis (DVT) is a condition where blood clots form in deep veins, particularly in the leg. When these clots break off and travel to the lungs, it is referred to as "pulmonary embolism" (PE). These complications are usually rare, affecting only 0.09 percent of all patients undergoing plastic surgery. However, these clots can be fatal.

Abdominoplasty procedures have a slightly higher rate of DVT and PE, affecting less than 1 percent of patients. The risk of clots is five times higher for people having multiple procedures than it is for people having only one procedure.

Organ Damage

Liposuction can tend to be traumatic for the internal organs. Visceral perforations (punctures) can occur when the surgical probe comes into contact with internal organs. Repairing these injuries can require additional surgery, and the perforations may also be fatal.

Scarring

Hypertrophic scarring is an abnormally red and thick raised scar that can occur after a plastic surgery procedure. It happens in 1 to 3.7 percent of tummy tucks along with smooth or hard keloid scars.

General Appearance Dissatisfaction

People undergoing breast surgery may end up with contouring or asymmetry problems, while those undergoing facial surgeries could be dissatisfied with the result.

Complications of Anesthesia

Anesthesia is the use of medication to make the patient unconscious during surgery. General anesthesia can lead to complications such as lung infections, stroke, heart attacks, and even death. Anesthesia awareness (waking up in the middle of surgery), is a very rare occurrence but possible.

According to a 2018 review of over 25,000 cases, complications have occurred in less than one percent of outpatient surgeries. Plastic surgery complications are more common in smokers, older adults, and people who are obese.

The risk of unwanted side effects can be reduced by thoroughly checking out the doctor and their credentials. Self-educating about the procedure and possible risks and discussing the concerns with a doctor, will also help manage the expectations and reduce the risk of complications.

References

1. "What Is Plastic Surgery: An Overview," DocDoc, March 14, 2015.
2. "10 of the Most Common Plastic Surgery Complications," Healthline, April 25, 2019.
3. Whitlock, Jennifer. "The 10 Most Common Plastic Surgery Procedures," December 3, 2019.
4. "Overview of Plastic Surgery," UCHealth, March 20, 2020.

Section 40.2 | Head and Face Reconstruction

"Head and Face Reconstruction," © 2020 Omnigraphics. Reviewed April 2020.

Surgery that is done to repair or reshape deformities of the head and face is known as "head and face reconstruction" or "craniofacial reconstruction." The medical term for this surgery is known as "orbital-craniofacial surgery." This type of surgery involves the reconstruction of the skull (cranium), bones and skin of the face, brain, nerves, ears, mouth, and the eyes. Plastic surgeons and neurosurgeons work together, along with head and neck surgeons to perform craniofacial reconstruction operations.

THE PROCEDURE

Craniofacial surgery is done while the patient is under general anesthesia and it may take 4 to 12 hours or more. A few selected bones of the face are cut and moved, while tissues are transplanted and blood vessels and nerves are reconnected using microscopic surgery techniques.

Bone grafts (pieces of bone) may be removed from the ribs, pelvis, or skull to fill in spaces where bones of the face and head were moved. Small screws and plates made of titanium or a fixation device made of absorbable material may be used to keep the bones in place. Implants may also be used. The jaws may be wired together to hold the new bones in place, and to cover the holes, flaps may be taken from the hand, buttocks, chest wall, or thigh.

WHY IS A CRANIOFACIAL RECONSTRUCTION PERFORMED?

Craniofacial reconstruction is usually done to fix:
- Birth defects and deformities such as cleft lip or palate, and genetic disorder featuring skeletal abnormalities, such as craniosynostosis and Apert syndrome
- Deformities caused by surgery done to treat tumors
- Injuries to the face, head, or jaw
- Tumors
- Reverse the signs of aging, remove contour irregularities, or make the features of the face look natural and in proportion with one another

RISK FACTORS

General risks of anesthesia and surgery include:
- Trouble breathing
- Reactions to medicines
- Blood clots, bleeding, and infection

Risks involved in surgery to the head and face are:
- Nerve (cranial nerve dysfunction) or brain damage
- Necessity for a follow-up surgery, particularly in growing children
- Partial or complete loss of bone grafts
- Permanent scarring

The above mentioned complications are more common in people who:

- Smoke
- Have poor nutrition
- Have other medical conditions, such as lupus
- Have poor blood circulation
- Have prior nerve damage

Further complications arising from the surgery include swelling of the face, mouth, or neck that lasts for weeks, which can further result in obstruction of the airway. This requires a tracheostomy (a small hole made in the neck) through which a tube (endotracheal tube) is placed in the trachea (airway), allowing the patient to breathe. The patient is required to spend the first two days after surgery in the intensive care unit. If there is no complication after the surgery, the patient can be discharged from the hospital within one week. Complete healing may require six weeks or more, and swelling will gradually reduce over the following months.

OUTCOME OF THE CRANIOFACIAL RECONSTRUCTION SURGERY

People can anticipate a more normal appearance after surgery. Some people might require follow-up procedures during the next one to four years. It is not advisable to play contact sports for two to six months after surgery.

People who have had a severe injury often need to work through the emotional issues of the trauma and the change in their appearance. Children and adults who have had a serious injury may have depression, posttraumatic stress disorder (PTSD), and anxiety disorders. It is recommended to talk to a mental-health professional or join a support group as they can be quite helpful.

References

1. "Head and Face Reconstruction," A.D.A.M. Medical Encyclopedia, May 15, 2019.
2. "Craniofacial reconstruction," The Encyclopedia of Surgery, October 24, 2005.

Section 40.3 | **Blepharoplasty (Eye Lift)**

Eyelid surgery, also referred to as "blepharoplasty" or "eye lift," reduces bagginess from the lower eyelids and removes excess skin from the upper eyelids. This surgery is usually done for cosmetic reasons. It is also an effective way to improve sight in older people whose sagging upper eyelids obstructs their vision. It is often done along with other procedures such as filler injections, laser resurfacing, or forehead lifts. An eye lift does not remove crow's feet (wrinkles around the eyes), dark circles under the eyes, or other facial wrinkles.

Certain medical conditions that may require an eyelid surgery include:

- Irritation due to excess folds of eyelid skin rubbing together
- Headaches caused by overuse of muscles straining to lift sagging skin in the eyelid area
- Ptosis, a condition that causes excessive drooping of the upper eyelid

Several types of surgeons can perform blepharoplasty. Ophthalmologists and oculoplastic surgeons (a surgical subspecialty of ophthalmology) are usually known to perform these types of procedures. However, plastic surgeons, oral and maxillofacial surgeons, and ear, nose and throat surgeons can also perform an eyelid surgery.

THE EYELID AGING PROCESS

Aging causes the skin to gradually lose its elasticity. A lack of elasticity plus the constant pull due to gravity leads to excessive skin being accumulated on the upper and lower eyelids. Excess skin on the lower eyelids leads to wrinkles and bulges, and the fat that cushions the eyeball from the skull can also result in bulges in the upper and lower eyelids due to the thin membrane holding the fat in place weakening with age.

THE PROCEDURE

Blepharoplasty is done on the upper, lower, or both eyelids simultaneously. An eyelift usually takes about two hours if both upper and lower eyelids are operated on simultaneously. Local anesthesia (a painkiller injected around the eye) with oral sedation is used by the physician. If the procedure is done at a hospital or surgical center, the patient will most likely receive intravenous (IV) sedation.

Eyelift surgery is done by making incisions in the natural folds of the eyelid, in the fold of the upper eyelid and just underneath the lashes or inside the lower eyelid. This is done so that incisions are virtually unnoticeable once they heal.

The surgeon will make precise markings to designate where excess skin and fat pads need to be removed. Some underlying muscles may also be removed. These tissues are removed with surgical instruments such as surgical scissors, scalpels, radio-frequency cutting devices, and lasers. Sutures or tissue adhesives (glue) are then carefully applied to smoothen and reconfigure the portions around the eyebrows and eyelids.

During the procedure, the surgeon decides the amount of skin, muscle and/or fat to remove, based on a preoperative evaluation of factors such as the patient's underlying facial muscle structure, bone structure, and the symmetry of the eyebrows. Less tissue is to be removed, in case of a patient with dry eye, to avoid causing the symptoms of dry eye to worsen.

A carbon dioxide (CO_2) laser is sometimes used to enhance the procedure by smoothing out any remaining wrinkles and resurfacing the skin in the eyelid and eyebrow area.

RECOVERY AFTER EYELID SURGERY

After eyelid surgery, there are stitches in both lids that remain for as long as a week. It is common to have swelling and, occasionally, bruising, but the eyelids should look normal within a week or two.

Upper eyelid surgery can last for at least five to seven years. Lower eyelid surgery rarely needs to be repeated. The eyes are prone to age even after the procedure. If the lids sag again, a forehead lift rather than another eye lift is preferred.

COMPLICATIONS FROM EYELID SURGERY

Complications due to an eye lift is quite rare, but sometimes they do occur that includes:

- Bleeding
- Infection
- Dry eyes
- Abnormal coloring of the eyelids
- Eyelid skin that folds in or out unnaturally
- Not being able to fully close the eyes
- A pulled-down lower lid lash line
- Possible loss of vision

References

1. "Eyelid Surgery," WebMD, May 15, 2019.
2. "Eyelid Surgery (Blepharoplasty) for a More Youthful Appearance," All About Vision, November 2016.

Section 40.4 | Otoplasty

"Otoplasty," © 2020 Omnigraphics. Reviewed April 2020.

Otoplasty, or cosmetic ear surgery, is a procedure to change the shape, position, or size of the ears. It can be done at any age after the ears have reached their full size, usually after five years of age and through adulthood. However, in some cases, the surgery is done as early as three years of age.

Otoplasty is considered if:

- The ear(s) stick out too far from the head
- The ears are large in proportion to the head
- Dissatisfied with a previous ear surgery
- Ear(s) are misshaped due to an injury or birth defect

Otoplasty is typically done on both ears to maintain symmetry. Otoplasty does not change the location of the ears or alter the ability to hear.

TYPES OF OTOPLASTY

The different types of otoplasty performed are:

- **Ear augmentation.** Some people may have small ears or ears that are not fully developed. In these cases, otoplasty is done to increase the size of their outer ear.
- **Ear pinning.** This procedure involves drawing the ears closer to the head. It is performed on individuals whose ears extend conspicuously from the sides of their head.
- **Ear reduction.** Macrotia is a condition where the ears are larger than normal, and otoplasty is done to reduce the size of the individual's ears.

DURING THE PROCEDURE

Otoplasty techniques vary based on the type of correction required. The specific technique that a plastic surgeon chooses will determine the location of the incisions and resulting scars. Your doctor might make incisions on the back of the ears or within the inner creases of the ears. After making incisions, excess cartilage and skin might be removed. The cartilage is then folded into the proper position and secured with internal stitches. Additional stitches will be used to close the incisions. This procedure typically takes about two hours.

AFTER THE PROCEDURE

After otoplasty, the ears will be covered in bandages for protection and support. Slight discomfort and itching are experienced. Pain medication should be taken as recommended by the doctor. To keep pressure off the ears, sleeping on side should be avoided. It is also necessary to avoid rubbing or placing excessive force on the incisions. It is recommended to wear button-down shirts or shirts with loose-fitting collars.

The ears will likely be swollen and red after the surgery. A loose headband that covers the ears is required to be worn at night for two to six weeks. This will help the patients from pulling the ears forward when rolling over in bed.

RESULTS

After the bandages are removed, an immediate change in the appearance of the ears is noticeable. These changes are permanent. If not satisfied with the results, there is a possibility of revision surgery.

RISKS OF OTOPLASTY

Otoplasty poses various risks, such as:

- **Scarring.** While scars are permanent, they will likely be hidden behind the ears or within the creases of the ears.
- **Asymmetry in ear placement.** The asymmetrical positioning of ears could occur due to the changes during the healing process. Also, surgery might not be able to successfully correct the preexisting asymmetry.
- **Changes in skin sensation.** During otoplasty, the repositioning of the ears can temporarily affect skin sensation in the area. These changes are rarely permanent.
- **Problems with stitches.** Stitches that were used to secure the ear's new shape might break out onto the surface of the skin, causing inflammation and might require additional surgery to remove.
- **Overcorrection.** Otoplasty can also result in unnatural contours that make ears appear to be pinned back.

Similar to other surgeries, otoplasty poses a risk of bleeding, infection, and any adverse reaction to anesthesia. An allergic reaction to the surgical tape or other materials used during or after the procedure is also possible.

References

1. "Otoplasty," Mayo Clinic, Mayo Foundation for Medical Education and Research (MFMER), August 14, 2018.
2. "All about Otoplasty (Cosmetic Ear Surgery)," Healthline, February 26, 2020.

Section 40.5 | **Nose Reshaping Surgery (Rhinoplasty)**

DEVIATED SEPTUM

Inside the nose is a hollow cavity called the "nasal cavity," which is separated into two parts by a wall-like structure called the "septum." The septum extends from the nostril to the back of the nose and is made of bone and cartilage. It is positioned in the middle of the nose and is intended to be straight to give good support to the nose and also to maintain the facial features of an individual cosmetically. The condition in which the nasal septum deviates from the center or looks bent or crooked, which can lead to a disfigurement of the nose, is referred to as a "deviated septum."

Displacement of the septum ranges from minor to major—when one nostril becomes tighter than the other. When the degree of deviation is severe, it can even block one side of the breathing passage and cause difficulty breathing due to reduce air flow; this is called a "nasal obstruction."

CAUSES OF DEVIATED SEPTUM

Septal deviation can be a result of:
- **Trauma**—injury to the nose or a broken nose caused by:
  - Injury during childbirth that resulted in septal displacement
  - Accidental injury to the nose from contact sports, roughhousing, active play, or automobile accidents
  - An intentional injury that may result from getting hit in the nose with force
- **Birth defect (congenital)**—in which the fetus develops a nasal septal deviation (defect) that becomes apparent at birth

SYMPTOMS OF DEVIATED SEPTUM

In most people, the deviated septum may not cause problems but in some, it can cause any of the following symptoms:

- Nosebleeds
- Postnasal drip accompanied by headache
- Recurrent sinus infections
- Nasal congestion, or a stuffy nose, more severe on one side than the other
- Difficulty breathing through the nose
- Sleep problems that contribute to loud breathing (snoring) or sleep apnea

The symptoms, as well as the degree of septal deviation, worsens:

- With age—the aging process worsens septal deviation over time
- With infection of the nose (rhinitis/rhinosinusitis)— infection leads to swelling of nasal tissues, which accentuates the narrowing of the nasal passage from a deviated septum

DIAGNOSIS OF DEVIATED SEPTUM

Deviated septum can be easily diagnosed during a physical examination. Your doctor will open the nostril with a nasal speculum (a medical tool for investigating body orifices) and use a bright light to examine your nasal septum. The doctor may need to view deeper deviations with the aid of an endoscope or small telescope. The doctor or a medical professional will use computed tomography (CT) of the nose in some cases to view the extent of the deviation or to rule out other associated findings.

TREATMENT OF A DEVIATED SEPTUM

Septal deviation is an extremely common condition that does not need treatment in most cases. Septal repair may be suggested if the deviation is severe enough to cause breathing problems and contribute to sleep apnea and snoring. For children with a deviated septum, it is best to opt for surgery after the nose has completely grown (i.e., around or after 15 years of age).

Symptoms, such as postnasal drip or stuffy nose/nasal congestion (blocked nose) can be treated using decongestants, antihistamines, or nasal sprays.

The surgical method of repairing a malpositioned septum is called "septoplasty." The surgeon makes a small cut in the nasal septum and then trims the cartilage or bone to even out the breathing space of the nostrils. Septoplasty can also be performed in combination with sinus surgery when there is damage to the sinuses.

"Rhinoplasty," or a "nose job," is performed on occasion along with the septoplasty in order to achieve a better cosmetic outcome of the nasal appearance. This procedure is called "septorhinoplasty."

Other surgical septal corrections, such as septal reconstruction and submucous resection of the septum can also be done in some cases.

Septoplasty and Turbinate Reduction

Septoplasty is a procedure that is performed as a treatment option for conditions that block the breathing passage such as:

- Deviated septum or septal deviation
- Chronic sinusitis
- Nasal polyp removal
- Recurrent nosebleeds (sometimes)

Risks and complications of the surgery include:

- Bleeding
- Infection
- Hole (perforation) of the septum
- Loss of ability to smell (rare) or decreased sense of smell (rare)

This procedure is done under local or general anesthesia in an outpatient setting. The procedure takes around one to two hours, depending on the severity of the deviation and the need to combine other procedures for a better outcome.

During the surgery, the surgeon will first lift the mucosa that covers the cartilage and bone, then attempt to straighten the septum by trimming or shaving the cartilage or bone.

Balloon septoplasty may also be performed for mild cases; this procedure is also performed in an office setting and is not a surgical procedure.

In some cases, enlarged bone structures (turbinates) can cause blockage of the breathing passage. In such cases, the surgeon may perform a septoplasty as well as a turbinate correction to remove a portion of the turbinate, or reduce the enlargement, using radiofrequency. This is called "turbinate reduction."

Once the reshaping has been performed, the surgeon will put the mucosal lining back in place. A dressing of soft packing material will be applied to avoid excess postsurgical bleeding. Patients may need to breathe through their mouths immediately after the surgery as both nostrils will be packed with dressing to support the healing process.

The dressing will be removed by the nurse three to four hours after postoperative recovery. Then the doctor will inspect the site. If the surgical site is stable, then the patient will be sent home.

Rarely, internal splints will be put in place in the appropriate position to help the septum heal; in such cases, a follow-up appointment will be scheduled after seven days for removal of the splints.

If a septoplasty is only performed, there will be little to no swelling or bruising after surgery. If septoplasty in combination with sinus surgery or rhinoplasty is performed, mild swelling along with bruising will remain for a week or two after surgery, which is normal.

For a safe and speedy recovery, it is best to avoid:
- Blowing the nose for three to four days
- Using alcohol
- Smoking (or coming into contact with secondhand smoke)
- Returning to work too soon
- Crowds or individuals who have a cough or cold, which will increase the chances of the patient getting sick

Rhinoplasty, or a "Nose Job"

This surgery is performed to change the shape and size of the nose and can be done for:

- **Medical reasons**—to correct breathing problems or disfigurement due to trauma or a birth defect
- **Cosmetic reasons**—to change the shape of the nose and enhance facial appearance

Once the patient is placed under general or local anesthesia, the surgeon makes a small cut (incision) inside the nostrils or externally at the base of the nose and then reshapes the cartilage and bones in order to obtain a pleasing anatomical structure of the nose.

For small changes, the surgeon may use cartilage inside the nose for reshaping. For large changes, the surgeon may remove cartilage from the ribs or bones from other parts of the body, or sometimes use implants placed inside the nose for reshaping. The amount of work performed depends on the availability of materials and the amount of reshaping needed.

Once the reshaping is complete, the surgeon will stitch the incision closed and pack the nostrils with a dressing that reduces excess bleeding. A protective splint may also be used to support and maintain the shape of the nose as it heals. The patient may feel swelling inside the nose due to the presence of the splint. The dressing and splint will be removed in seven days during a post-surgical follow-up appointment. A "drip pad"—a small piece of gauze held with tape—will then be placed in the nose to absorb further drainage.

POSTSURGERY DO'S AND DONT'S

- Do not blow the nose.
- Avoid extreme facial expressions, such as laughing or wide smiling.
- Avoid strenuous activities, such as jogging or aerobics.
- Do not use ice/cold packs after surgery to reduce swelling of the nose, which could take a longer time to heal. Also, do not panic if you notice black-and-blue discoloration of the eyelids due to nasal swelling; this is normal.

- Take baths instead of showers to accommodate the bandaged nose.
- Brush teeth gently to avoid vigorous movement of the upper lip.
- Do not wear clothing that needs to be removed over the head; instead, wear clothes that fasten in the front.
- Do not rest eyeglasses or sunglasses on the nose for at least a month after surgery. If you have to wear glasses, use cheek rests or tape the glasses on the forehead.
- Use SPF30 sunscreen, especially on the nose, while in sun to avoid permanent discoloration of the nose.
- Limit dietary intake of sodium to help the swelling heal faster.
- Eat a high-fiber diet to avoid constipation, as this will put pressure on the surgical site.

HOW IS RHINOPLASTY DIFFERENT FROM SEPTOPLASTY?

Rhinoplasty is performed to change the way that the nose looks (the cosmetic shape of the nose) or to improve breathing through the nose. Septoplasty is done to straighten the wall (septum) that divides nasal passages inside the nose when it is crooked and makes it harder to breathe through the nose. Often a septoplasty is combined with rhinoplasty.

References

1. Cunha, John P DO, FACOEP; Balentine, Jerry R DO, FACEP. "Deviated Septum Facts," MedicineNet, May 7, 2011.
2. Robinson, Jennifer MD. "Deviated Septum," WebMD, December 12, 2018.
3. "Septoplasty," Mayoclinic, January 3, 2018.

Section 40.6 | Liposuction and Abdominoplasty

The liposuction and abdominoplasty (tummy tuck) are two different surgical procedures done to change the appearance of the abdomen (midsection). Both procedures are supposed to make the stomach appear flatter, tighter, and smaller. These procedures are performed by plastic surgeons, and are considered "cosmetic," and therefore, they are not covered by health insurance. However, there are some important differences between them.

WHAT IS LIPOSUCTION?

Liposuction is suitable when there is a need to remove small fat deposits that are usually found in the hips, thighs, buttocks, or stomach area. This procedure will remove fat deposits from the targeted area, reducing bulges and enhancing contour. There are two major types of liposuction known as "ultrasound-assisted liposuction" (UAL); and "laser-assisted liposuction," or "SmartLipo." However, liposuction is not recommended as a weight-loss tool for people who are obese.

WHAT IS ABDOMINOPLASTY?

The abdominoplasty, removes excess fat from the abdomen, along with the removal of excess skin. Pregnancy or significant shifts in weight can stretch out the skin that surrounds the stomach. The appearance of a flat and contoured midsection can be achieved using abdominoplasty. This procedure may involve bringing the rectus abdominis (sit-up muscles) back together if they have been stretched or separated during pregnancy.

Abdominoplasty is not to be considered if a person:
- Has body mass index over 30
- Is considering getting pregnant
- Is actively trying to lose weight
- Has a chronic heart condition

THE PROCEDURES
Liposuction Surgery Procedure
The patient is either intravenously (IV) sedated for this procedure or a local anesthetic is administered in the abdomen. Once the area is numb, small incisions are made around the site of the fat deposits. A thin tube (cannula) will be inserted underneath the skin to loosen the fat cells. A medical vacuum is then used to suction out the dislodged fat deposits. Several sessions might be required to achieve the desired result.

Abdominoplasty Surgery Procedure
The patient is sedated using general anesthesia, and an incision is made at the bottom of the skin that covers the abdominal wall. Once the muscles are exposed, the muscles in the abdominal wall are sewn together if they have become stretched out. The skin over the abdomen is then pulled tight, the excess skin is trimmed off, and finally, the incision is closed with sutures. It is done in one procedure, and the entire surgery usually takes two to three hours.

OUTCOMES OF THE PROCEDURES
Although liposuction and abdominoplasty have permanent results, significant weight gain after either procedure can alter this outcome.

Liposuction Outcomes
Liposuction tends to give the appearance of a flatter, more proportioned abdomen, following recovery from the procedure. These outcomes are expected to be permanent. However, studies show that up to a year after the procedure, if there is weight gain, fat will reaccumulate in the body, though not typically in the areas that were suctioned.

Abdominoplasty Outcomes
After the abdominoplasty, the results are considered to be permanent. The abdominal wall will be more stable and strong. The excess

skin that has been removed does not return unless fluctuation in weight or a subsequent pregnancy stretches out the area again.

COMPLICATIONS OF THE PROCEDURES

Side effects occur as a result of any form of surgery; however, each procedure poses different risks.

Liposuction Complications

With liposuction, the risk of complications increases if it is performed in a large area of the body. Performing multiple procedures during the same operation can also increase the risk.

Possible risks include:

- **Numbness.** The affected area might feel numb for a while; however, it may become permanent over time.
- **Contour irregularities.** The fat that is removed creates a jagged or wavy impression on the epidermis (top layer of the skin), making the skin appear less smooth.
- **Fluid accumulation or seromas.** Temporary pockets of fluid may form under the skin.

Rare risks include:

- **Infection.** There is a possibility of infection occurring at the site of the incision.
- **Internal organ puncture.** An organ might be punctured if the cannula penetrates too deeply.
- **Fat embolism.** A loosened piece of fat breaks away, and gets trapped in a blood vessel travelling to the lungs or brain.

Abdominoplasty Complications

Abdominoplasty has been shown to have more complication risks than other cosmetic procedures. Studies show that 8.5 percent of people who had a tummy tuck needed to return to the hospital because of some kind of complication. Wound complications and infections were among the most common reasons for readmission.

Other possible risks include:
- **Changes in sensation.** Repositioning the abdominal tissue may affect the superficial sensory nerves in this area, as well as in the upper thighs, which causes a feeling of numbness in those areas.
- **Fluid accumulation.** Temporary pockets of fluid may form under the skin, similar to liposuction.
- **Tissue necrosis.** Fatty tissue deep within the abdominal area may get damaged in some cases. Tissue that dies or does not heal must be removed by the surgeon.

References

1. "Liposuction versus Tummy Tuck: Which Option Is Better," Healthline, February 26, 2019.
2. "Liposuction: What You Should Know," WebMD, August 6, 2018.

Section 40.7 | Skin Grafting

Skin grafting is a surgical procedure through which skin from one area of the body is removed and transplanted to a different area of the body.

Common reasons for a skin graft include:
- Skin infections
- Deep burns
- Large, open wounds
- Venous ulcers, pressure ulcers (bed sores), or diabetic ulcers that do not heal properly
- Skin cancer surgery
- Vitiligo
- Contracture (when skin becomes too tight while healing from an injury and limits joint movements)

TYPES OF SKIN GRAFT

Depending on the donor type (origin), skin grafts can be classified into:

- **Autograft or autologous graft**—Skin obtained from a different part of the patient's body.
- **Allograft or heterologous graft**—Skin obtained from another person or from a cadaver.
- **Xenograft or heterograft**—Skin taken from other species, especially pigs.
- **Synthetic skin substitutes**—Artificial skin manufactured in laboratory. They can be epidermal (keratinocyte cultures), dermal, or dermo epidermal (artificial skin).

Depending on the thickness of the graft, skin grafts can be classified into:

- **Split-thickness grafts**
  A split-thickness graft involves removing the top layer of the skin (epidermis) along with a portion of the deeper layer of the skin (dermis). These layers are taken from the "donor site," the area where healthy skin is found. Common donor sites are front or outer thigh, abdomen, buttocks, or back.
  Split-thickness grafts are used to cover large areas. These grafts are fragile and typically have a shiny or smooth appearance. They may also look paler compared to the adjoining skin. Split-thickness grafts do not grow as readily as normal skin; therefore, children who get them may require additional grafts as they grow older.
- **Full-thickness grafts**
  A full-thickness graft is done by removing all of the epidermis and dermis from the donor site. These are usually harvested from the abdomen, forearm, groin, or the collarbone. They tend to be smaller pieces of skin, as the donor site is usually pulled together and closed in a straight-line incision with stitches or staples.

Full-thickness grafts are generally used for small wounds on highly visible parts of the body, particularly the face. Full-thickness grafts blend well with the skin around it and usually, presents a better cosmetic result.

THE PROCEDURE

A surgeon will begin by removing the healthy skin from the donor site and placing it over the transplant area and securing it with a surgical dressing, stitches, or staples. The doctor also covers the donor area with a dressing that will cover the wound without sticking to it. A pressure bandage is applied over the transplanted graft. A vacuum apparatus known as a "wound VAC" may be placed over the area for the first three to five days to control drainage and enhance the chances of survival for the graft.

THE HEALING PROCESS

Split-thickness skin grafting requires lesser time to heal when compared to full-thickness grafts. The graft should begin to grow new blood vessels within the first 36 hours after surgery, which then attaches to the skin that surrounds it.

The following steps are to be taken to protect a skin graft after the surgery:

- Wearing a dressing for one or two weeks, and avoiding getting it wet
- Protecting the graft from trauma for three to four weeks, including avoiding being hit or doing any exercise that might stretch or injure the graft
- Getting physical therapy, if the surgeon recommends it

COMPLICATIONS OF SKIN GRAFTING

Risks due to a skin grafting include:

- Bleeding
- Chronic pain (rare occurrence)
- Infection
- Losing or rejection of the grafted skin

- Increased reduction or loss of skin sensation
- Scarring
- Skin discoloration
- Uneven skin surface

References

1. "Skin Graft," Healthline, May 30, 2017.
2. "Skin Graft," URAC, March 12, 2019.
3. "What to Expect from a Skin Graft," March 4, 2020.
4. Conde, Elena "Types of Skin Grafts to Cover Chronic Wounds: Which One Should You Choose," Elena Conde Montero, January 17, 2019.

Part 4 | Managing Pain and Surgical Complications

Chapter 41 | **Managing Pain after Surgery**

PAIN MANAGEMENT
What Is Pain?

Pain is an uncomfortable feeling that tells you something may be wrong in your body. When there is an injury to your body (e.g., surgery, broken bones) or if you have a painful disease or condition (e.g., sickle-cell disease, arthritis, cancer), tiny nerve cells send messages to your brain. Pain medicine blocks or lessens these messages.

Why Is Pain Control Important?

Pain can affect your activity, appetite, sleep, energy, mood, and relationships. It can also affect your rate of recovery from the surgery. Pain relief allows you to start walking and doing your breathing exercises so that you can get your strength back faster and leave the hospital sooner after surgery. Pain relief helps you avoid problems such as pneumonia and blood clots, enjoy greater comfort while you heal, and may help you heal faster.

Can Pain Be Relieved?

Pain in almost all cases can be controlled. Although pain is a common experience after surgery and with many types of illness, most patients with postoperative pain can be kept comfortable with simple treatment.

This chapter includes text excerpted from "VHA/DoD Clinical Practice Guideline for the Management of Postoperative Pain in the Primary Care Settings," U.S. Department of Veterans Affairs (VA), May 2002.

If You Are Taking Pain Medications Already, Does It Make a Difference?

Be sure to notify your healthcare provider if you are already taking pain medications. You may require a higher dose of pain medicine to relieve your pain.

How Can You Help the Doctors and Nurses "Measure" Your Pain?

Use a pain scale to communicate your pain. For pain management to work, we need to have some way to help your doctors and nurses understand how much you are hurting. You will be asked to use a "pain rating scale" to do this. For example, on a scale of 0 to 10, with 0 being no pain, and 10 being the worst pain you can imagine, how much pain do you have right now?

PAIN RELIEF GOAL

Talk to your doctors and nurses about setting a pain control goal (such as having no pain that's worse than 3 on the scale and being able to turn, cough, take deep breaths, walk, take care of yourself at home etc.). The goal is to relieve your pain without causing too many side effects. It may not be possible to eliminate all your pain after surgery. Our goal is to control your pain so that you are able to function well enough to walk, cough, and deep breathe after surgery. This will allow you to recover more easily following surgery.

When Should You Ask for Pain Medication?

Ask for pain medication when your pain first begins. If you know your pain will worsen when walking or doing breathing exercises, ask for pain medication first. It is harder to ease pain once it has taken hold. This is a key step in proper pain control.

How Soon after You Take Medicine Should Your Pain Be Relieved?

Your pain should be relieved within 30 to 45 minutes of taking pain medication. If it is not relieved, report this to your nurse or physician so that they can make prompt adjustments to your pain treatment plan.

Will You Become Addicted to the Pain Medicine?

It is very unlikely that you will become addicted to pain medication when used as prescribed by your physician. Studies have shown that becoming addicted to pain medication is very rare unless you already have a problem with substance abuse.

How Can Your Pain Be Controlled?

Both drug and nondrug methods can be successful in helping to prevent and control pain. The most common methods are described below. You, your doctor, and your nurse will decide which ones are right for you.

MEDICINES FOR PAIN RELIEF
Nonsteroidal Anti-Inflammatory Drugs

Acetaminophen (e.g., Tylenol) will relieve mild to moderate pain and soreness. Aspirin and ibuprofen (e.g., Motrin) will reduce swelling and soreness and relieve mild to moderate pain.

BENEFITS

- These medicines can lessen or eliminate the need for stronger medicines (e.g., morphine or another opioid).

RISKS

- Most nonsteroidal anti-inflammatory drugs (NSAIDs) interfere with blood clotting. They may cause nausea, stomach bleeding, or kidney problems. For severe pain, an opioid usually must be added.

Opioids

Morphine, oxycodone, codeine, and other opioids are most often used for acute pain such as short-term pain after surgery.

BENEFITS

- These medicines are effective for severe pain and they do not cause bleeding in the stomach or elsewhere.
- It is rare for a patient to become addicted as a result of taking opioids for postoperative pain.

RISKS

- Opioids may cause drowsiness, nausea, constipation, itching or interfere with breathing or urination.

Local Anesthetics

These drugs (e.g., bupivacaine) are given either near the incision, near nerves or through a small tube in your back to block the nerves that transmit pain signals.

BENEFITS

- Local anesthetics are effective for severe pain.
- Injections or infusions at the incision site block pain from that site.
- There is little or no risk of drowsiness, constipation, or breathing problems.
- Local anesthetics reduce the need for opioid use.

RISKS

- Repeated injections or continuous infusions are needed to maintain pain relief.
- Average epidural doses may cause some patients to have weakness in their legs or dizziness.

NONDRUG MEASURES FOR PAIN RELIEF
Education

Learning about the operation and the pain expected afterward may reduce anxiety and pain

BENEFITS
- Reduces anxiety; no equipment needed.
- There are no risks; however, patient attention and cooperation with staff are required.

Relaxation
Simple techniques such as abdominal breathing and jaw relaxation can help to increase your comfort after surgery.

BENEFITS
- Relaxation techniques are easy to learn, and they can help to reduce anxiety.
- After instruction, you can use relaxation at any time.
- No equipment is needed.

RISKS
- There are no risks, but you will need instruction from your healthcare provider.

EXAMPLE: SLOW RHYTHMIC BREATHING FOR RELAXATION
1. Breathe in slowly and deeply.
2. As you breathe out slowly, feel yourself beginning to relax; feel the tension leaving your body.
3. Now breathe in and out slowly and regularly, at whatever rate is comfortable for you. You may wish to try abdominal breathing. If you do not know how to do abdominal breathing, ask your nurse for help.
4. To help you focus on your breathing and breathe slowly and rhythmically: Breathe in as you say silently to yourself, "in, two, three." Breathe out as you say silently to yourself: "out, two, three." Or:
5. Each time you breathe out, say silently to yourself a word such as 'peace' or 'relax.'

6. You may imagine that you are doing this in a place that is very calming and relaxing for you, such as lying in the sun at the beach.
7. Do steps 1 through 4 only once or repeat steps 3 and 4 for up to 20 minutes.
8. End with a slow deep breath. As you breathe out say to yourself, "I feel alert and relaxed."

Additional Points

If you intend to do this for more than a few seconds, try to get in a comfortable position in a quiet place. You may close your eyes or focus on an object. This breathing exercise may be used for only a few seconds or up to 20 minutes.

Physical Agents

Cold packs, support of surgical site while moving, mild exercise such as walking, massage, rest, heat, and transcutaneous electrical nerve stimulation (TENS) are some nondrug pain relief methods that might be used following surgery.

BENEFITS

- In general, physical agents are safe and have no side effects.
- TENS, which stands for transcutaneous electrical nerve stimulation is often helpful; it is quick to act and can be controlled by the patient.
- Walking is very beneficial in relieving gas pains.

RISKS

- There are few risks related to the use of physical techniques.
- Your physician should approve the use of heat or cold after surgery.
- If TENS is used, there is some cost and staff time involved for purchasing the machine and instructing patients in its use.

Distraction

Distraction prevents or lessens the perception of pain by focusing attention on sensations unrelated to pain. The goals of distraction are to increase pain tolerance and perceived control and to decrease pain intensity. This technique can involve all the senses.

BENEFITS
- Distraction is safe and has no side effects.
- It can be individualized to each person's interests.
- It can include music, videos, reading, humor, and television.

RISKS
- There are no risks related to the use of distraction for pain control.

Hypnosis

Hypnosis is a state of focused attention to allow distraction from external stimuli. The induction of this state has been shown to improve pain management.

BENEFITS
- Hypnosis is safe and decreases anxiety.

RISKS
- There is a need for a professional trained in hypnosis to assist this procedure.
- It does not work with all patients.

HOW ARE PAIN MEDICINES GIVEN?
Oral Medication

Pills (tablets or capsules) and liquid taken by mouth.

BENEFITS
- Tablets and liquids cause less discomfort than injections into muscle or fat, and they can work just as well.

- They are inexpensive, simple to give, and easy to use at home.

RISKS
- These medicines cannot be used if nothing can be taken by mouth or if you are nauseated or vomiting.
- There may be a delay in pain relief since you must ask for the medicine and wait for it to be brought to you. Also, these medicines take time (30 to 60 minutes) to take full effect.

Intramuscular or Subcutaneous
An injection or "shot" of medicine given into a muscle or fat.

BENEFITS
- Medicine given by injection into fat or muscle is effective even if you are nauseated or vomiting;
- Injections are simple to give.
- They do not require intravenous access.
- This technique is successfully used to control moderate to severe pain in all regions of the body.

RISKS
- The injection site is usually painful for a short time.
- There are possibilities of infection, sterile abscess, or peripheral nerve injury.
- Medicines given by injection are more expensive than tablets or liquids.
- Pain relief may be delayed while you ask the nurse for medicine and wait for the shot to be drawn up and given.
- Due to the variable absorption and the time and staff necessary to administer, other routes are preferred.

Patient-Controlled Analgesia or Intravenous
Intravenous (IV) is an injection or "shot" of medication given into a vein. IV patient-controlled analgesia (PCA) allows you to control

when you get IV pain medication. When you begin to feel pain, you press a button to inject the pain medicine through the IV into your vein.

BENEFITS
- Medicines given by injection into a vein are fully absorbed and act quickly.
- This method is well suited for the relief of brief episodes of pain.
- When an IV PCA pump is used you can control your doses of pain medicine.

RISKS
- A small tube must be inserted in a vein.
- You must want to use the pump and learn how and when to give yourself doses of medicine if you use IV PCA.

Regional Analgesia
Local anesthetics injections along a nerve that provide pain relief to a specific area of the body and a decrease in systemic side effects.

BENEFITS
- Limiting the analgesia to a region of the body may allow for reducing or eliminating other types of pain medication.
- Reducing the need for other types of pain medication may reduce the incidence of adverse effects.

RISKS
- This technique requires knowledgeable providers and specialized equipment.
- If a single administration is used, there is a limited duration of action, so these patients may require some of the other methods of pain relief also.

Epidural or Spinal

Medication is given by injection or through a small tube placed in your back (epidural space or into the spinal fluid). The tube may be connected to a pump, which delivers pain medicine. Some pumps allow you to press a button to inject the pain medicine while others provide a continuous flow of medication.

BENEFITS

- This method works well when you have chest surgery or an operation on the lower parts of your body.
- These methods provide excellent pain relief with minimal side effects from the medications because they are given in lower doses.

RISKS

- Staff must be specially trained to place a small tube in the back and to watch for problems that can appear hours after pain medicine is given.
- A spinal anesthetic may only provide relief for the duration of the operation and you may require medications by other routes after the operation.
- You may not be allowed to walk or required to walk with assistance only while an epidural catheter is in place.
- You may also experience difficulty urinating that may require a urinary catheter to be placed.

Rectal

Medication in a suppository placed into the rectum.

BENEFITS

- This method is inexpensive, simple to give, and easy to use at home.

RISKS

- Some people do not like this route.

Managing Pain after Surgery

- There may be a delay in pain relief since you must ask for the medicine and wait for it to be brought to you.
- Also, these medicines take time (30 to 60 minutes) to take full effect.

Chapter 42 | **Postoperative Complications**

There are instances where patients have experienced complications postsurgery. There are a few discomforts and complication discomforts that are most common after undergoing a surgery.

WHAT ARE POSTSURGERY DISCOMFORTS?

The following are some discomforts experienced by patients postsurgery:

- Nausea or vomiting after being subjected to general anesthesia
- The tube that is used in the windpipe to support breathing during surgery causes sore throat
- Swelling and pain around the incision area
- Feeling restless and sleepless during the first few days after surgery due to pain
- Feeling thirsty
- Constipation and gas formation

WHAT ARE POSTSURGERY COMPLICATIONS?
Shock

Shock happens due to low blood pressure that slows down the blood flow throughout the body. Spine injury, blood loss, metabolic problems, and infection causes shock. Treatment for shock includes:

- Reducing heat loss
- Support with a breathing machine

- Stopping blood loss
- Giving intravenous (IV) fluids or blood

Bleeding

Swift blood loss from the surgical site can lead to shock. Treatments may include:

- Blood transfusion
- Additional surgery to control the bleeding
- IV fluids or blood plasma

Wound Infection

Infection occurs when bacteria enter the site of surgery. Infections can delay healing and can spread to nearby organs or tissues or distant areas through the bloodstream. Treatments include:

- Antibiotics
- Performing another surgery to clean or drain the infected area

Deep Vein Thrombosis

A blood clot in a large vein deep inside an arm, leg, or other such parts of the body is called "deep vein thrombosis" (DVT). Symptoms of DVT include pain, swelling, tenderness, and skin redness in leg, arm, or other areas. Call your healthcare provider if you have such symptoms. Compression stockings are used to prevent DVT and these stockings are used for treatment as well.

Lung Problems

Lung problems occur when patients are not able to breath and cough within 48 hours of surgery. The other reasons may include pneumonia or from inhaling food or fluids into the airways. The symptoms of lung problems are:

- Wheezing
- Chest pain
- Shortness of breath
- Fever
- Cough

Pulmonary Embolism

Pulmonary embolism is when the clot can break away from the vein and travel to the lungs. These clots in the lungs can cut off the blood flow, which is a serious medical emergency and can even cause death. The symptoms of pulmonary embolism include:

- Chest pain
- Troubled breathing
- Coughing up blood
- Sweating
- Very low blood pressure
- Rapid heartbeat
- Fainting and light headedness

Treatment varies depending on the size and location of the blood clot. Treatments may include:

- Blood-thinner medicines to prevent clots
- Thrombolytic medicines to dissolve clots
- Surgery

Urinary Retention

Urinary retention is when the patient is not able to empty their urinary bladder. Surgeries or certain anesthesia can causes this and it is often treated by using a catheter (thin tube) to drain the urine. The tube is kept in place till bladder control is regained. Medicines to stimulate the bladder may be prescribed to patients at times.

Reaction to Anesthesia

Reaction to anesthesia happens but it is rare. The symptoms vary and they can range from severe to mild. Treatments to allergic reactions caused due to anesthesia include prescribing other medicines to treat allergies.

Make sure to inform the healthcare team about any allergies before surgery to minimize the risk postsurgery.

HOW TO PREVENT POSTOPERATIVE COMPLICATIONS

There are a few basic principles that can be followed to prevent postoperative complications.

The preventive measures are:

- Weight control
- Quitting smoking
- Following a healthy diet with supplements to correct any deficiencies, such as anemia
- Stopping any medication well in advance if your healthcare provider has advised to stop
- Making sure to follow the instructions about when to have the last food and drink before surgery

The following are certain aspects that the surgeon and anesthetist should monitor to avoid postoperative complications:

- Preoperative checkups to analyze for medical conditions, such as anemia or high blood pressure that could be corrected prior to surgery
- To evaluate and discuss the importance of fitness and to make a plan for fitness after surgery
- An action plan to reduce the risk of thrombosis
- Antibiotics should be prescribed to "cover" surgery with chances for risk of infection
- Specialist postoperative nurses and doctors to monitor the patients after the surgery
- Careful observation of fluid balance and pain relief during and after surgery
- Early mobilization

References

1. "After Surgery: Discomforts and Complications," University of Rochester Medical Center, February 17, 2019.
2. Loweth, Mary. "Common Postoperative Complications," Patientinfo, July 30, 2017.

Chapter 43 | Infection and Surgery

Chapter Contents

Section 43.1 | Surgical Site Infections (SSIs)

This section includes text excerpted from "Frequently Asked Questions about Surgical Site Infections," Centers for Disease Control and Prevention (CDC), May 9, 2019.

WHAT IS A SURGICAL SITE INFECTION?

A surgical site infection (SSI) is an infection that occurs after surgery in the part of the body where the surgery took place. Surgical site infections may sometimes be superficial infections involving the skin only. Other surgical site infections are more serious and may involve tissues under the skin, organs, or implanted material.

Symptoms include:
- Redness and pain around the area where you had surgery
- Drainage of cloudy fluid from your surgical wound
- Fever

CAN SURGICAL SITE INFECTIONS BE TREATED?

Yes. Most SSIs can be treated with antibiotics. The type of antibiotic given depends on the bacteria (germs) causing the infection. Sometimes patients with SSIs also need another surgery to treat the infection.

WHAT ARE SOME OF THE THINGS THAT HOSPITALS ARE DOING TO PREVENT SURGICAL SITE INFECTIONS?

To prevent SSIs, doctors, nurses, and other healthcare providers should follow the Centers for Disease Control and Prevention's (CDC) infection prevention guidelines including:
- Cleaning their hands and arms up to their elbows with an antiseptic agent just before the surgery
- Cleaning their hands with soap and water or an alcohol-based hand rub before and after caring for each patient
- If indicated, removing some of your hair immediately before your surgery using electric clippers if the hair is in the same area where the procedure will occur

- Wearing special hair covers, masks, gowns, and gloves during surgery to keep the surgery area clean
- When indicated, giving you antibiotics before your surgery starts. In most cases, you should get antibiotics within 60 minutes before the surgery starts and the antibiotics should be stopped within 24 hours after surgery
- Cleaning the skin at the site of your surgery with a special soap that kills germs

WHAT CAN YOU DO TO HELP PREVENT SURGICAL SITE INFECTIONS?
Before Surgery

- **Tell your doctor about other medical problems you may have**. Health problems such as allergies, diabetes, and obesity could affect your surgery and your treatment.
- **Quit smoking**. Patients who smoke get more infections. Talk to your doctor about how you can quit before your surgery.
- **Do not shave near where you will have surgery**. Shaving with a razor can irritate your skin and make it easier to develop an infection.

At the Time of Surgery

Speak up if someone tries to shave you with a razor before surgery. Ask why you need to be shaved and talk with your surgeon if you have any concerns.

After Surgery

- If you do not see your healthcare providers clean their hands, please ask them to do so.
- Family and friends who visit you should not touch the surgical wound or dressings.
- Family and friends should clean their hands with soap and water or an alcohol-based hand rub before and after

visiting you. If you do not see them clean their hands, please ask them to do so.

- Make sure you understand how to care for your wound before you leave the hospital.
- Always clean your hands before and after caring for your wound.
- Make sure you know who to contact if you have questions or problems after you get home.
- If you have any symptoms of an infection such as redness and pain at the surgery site, drainage, or fever, call your doctor immediately.

Section 43.2 | Catheter-Associated Urinary Tract Infections (CAUTIs)

This section contains text excerpted from the following sources: Text in this section begins with excerpts from "Catheter-Associated Urinary Tract Infections (CAUTI)," Centers for Disease Control and Prevention (CDC), October 16, 2015. Reviewed April 2020; Text beginning with the heading "What Is a Urinary Catheter?" is excerpted from "Frequently Asked Questions about Catheter-Associated Urinary Tract Infections," Centers for Disease Control and Prevention (CDC), November 24, 2010. Reviewed April 2020.

A urinary tract infection (UTI) is an infection involving any part of the urinary system, including urethra, bladder, ureters, and kidney. Some of the common symptoms of a urinary tract infection are burning or pain in the lower abdomen (that is, below the stomach), fever, burning during urination, or an increase in the frequency of urination. UTIs are the most common type of healthcare-associated infection (HAI) reported to the National Healthcare Safety Network (NHSN). Among UTIs acquired in the hospital, approximately 75 percent are associated with a urinary catheter, which is a tube inserted into the bladder through the urethra to drain urine. Between 15 to 25 percent of hospitalized patients receive urinary catheters during their hospital stay. The most important risk factor for developing a catheter-associated UTI (CAUTI) is prolonged use of the urinary catheter. Therefore, catheters should only be used for appropriate indications and should be removed as soon as they are no longer needed.

WHAT IS A URINARY CATHETER?

A urinary catheter is a hollow, partially flexible tube that collects urine from the bladder and leads to a drainage bag. There are three types of urinary catheters: indwelling catheters (urethral or suprapubic catheter), intermittent catheters, and external catheters (condom catheter).

An indwelling or a suprapubic urinary catheter is a drainage tube that is inserted into the urinary bladder through the urethra, is left in place, and is connected to a closed collection system. It is surgically inserted into the bladder through an incision above the pubis. Alternative methods of urinary drainage may be employed in some patients. Intermittent ("in-and-out") catheterization involves brief insertion of a catheter into the bladder through the urethra to drain urine at intervals. An external catheter is a urine containment device that fits over or adheres to the genitalia and is attached to a urinary drainage bag. The most commonly used external catheter is a soft flexible sheath that fits over the penis ("condom" catheter).

WHAT IS A CATHETER-ASSOCIATED URINARY TRACT INFECTION?

A catheter-associated urinary tract infection (CAUTI) occurs when germs (usually bacteria) enter the urinary tract through the urinary catheter and cause infection. CAUTIs have been associated with increased morbidity, mortality, healthcare costs, and length of stay. The risk of CAUTI can be reduced by ensuring that catheters are used only when needed and removed as soon as possible; that catheters are placed using proper aseptic technique; and that the closed sterile drainage system is maintained.

CAN CATHETER-ASSOCIATED URINARY TRACT INFECTIONS BE TREATED?

Yes, most CAUTIs can be treated with antibiotics and/or removal or change of the catheter. The healthcare provider will determine the best treatment for each patient.

WHAT ARE SOME OF THE THINGS THE HOSPITALS ARE DOING TO PREVENT CATHETER-ASSOCIATED URINARY TRACT INFECTION

Hospitals emphasizes the proper use, insertion, and maintenance of urinary catheters in different healthcare settings. It also presents effective quality improvement programs that healthcare facilities can use to prevent CAUTIs.

WHAT CAN PATIENTS TO DO HELP PREVENT CATHETER-ASSOCIATED URINARY TRACT INFECTION?

Patients with a urinary catheter can take the following precautions to prevent CAUTI:

- Understand why the catheter is needed and ask the healthcare provider frequently if the catheter is still needed.
- If the patient has a long-term catheter, they must clean their hands before and after touching the catheter.
- Check the position of the urine bag; it should always be below the level of the bladder.
- Do not tug or pull on the tubing.
- Do not twist or kink the catheter tubing.

Section 43.3 | Central Line-Associated Bloodstream Infection (CLABSI)

This section includes text excerpted from "Central Line-Associated Bloodstream Infections: Resources for Patients and Healthcare Providers," Centers for Disease Control and Prevention (CDC), February 7, 2011. Reviewed April 2020.

Central line-associated bloodstream infections (CLABSIs) result in thousands of deaths each year and billions of dollars in added costs to the United States healthcare system, yet these infections are preventable. The Centers for Disease Control and Prevention (CDC) is providing guidelines and tools to the healthcare community to help end CLABSIs.

WHAT IS A CENTRAL LINE?

A central line (also known as a "central venous catheter") is a catheter (tube) that doctors often place in a large vein in the neck, chest, or groin to give medication or fluids or to collect blood for medical tests. You may be familiar with intravenous catheters (also known as "IVs") that are used frequently to give medicine or fluids into a vein near the skin's surface (usually on the arm or hand), for short periods of time. Central lines are different from IVs because central lines access a major vein that is close to the heart and can remain in place for weeks or months and be much more likely to cause serious infection. Central lines are commonly used in intensive care units.

WHAT IS A CENTRAL LINE-ASSOCIATED BLOODSTREAM INFECTION?

A CLABSI is a serious infection that occurs when germs (usually bacteria or viruses) enter the bloodstream through the central line. Healthcare providers must follow a strict protocol when inserting the line to make sure the line remains sterile and a CLABSI does not occur. In addition to inserting the central line properly, healthcare providers must use stringent infection control practices each time they check the line or change the dressing. Patients who get a CLABSI have a fever, and might also have red skin and soreness around the central line. If this happens, healthcare providers can do tests to learn if there is an infection present.

WHAT ARE SOME OF THE THINGS THAT HEALTHCARE PROVIDERS ARE DOING TO PREVENT CENTRAL LINE-ASSOCIATED BLOODSTREAM INFECTION?

Healthcare providers can take the following steps to help prevent CLABSIs:
- Follow recommended central line insertion practices to prevent infection when the central line is placed, including:
  - Perform hand hygiene.
  - Apply appropriate skin antiseptic.

- Ensure that the skin prep agent has completely dried before inserting the central line.
- Use all five maximal sterile barrier precautions:
  - Sterile gloves
  - Sterile gown
  - Cap
  - Mask
  - Large sterile drape
- Once the central line is in place:
  - Follow recommended central line maintenance practices.
  - Wash their hands with soap and water or an alcohol-based hand rub before and after touching the line.
- Remove a central line as soon as it is no longer needed. The sooner a catheter is removed, the less likely the chance of infection.

WHAT CAN PATIENTS DO TO HELP PREVENT CENTRAL LINE-ASSOCIATED BLOODSTREAM INFECTION?

Here are some ways patients can protect themselves from CLABSI:

- Research the hospital, if possible, to learn about its CLABSI rate.
- Speak up about any concerns so that healthcare personnel are reminded to follow the best infection prevention practices.
- Ask a healthcare provider if the central line is absolutely necessary. If so, ask them to help you understand the need for it and how long it will be in place.
- Pay attention to the bandage and the area around it. If the bandage comes off or if the bandage or area around it is wet or dirty, tell a healthcare worker right away.
- Do not get the central line or the central line insertion site wet.
- Tell a healthcare worker if the area around the catheter is sore or red or if the patient has a fever or chills.
- Do not let any visitors touch the catheter or tubing.

- The patient should avoid touching the tubing as much as possible.
- In addition, everyone visiting the patient must wash their hands—before and after they visit.

Section 43.4 | Steps to Reduce Healthcare-Associated Infections (HAIs)

This section includes text excerpted from "Healthcare-Associated Infections," Office of Disease Prevention and Health Promotion (ODPHP), U.S. Department of Health and Human Services (HHS), February 6, 2016. Reviewed April 2020.

Healthcare-associated infections (HAIs) are infections that patients get while receiving treatment for medical or surgical conditions, and many HAIs are preventable. Modern healthcare employs many types of invasive devices and procedures to treat patients and to help them recover. Infections can be associated with procedures (like surgery) and the devices used in medical procedures, such as catheters or ventilators. HAIs are important causes of morbidity and mortality in the United States and are associated with a substantial increase in healthcare costs each year. At any one time in the United States, 1 in every 25 hospitalized patients are affected by an HAI.

HAIs occur in all types of care settings, including:
- Acute care hospitals
- Ambulatory surgical centers
- Dialysis facilities
- Outpatient care (e.g., physicians' offices and healthcare clinics)
- Long-term care facilities (e.g., nursing homes and rehabilitation facilities)

The establishment of the Healthcare-Associated Infections objectives for Healthy People 2020 reflects the commitment of the U.S. Department of Health and Human Services (HHS) to preventing HAIs. These high-priority objectives address central line-associated bloodstream infections (CLABSI) and methicillin-resistant *Staphylococcus aureus* (MRSA) infections.

- A central line-associated bloodstream infection (CLABSI) is a serious HAI that occurs when germs (e.g., bacteria) enter the bloodstream through the central line (a long flexible tube placed in a large vein that empties out near the heart). These infections result in thousands of deaths each year and several million dollars in added costs to the U.S. healthcare system.
- Methicillin-resistant *Staphylococcus aureus* is a type of bacteria that is resistant to many antibiotics. In medical facilities, MRSA causes life-threatening bloodstream infections, pneumonia, and surgical site infections.
- Besides these sources of HAIs, several other sources have been identified as major contributors to HAI-related illness and deaths in the National Action Plan to Prevent Healthcare-Associated Infections: Roadmap to Elimination.

Common types of HAIs include:
- Catheter-associated urinary tract infections
- Surgical site infections
- Bloodstream infections
- Pneumonia
- *Clostridium difficile* infection

WHY ARE HEALTHCARE-ASSOCIATED INFECTIONS IMPORTANT?

Healthcare-associated infections are a significant source of complications across the continuum of care and can be transmitted between different healthcare facilities. However, studies suggest that implementing existing prevention practices can lead up to a 70 percent reduction in certain HAIs. Likewise, modeling data suggests that substantial reductions in resistant bacteria, like MRSA, can be achieved through coordinated activities between healthcare facilities in a given region. The financial benefit of using these prevention practices is estimated to be $25 billion to $31.5 billion in medical cost savings.

Risk factors for HAIs can be grouped into three general categories: medical procedures and antibiotic use, organizational factors, and patient characteristics. The behaviors of healthcare providers and their interactions with the healthcare system also influence the rate of HAIs.

Studies have shown that proper education and training of healthcare workers increases compliance with and adoption of best practices (e.g., infection control, hand hygiene, attention to safety culture, and antibiotic stewardship) to prevent HAIs. Examples of best practices by a healthcare provider include careful insertion, maintenance, and prompt removal of catheters, as well as the careful use of antibiotics. Another example of a best practice is decolonization of patients with an evidence-based method to reduce transmission of MRSA in hospitals.

EMERGING ISSUES IN HEALTHCARE-ASSOCIATED INFECTIONS

Healthy People 2020 objectives measure progress toward reducing the incidence of CLABSI and invasive MRSA infections. However, more work needs to be done. In addition, there are other major types of HAIs that HHS is working to prevent, including those caused by antibiotic-resistant pathogens:

- Catheter-associated urinary tract infections
- Surgical site infections
- Ventilator-associated events/ventilator-associated pneumonia
- *Clostridium difficile* infections

Research suggests that many of these infections are preventable. Efforts are underway to expand implementation of strategies known to prevent HAIs, advance development of effective prevention tools, and explore new prevention approaches. Many efforts to prevent HAIs have focused on acute care settings. Increasingly, healthcare delivery, including complex procedures, is being shifted to outpatient settings such as ambulatory surgical centers, end-stage renal disease facilities, and long-term care facilities. These settings often have limited capacity for oversight and infection control compared to hospital-based settings. Because patients with HAIs, including HAIs caused by antibiotic-resistance organisms, often move between various types of healthcare facilities, prevention efforts must also expand across the continuum of care. Moreover, the challenges posed by antibiotic-resistant organisms and *C. difficile* are best addressed through coordinated action among healthcare facilities in a given region.

The National Action Plan to Prevent Healthcare-Associated Infections: Roadmap to Elimination contains strategies on preventing HAIs in nonacute care hospital settings and supports further research on how to identify and control HAIs in these settings and apply evidence-based approaches for reducing HAIs.

Section 43.5 | Sepsis (Bloodstream Infection)

This section includes text excerpted from "Inpatient Care for Septicemia or Sepsis: A Challenge for Patients and Hospitals," Centers for Disease Control and Prevention (CDC), June 2011. Reviewed April 2020.

Septicemia and sepsis are serious bloodstream infections that can rapidly become life-threatening. They arise from various infections, including those of the skin, lungs, abdomen, and urinary tract. Patients with these conditions are often treated in a hospital's intensive care unit. Early aggressive treatment increases the chance of survival. In 2008, an estimated $14.6 billion was spent on hospitalizations for septicemia, and from 1997 through 2008, the inflation-adjusted aggregate costs for treating patients hospitalized for this condition increased annually on an average by 11.9 percent.

Despite high treatment expenditures, septicemia and sepsis are often fatal. Those who survive severe sepsis are more likely to have permanent organ damage, cognitive impairment, and physical disability. Septicemia is a leading cause of death.

RECENT TRENDS IN CARE FOR HOSPITAL INPATIENTS WITH THESE DIAGNOSES

The hospitalization rate of those with a principal diagnosis of septicemia or sepsis more than doubled from 2000 through 2008, increasing from 11.6 to 24.0 per 10,000 population. During the same period, the hospitalization rate for those with septicemia or sepsis as a principal or as a secondary diagnosis increased by 70 percent from 22.1 to 37.7 per 10,000 population. Reasons for these increases may include an aging population with more chronic illnesses; greater use of invasive procedures, immunosuppressive drugs, chemotherapy, and transplantation; and increasing microbial resistance to antibiotics. Increased coding of these conditions due to greater clinical awareness of septicemia or sepsis may also have occurred during the period studied.

Septicemia or sepsis treatment involves caring for sicker patients who have longer inpatient stays than those with other diagnoses. Total nationwide inpatient annual costs of treating those hospitalized for septicemia had been rising and were estimated to be $14.6 billion in 2008. Even with this expenditure, the death rate was high. Patients who do survive severe cases are more likely to have negative long-term effects on health and on cognitive and physical functioning.

The "Surviving Sepsis Campaign" was an international effort organized by physicians that developed and promoted widespread adoption of practice improvement programs grounded in evidence-based guidelines. The goal was to improve diagnosis and treatment of sepsis. Included among the guidelines were sepsis screening for high-risk patients; taking bacterial cultures soon after the patient arrived at the hospital; starting patients on broad-spectrum intravenous antibiotic therapy before the results of the cultures are obtained; identifying the source of infection and taking steps to control it (e.g., abscess drainage); administering intravenous fluids to correct a loss or decrease in blood volume; and maintaining glycemic (blood sugar) control. These and similar guidelines have been tested by a number of hospitals and have shown potential decrease in hospital mortality due to sepsis.

Chapter 44 | Gram-Negative Bacteria in Healthcare Settings

Chapter Contents

Section 44.1 | *Acinetobacter* in Healthcare Settings

This section contains text excerpted from the following sources: Text in this section begins with excerpts from "Gram-Negative Bacteria Infections in Healthcare Settings," Centers for Disease Control and Prevention (CDC), January 17, 2011. Reviewed April 2020; Text beginning with the heading "About *Acinetobacter*" is excerpted from "*Acinetobacter* in Healthcare Settings," Centers for Disease Control and Prevention (CDC), November 13, 2019.

Gram-negative bacteria cause infections including pneumonia, bloodstream infections, wound or surgical site infections, and meningitis in healthcare settings. Gram-negative bacteria are resistant to multiple drugs and are increasingly resistant to most available antibiotics. These bacteria have built-in abilities to find new ways to be resistant and can pass along genetic materials that allow other bacteria to become drug-resistant as well. The Centers for Disease Control and Prevention's (CDC) aggressive recommendations, if implemented, can prevent the spread of gram-negatives.

Gram-negative infections include those caused by *Klebsiella*, *Acinetobacter*, *Pseudomonas aeruginosa*, and *E. coli.*, as well as many other less common bacteria.

ABOUT *ACINETOBACTER*

Acinetobacter is a group of bacteria (germs) commonly found in the environment, like in soil and water. While there are many types, the most common cause of infections is *Acinetobacter baumannii*, which accounts for most *Acinetobacter* infections in humans.

Acinetobacter baumannii can cause infections in the blood, urinary tract, and lungs (pneumonia), or in wounds in other parts of the body. It can also "colonize" or live in a patient without causing infections or symptoms, especially in respiratory secretions (sputum) or open wounds.

These bacteria are constantly finding new ways to avoid the effects of the antibiotics used to treat the infections they cause. Antibiotic resistance occurs when the germs no longer respond to the antibiotics designed to kill them. If they develop resistance to the group of antibiotics called "carbapenems," they become carbapenem-resistant. When resistant to multiple antibiotics, they are multidrug-resistant. Carbapenem-resistant *Acinetobacter* are usually multidrug-resistant.

HOW COMMON ARE THESE INFECTIONS?

In 2017, carbapenem-resistant *Acinetobacter* caused an estimated 8,500 infections in hospitalized patients and 700 estimated deaths in the United States.

WHO ARE AT RISK?

Acinetobacter infections typically occur in people in healthcare settings. People most at risk include patients in hospitals, especially those who:
- Are on breathing machines (ventilators)
- Have devices, such as catheters
- Have open wounds from surgery
- Are in intensive care units
- Have prolonged hospital stays

In the United States, *Acinetobacter* infections rarely occur outside of healthcare settings. However, people who have weakened immune systems, chronic lung disease, or diabetes may be more susceptible.

HOW DOES IT SPREAD?

Acinetobacter can live for long periods of time on environmental surfaces and shared equipment if they are not properly cleaned. The germs can spread from one person to another through contact with these contaminated surfaces or equipment or though person to person spread, often via contaminated hands.

HOW CAN YOU AVOID GETTING AN INFECTION?

Patients and caregivers should:
- Keep their hands clean to avoid getting sick and spreading germs that can cause infections
  - Wash their hands with soap and water or use alcohol-based hand sanitizer, particularly before and after caring for wounds or touching a medical device

- Remind healthcare providers and caregivers to clean their hands before touching the patient or handling medical devices
- Allow healthcare staff to clean their room daily when in a healthcare setting

In addition to hand hygiene, healthcare providers should pay careful attention to recommended infection control practices, including rigorous environmental cleaning (e.g., cleaning of patient rooms and shared equipment), to reduce the risk of spreading these germs to patients.

HOW ARE THESE INFECTIONS TREATED?

Acinetobacter infections are generally treated with antibiotics. To identify the best antibiotic to treat a specific infection, healthcare providers will send a specimen (often called a "culture") to the laboratory and test any bacteria that grow against a set of antibiotics to determine which are active against the germ. The provider will then select an antibiotic based on the activity of the antibiotic and other factors, like potential side effects or interactions with other drugs.

Unfortunately, many *Acinetobacter* germs are resistant to many antibiotics, including carbapenems, which makes them difficult to treat with available antibiotics.

Section 44.2 | *Pseudomonas aeruginosa* in Healthcare Settings

This section includes text excerpted from "*Pseudomonas aeruginosa* in Healthcare Settings," Centers for Disease Control and Prevention (CDC), November 13, 2019.

ABOUT *PSEUDOMONAS AERUGINOSA*

Pseudomonas is a type of bacteria (germ) that is found commonly in the environment, like in soil and in water. Of the many different types of *Pseudomonas*, the one that most often causes infections in humans is called "*Pseudomonas aeruginosa*," which can cause infections in the blood, lungs (pneumonia), or other parts of the body after surgery.

These bacteria are constantly finding new ways to avoid the effects of the antibiotics used to treat the infections they cause. Antibiotic resistance occurs when the germs no longer respond to the antibiotics designed to kill them. If they develop resistance to several types of antibiotics, these germs can become multidrug-resistant.

HOW COMMON ARE THESE INFECTIONS?
In 2017, multidrug-resistant *Pseudomonas aeruginosa* caused an estimated 32,600 infections among hospitalized patients and 2,700 estimated deaths in the United States.

WHO ARE AT RISK?
Those most at risk include patients in hospitals, especially those:
- On breathing machines (ventilators)
- With devices, such as catheters
- With wounds from surgery or burns

HOW DOES IT SPREAD?
Pseudomonas aeruginosa lives in the environment and can be spread to people in healthcare settings when they are exposed to water or soil that is contaminated with these germs. Resistant strains of the germ can also spread in healthcare settings from one person to another through contaminated hands, equipment, or surfaces.

HOW CAN YOU AVOID GETTING AN INFECTION?
Patients and caregivers should:
- Keep their hands clean to avoid getting sick and spreading germs that can cause infections
  - Wash their hands with soap and water or use alcohol-based hand sanitizer, particularly before and after caring for wounds or touching a medical device

- Remind healthcare providers and caregivers to clean their hands before touching the patient or handling medical devices
- Allow healthcare staff to clean their room daily when in a healthcare setting

Healthcare providers should pay careful attention to recommended infection control practices, including hand hygiene and environmental cleaning (e.g., cleaning of patient rooms and shared equipment) to reduce the risk of spreading these germs to patients.

Healthcare facilities should have water management plans that help ensure water quality and reduce the risk of exposure to potentially harmful germs like *Pseudomonas aeruginosa*.

HOW ARE THESE INFECTIONS TREATED?

Pseudomonas aeruginosa infections are generally treated with antibiotics. Unfortunately, in people exposed to healthcare settings like hospitals or nursing homes, *Pseudomonas aeruginosa* infections are becoming more difficult to treat because of increasing antibiotic resistance.

To identify the best antibiotic to treat a specific infection, healthcare providers will send a specimen (often called a "culture") to the laboratory and test any bacteria that grows against a set of antibiotics to determine which are active against the germ. The provider will then select an antibiotic based on the activity of the antibiotic and other factors, like potential side effects or interactions with other drugs. For some multidrug-resistant types of *Pseudomonas aeruginosa*, treatment options might be limited.

Chapter 45 | Common Multidrug-Resistant Organisms in Healthcare Settings

Chapter Contents

Section 45.1 | Methicillin-Resistant *Staphylococcus aureus*

This section includes text excerpted from "Methicillin-Resistant *Staphylococcus aureus* (MRSA)—Healthcare Settings," Centers for Disease Control and Prevention (CDC), February 28, 2019.

HOW DOES METHICILLIN-RESISTANT *STAPHYLOCOCCUS AUREUS* SPREAD IN HEALTHCARE SETTINGS?

Methicillin-resistant *Staphylococcus aureus* (MRSA) is usually spread by direct contact with an infected wound or from contaminated hands, usually those of healthcare providers. Also, people who carry MRSA, but do not have signs of infection can spread the bacteria to others (i.e., people who are colonized).

HOW DO YOU KNOW IF METHICILLIN-RESISTANT *STAPHYLOCOCCUS AUREUS* IS THE CAUSE OF AN INFECTION?

The only way to know if MRSA is the cause of an infection is to perform a culture (a laboratory test) of the bacteria. Obtaining bacteria to culture is a procedure done by a healthcare provider.

HOW COMMON IS METHICILLIN-RESISTANT S*TAPHYLOCOCCUS AUREUS?*

The Centers for Disease Control and Prevention (CDC) is engaged in several short- and long-term MRSA surveillance (infection tracking) projects that involve collaboration with health departments, individual hospitals, and academic medical centers, among others. Understanding the burden of MRSA infections—how much is occurring, where it is happening, and how it is being spread—is essential for developing effective prevention programs and measuring their impact.

Studies show that about one in three (33%) people carry *S. aureus* bacteria in their nose, usually without any illness. About two in every 100 people carry MRSA. Although many people carry MRSA bacteria in their nose, most do not develop serious MRSA infections.

Significant progress was made to reduce MRSA bloodstream infections in healthcare from 2005–2012, when the rates of MRSA bloodstream infections decreased by 17.1 percent each year. Declines in MRSA bloodstream infections slowed from 2013–2016, when no significant change was detected.

WHERE CAN YOU FIND INFORMATION ABOUT METHICILLIN-RESISTANT *STAPHYLOCOCCUS AUREUS* AT HOSPITALS NEAR YOU?

Information about MRSA rates in hospitals across the United States is available through the National Healthcare Safety Network (NHSN), the nation's most widely used healthcare-associated infection tracking system.

IS METHICILLIN-RESISTANT *STAPHYLOCOCCUS AUREUS* AN ANTIBIOTIC RESISTANCE PROBLEM?

Yes. *Staphylococcus aureus* (staph) have become resistant to several antibiotics, making MRSA and other types of resistant staph major antibiotic-resistance problems.

CAN METHICILLIN-RESISTANT *STAPHYLOCOCCUS AUREUS* INFECTIONS BE PREVENTED?

Yes. Numerous studies, including a 2019 publication about Veterans Affairs Medical Centers, demonstrate that MRSA prevention efforts can reduce infections.

Successful MRSA prevention requires action both at the healthcare facility level, among healthcare providers and healthcare leadership.

Healthcare facilities can make prevention of MRSA infections a priority, assess their relevant data, implement prevention actions and, evaluate progress.

Healthcare providers can follow current prevention recommendations for device-and procedure-related infections, treat infections appropriately and rapidly if they do occur, and educate patients about ways to avoid infection and spread, and about early signs of sepsis.

Section 45.2 | Carbapenem-Resistant *Enterobacteriaceae*

This section includes text excerpted from "Healthcare Facilities: Information about CRE," Centers for Disease Control and Prevention (CDC), November 4, 2019.

HEALTHCARE FACILITIES: INFORMATION ABOUT CARBAPENEM-RESISTANT *ENTEROBACTERIACEAE*

Carbapenem-resistant *Enterobacteriaceae* (CRE) are a serious threat to public health. Infections with CRE are difficult to treat and have been associated with mortality rates of up to 50 percent for hospitalized patients. Due to the movement of patients throughout the healthcare system, if CRE is a problem in one facility, then typically they are a problem in other facilities in the region as well.

Healthcare Facilities Should

- Recognize these organisms as important to patient safety and adhere to public-health guidance for CRE detection, tracking, and reporting
- Ensure their clinical laboratory can accurately identify CRE and has a policy to immediately alert clinical and infection prevention staff when CRE are identified
- Understand the local epidemiology of carbapenemase-producing CRE, including prevalence in the facility and in the region. If your laboratory does not perform testing for carbapenemases, talk to your HAI coordinator about getting isolates tested through the AR Laboratory Network.
- Ensure precautions are implemented for CRE colonized or infected patients. These include:
  - Whenever possible, place patients currently or previously colonized or infected with CRE in a private room with a bathroom and dedicate noncritical equipment (e.g., stethoscope, blood pressure cuff) to CRE patients.
  - Have and enforce a policy for using gown and gloves when caring for patients with CRE.

- Have and enforce policies for healthcare personnel hand hygiene before and after contact with patient or their environment, and increase emphasis on hand hygiene on a unit caring for a patient or resident with CRE.
- Healthcare personnel should follow standard hand hygiene practices, which include use of alcohol-based hand sanitizer or, if hands are visibly soiled, washing with soap and water.
- When a patient with an unusual type of carbapenemase-producing CRE is identified in your facility, work with public health to prevent spread, including following the guidance to assess for ongoing transmission.
- Have a system to assess, at admission, if a patient has received medical care somewhere else, including other facilities or other countries. Screen patients who have had an overnight stay in a healthcare facility outside the United States in the prior six months for the presence of carbapenemase-producing CRE. Admission screening is available free of charge through the AR Lab Network. Contact your HAI coordinator for more information on accessing AR Lab Network testing.
- When transferring a patient or resident, require staff to notify the receiving facility about infection or colonization with CRE and other multidrug-resistant organisms.
- Support healthcare providers prescribing and using antibiotics appropriately.
- Participate in regional and facility-based prevention efforts designed to stop the transmission of these organisms.

Chapter 46 | **Ventilator-Associated Pneumonia**

WHAT IS A VENTILATOR-ASSOCIATED PNEUMONIA?

Ventilator-associated pneumonia (VAP) is a lung infection that develops in a person who is on a ventilator. A ventilator is a machine that is used to help a patient breathe by giving oxygen through a tube placed in a patient's mouth or nose, or through a hole in the front of the neck. An infection may occur if germs enter through the tube and get into the patient's lungs.

WHY DO PATIENTS NEED A VENTILATOR?

A patient may need a ventilator when she or he is very ill or during and after surgery. Ventilators can be life-saving, but they can also increase a patient's chance of getting pneumonia by making it easier for germs to get into the patient's lungs.

WHAT ARE SOME OF THE THINGS THAT HOSPITALS ARE DOING TO PREVENT VENTILATOR-ASSOCIATED PNEUMONIA?

To prevent VAP, doctors, nurses, and other healthcare providers can do the following things:

- Keep the head of the patient's bed raised between 30 and 45 degrees unless other medical conditions do not allow this to occur.

This chapter includes text excerpted from "Frequently Asked Questions about Ventilator-Associated Pneumonia," Centers for Disease Control and Prevention (CDC), May 9, 2019.

- Check the patient's ability to breathe on her or his own every day so that the patient can be taken off of the ventilator as soon as possible.
- Clean their hands with soap and water or an alcohol-based hand rub before and after touching the patient or the ventilator.
- Clean the inside of the patient's mouth on a regular basis.
- Clean or replace equipment between use on different patients.

WHAT CAN PATIENTS DO TO HELP PREVENT VENTILATOR-ASSOCIATED PNEUMONIA?

Patients and family members can do the following things to help prevent VAP:

Patients

- **Quit smoking**. Patients who smoke get more infections. Seek information about how to quit smoking before surgery.
- If healthcare providers do not clean their hands, ask them to do so.

Family Members

- Ask about raising the head of the bed.
- Ask when the patient will be allowed to try breathing on her or his own.
- If healthcare providers do not clean their hands, ask them to do so.
- Ask about how often healthcare providers clean the patient's mouth.

CAN VENTILATOR-ASSOCIATED PNEUMONIA BE TREATED?

Most of the time, these infections can be treated with antibiotics. The choice of antibiotics depends on which specific germs are causing the infection. The healthcare provider will decide which antibiotic is best.

Chapter 47 | **Other Surgical Complications**

Chapter Contents

Section 47.1 | Abdominal Adhesions

This section includes text excerpted from "Abdominal Adhesions," National Institute of Diabetes and Digestive and Kidney Diseases (NIDDK), June 2019.

WHAT ARE ABDOMINAL ADHESIONS?

Abdominal adhesions are bands of scar-like tissue that form inside your abdomen. The bands form between two or more organs or between organs and the abdominal wall.

Normally, the surfaces of organs and your abdominal wall do not stick together when you move. However, abdominal adhesions may cause these surfaces to become adherent, or stick together.

Abdominal adhesions can kink, twist, pull, or compress the intestines and other organs in the abdomen, causing symptoms and complications, such as intestinal obstruction or blockage.

HOW COMMON ARE ABDOMINAL ADHESIONS?

Abdominal adhesions are common and often develop after abdominal surgery. In abdominal surgery, surgeons enter a patient's abdomen through an incision, or cut. Abdominal surgery may be laparoscopic or open.

In laparoscopic surgery, which is increasingly common, surgeons make small cuts in the abdomen and insert special tools to view, remove, or repair organs and tissues. In open surgery, surgeons make a larger cut to open the abdomen.

Abdominal adhesions develop in more than 9 in every 10 people who have surgery that opens the abdomen. However, a majority of people with abdominal adhesions do not develop symptoms or complications. Abdominal adhesions are less common after laparoscopic surgery than after open surgery.

WHO IS MORE LIKELY TO HAVE ABDOMINAL ADHESIONS?

People who have had abdominal surgery are more likely to have abdominal adhesions. Among people who have had abdominal surgery, adhesions and related complications are more common in people who:

- Had emergency abdominal surgery
- Had pelvic surgery or surgery that involved the lower digestive tract, including the colon and rectum

WHAT ARE THE COMPLICATIONS OF ABDOMINAL ADHESIONS?

Abdominal adhesions can cause intestinal obstruction and female infertility.

Intestinal Obstruction

Intestinal obstruction is the partial or complete blockage of the movement of food, fluids, air, or stool through the intestines. Abdominal adhesions are the most common cause of obstruction of the small intestine. Intestinal obstruction may lead to:

- Lack of blood flow to the blocked part of the intestine and death of the blood-starved intestinal tissues
- Peritonitis-an infection of the lining of the abdominal cavity

Intestinal obstruction can be life—threatening. People with symptoms of a complete blockage—which include abdominal pain and passing no fluids, stool, or gas—should seek medical attention right away.

Female Infertility

In women, abdominal adhesions in the pelvis or inside the uterus can compress or block parts of the reproductive system and cause infertility.

WHAT ARE THE SYMPTOMS OF ABDOMINAL ADHESIONS?

In many cases, abdominal adhesions do not cause symptoms. If they do cause symptoms, chronic abdominal pain is the most common symptom.

Abdominal adhesions may cause intestinal obstruction, which can be life-threatening. If you have symptoms of intestinal obstruction, seek medical help right away.

Symptoms of intestinal obstruction may include:
- Abdominal pain
- Bloating
- Constipation
- Not passing gas
- Nausea
- Vomiting

If intestinal obstruction cuts off the blood flow to the blocked part of the intestines or leads to peritonitis, you may develop additional symptoms, such a fast heart rate or fever.

WHAT CAUSES ABDOMINAL ADHESIONS

Abdominal surgery is the most common cause of abdominal adhesions. Adhesions caused by surgery are more likely to cause symptoms and complications than adhesions related to other causes. Symptoms and complications may start any time after surgery, even many years later.

Conditions that involve inflammation or infection in the abdomen may also cause adhesions. These conditions include Crohn disease, diverticular disease, endometriosis, pelvic inflammatory disease, and peritonitis.

Other causes of abdominal adhesions include long-term peritoneal dialysis to treat kidney failure and radiation therapy to treat cancer.

In some cases, abdominal adhesions are present at birth.

HOW DO DOCTORS DIAGNOSE ABDOMINAL ADHESIONS?

Doctors use medical history, physical exam, blood tests, imaging tests, and, in some cases, surgery to diagnose abdominal adhesions.

Medical History

A doctor will ask about your symptoms and your medical history, including your history of abdominal surgery or other conditions that may cause abdominal adhesions. A doctor will also ask about your history of other diseases and disorders that may cause symptoms similar to those of abdominal adhesions.

Physical Exam

During a physical exam, the doctor may tap on your abdomen to check for tenderness or pain and use a stethoscope to listen to sounds in your abdomen.

Blood Tests

A healthcare professional will take blood samples and send the samples to a lab. Although blood tests cannot be used to diagnose abdominal adhesions, doctors may order blood tests to rule out other health problems that could be causing your symptoms. If you have signs of an intestinal obstruction, blood tests can help doctors find out how severe the obstruction is.

Imaging Tests

Imaging tests most often cannot show abdominal adhesions. However, doctors can use imaging tests to diagnose intestinal obstruction caused by abdominal adhesions. Doctors may also use imaging tests to rule out other problems that may be causing your symptoms.

Imaging tests may include

- Computerized tomography (CT), which uses a combination of x-rays and computer technology to create images. A CT scan may help doctors diagnose intestinal obstruction and find the location, cause, and severity of the obstruction.
- X-rays, which use a small amount of radiation to create pictures of the inside of the body.
- X-rays with water-soluble contrast medium—a special liquid that makes the digestive tract more visible on x-rays. If adhesions are causing an intestinal obstruction, this imaging test can help doctors find out if you need surgery. The water-soluble contrast medium may also help relieve the obstruction.

- Lower GI series, which uses x-rays to view your large intestine.

Surgery

In some cases, doctors may recommend surgery to look inside the abdomen and check for adhesions or other problems that may be causing symptoms. Surgeons may check for abdominal adhesions with laparoscopic or open surgery.

In some cases, surgeons may be able to treat the problem during the procedure.

HOW DO DOCTORS TREAT ABDOMINAL ADHESIONS?

If abdominal adhesions do not cause symptoms or complications, they typically do not need treatment.

If abdominal adhesions cause symptoms or complications, doctors can release the adhesions with laparoscopic or open surgery. However, surgery to treat adhesions may cause new adhesions to form. If you have abdominal adhesions, talk with your doctor about the possible benefits and risks of surgery.

If abdominal adhesions cause intestinal obstruction, you will need treatment at a hospital right away. Doctors will examine you and may order tests to find out if you need emergency surgery. If you do, surgeons will release the adhesions, relieving the intestinal obstruction.

If you do not need emergency surgery, doctors may try to treat the obstruction without surgery. Healthcare professionals will give you intravenous (IV) fluids and insert a tube through your nose and into your stomach to remove the contents of your digestive tract above the obstruction. In some cases, the obstruction may go away. If the obstruction does not go away, surgeons will perform surgery to release the adhesions, relieving the intestinal obstruction.

CAN ABDOMINAL ADHESIONS BE PREVENTED?

When performing abdominal surgery, surgeons take steps to lower the chance that patients will develop abdominal adhesions and related complications after surgery. For example, surgeons may:

- Recommend laparoscopic surgery, if possible, instead of open surgery
- Handle tissues gently to prevent damage
- Take steps to keep foreign materials out of the abdomen, such as using powder-free gloves and lint-free tools
- Cover damaged tissues inside the abdomen with a special film-like barrier at the end of surgery. The barrier keeps tissues separated while they heal, and then the barrier is absorbed by the body.

CLINICAL TRIALS FOR ABDOMINAL ADHESIONS

The National Institute of Diabetes and Digestive and Kidney Diseases (NIDDK) and other components of the National Institutes of Health (NIH) conduct and support research into many diseases and conditions, including digestive disorders.

What Are Clinical Trials for Abdominal Adhesions?

Clinical trials—and other types of clinical studies—are part of medical research and involve people like you. When you volunteer to take part in a clinical study, you help doctors and researchers learn more about disease and improve healthcare for people in the future.

Researchers are studying many aspects of abdominal adhesions, such as improving diagnosis and treatment of adhesions.

What Clinical Studies for Abdominal Adhesions Are Looking for Participants?

You can find clinical studies on abdominal adhesions at www. ClinicalTrials.gov. In addition to searching for federally funded studies, you can expand or narrow your search to include clinical studies from industry, universities, and individuals; however, the NIH does not review these studies and cannot ensure they are safe. Always talk with your healthcare provider before you participate in a clinical study.

Section 47.2 | Cardiogenic Shock

This section includes text excerpted from "Cardiogenic Shock," National Heart, Lung, and Blood Institute (NHLBI), June 25, 2019.

Cardiogenic shock is a serious condition that occurs when your heart cannot pump enough blood and oxygen to the brain, kidneys, and other vital organs. Cardiogenic shock is considered a medical emergency and should be treated immediately.

The most common cause of cardiogenic shock is a heart attack. Other health problems that may lead to cardiogenic shock include heart conditions such as heart failure; chest injuries; medicine side effects; and conditions that prevent blood from flowing freely through your heart, such as a blood clot in the lungs.

Without oxygen-rich blood reaching the body's brain and other vital organs, your blood pressure drops, your pulse slows, and you may experience confusion, loss of consciousness, sweaty skin, and rapid breathing.

Treatment aims to restore blood flow and protect organs from damage. Options include medicines, heart procedures and surgery, and medical devices. Some people may need a heart transplant or a permanently implanted device to help maintain blood flow after cardiogenic shock. If cardiogenic shock was caused by problems in the lungs or by medicine side effects, your doctor will treat those problems. If not treated quickly, cardiogenic shock can lead to life-threatening organ failure or brain injury.

TREATMENT OF CARDIOGENIC SHOCK

Cardiogenic shock is life-threatening and requires rapid diagnosis and identification of the cause and emergency medical treatment. Treatments include medicines, heart procedures, and medical devices to support or restore blood flow in the body and prevent organ damage.

Because cardiogenic shock is a serious medical condition affecting multiple body organs, a team of medical specialists usually provides care. Some medical devices may be used temporarily to stabilize or support you until a permanent device can be implanted or until a heart transplant can be performed.

For people who have severe organ damage and may not survive after cardiogenic shock, palliative care or hospice care may help them have a better quality of life (QOL) with fewer symptoms.

Medicines

Medicine can help increase blood flow and protect against organ damage. Some medicines treat the underlying cause of cardiogenic shock, which is usually a heart attack. These medicines include:

- **Antiarrhythmia medicines** to restore a regular heartbeat
- **Blood thinners or antiplatelet medicines** to dissolve blood clots and reduce platelets that may be blocking the coronary arteries
- **Vasopressors and inotropes,** such as norepinephrine and dobutamine, to increase blood pressure and blood flow out of the heart

Procedures

The following medical procedures may be done right away to restore blood flow within your heart and throughout your body to prevent organ damage:

- **Percutaneous cardiac intervention (PCI)** to open coronary arteries that are narrowed or blocked by the buildup of plaque. A small mesh tube called a "stent" may be implanted after PCI to prevent an artery from narrowing again. Your doctor may repeat PCI later if any other coronary arteries are affected by plaque.
- **Coronary artery bypass grafting (CABG)** to improve blood flow to the heart. This procedure is usually done as soon as possible after a diagnosis of cardiogenic shock.

Medical Devices

You may need a medical device to aid, restore, or maintain blood flow, which may prevent organ damage from cardiogenic shock.

Temporary devices sometimes support people who are waiting for surgery to implant a permanent device or for a heart transplant.

- **Extracorporeal membrane oxygenation (ECMO)** circulates the blood and supplies oxygen to the body's organs through a heart-lung machine outside of the body. For ECMO devices, tubes connect to the large blood vessels near the base of the neck. The device draws blood from the right side of the heart, pumps it through the oxygenator, and then returns it to the left side of the heart so the oxygen-rich blood can be delivered throughout the body.
- **An intra-aortic balloon pump (IABP)** is no longer recommended to be used alone in cardiogenic shock, but it may improve survival when used along with ECMO. An IABP may also be used temporarily for people who have cardiogenic shock due to heart failure until another procedure can be done. An IABP helps the weakened heart muscle to pump as much blood as it can to vital organs. The IABP is placed in the aorta, and a balloon at the tip of the device inflates and deflates to match the heart's pumping rhythm.
- **Percutaneous circulatory assist devices (PCADs),** including ventricular assist devices (VADs), can help support your heart until it recovers or while you are waiting for a heart transplant. A PCAD can help your heart work better if you are not eligible for a heart transplant. Risks include blood clots, bleeding, infection, device malfunction, and right-sided heart failure if a left VAD was used.

Additional Emergency Treatment

Additional emergency treatments may include:

- **Continuous kidney dialysis** to filter wastes out of the blood if the kidneys were damaged
- **Fluids** given through an intravenous (IV) line inserted in one of your blood vessels to maintain normal blood volumes

- **Mechanical breathing support,** such as a ventilator to protect the airway and provide extra oxygen
- **Oxygen therapy** so that more oxygen reaches the lungs, the heart, and the rest of the body

Chapter 48 | Healthcare-Associated Venous Thromboembolism

WHAT IS HEALTHCARE-ASSOCIATED VENOUS THROMBOEMBOLISM?

People who are currently or recently hospitalized, recovering from surgery, or being treated for cancer are at increased risk of developing serious and potentially deadly blood clots in the form of venous thromboembolism (VTE). A blood clot that occurs as a result of hospitalization, surgery, or other healthcare treatment or procedure is called "healthcare-associated venous thromboembolism (HA-VTE)."

WHY IS HEALTHCARE-ASSOCIATED VENOUS THROMBOEMBOLISM A PUBLIC-HEALTH PROBLEM?

Each year VTE affects as many as 900,000 Americans, resulting in about 100,000 premature deaths. The associated healthcare costs $10 billion or more each year in the United States. More and more people living in the United States have factors that increase their risk for a VTE. Without improvements and consistent use of strategies to prevent VTE, the Centers for Disease Control and Prevention (CDC) expects the number of people affected by VTE to increase. Although anyone can develop a blood clot, over half

This chapter includes text excerpted from "Venous Thromboembolism (Blood Clots)—Learn about Healthcare-Associated Venous Thromboembolism," Centers for Disease Control and Prevention (CDC), February 7, 2020.

of blood clots are related to a recent hospitalization or surgery and most of these do not occur until after discharge.

An analysis of the National Hospital Discharge Survey (NHDS) found that each year during 2007–2009, there were on average nearly 550,000 U.S. hospitalizations of adults that had a discharge diagnosis of VTE. Fortunately, many cases of HA-VTE can be prevented. However, proven strategies to prevent HA-VTE are not being constantly or regularly applied across and within healthcare settings. Reports suggest that as many as 70 percent of cases of HA-VTE in patients could be prevented. Despite this finding, fewer than half of hospitalized patients receive appropriate prevention measures.

WHAT IS BEING DONE TO REDUCE HEALTHCARE-ASSOCIATED VENOUS THROMBOEMBOLISM?

Preventing HA-VTE in patients can result in a major decrease in overall VTE occurrence, illness, financial costs, and death. Reducing HA-VTE has been the subject of a number of patient safety and public-health programs developed and promoted by federal agencies including Healthy People 2020.

The CDC recognizes the need to improve, advance, and guide prevention efforts to ensure that VTE prevention is a priority across the nation's healthcare settings. This topic was the focus of the January 15, 2013, CDC Public Health Grand Rounds and the information presented was summarized in a subsequent Morbidity and Mortality Weekly Report. Nationally, CDC's work has guided and fostered VTE research and informed efforts throughout the country, including the Surgeon General's Call to Action on preventing VTE.

Currently, the CDC is focusing on three main areas to promote, translate, and implement strategies to prevent HA-VTE:

- **Strengthen Healthcare monitoring of HA-VTE.** Advance and promote methods and tools to improve and support monitoring of HA-VTE occurrence and prevention.
- **Identify and Promote Best Practices for HA-VTE Prevention.** Identify and share proven prevention tools and resources for partners and stakeholders.

- **Increase Education and Awareness of HA-VTE.** Share evidence-based education tools and strategies to increase awareness of risks for and prevention of HA-VTE.

THE CENTERS FOR DISEASE CONTROL AND PREVENTION ACTIVITIES

The Centers for Disease Control and Prevention (CDC) has worked with two pilot programs at Duke University Medical Center and University of Oklahoma Health Sciences Center to assess and better understand VTE occurrence. These two pilot programs will help CDC:

- Develop and evaluate methods and electronic tools to monitor the occurrence of VTE including those that are healthcare-associated
- Provide a more accurate picture of the health and economic impact of VTE (and HA-VTE), which will include identifying high-risk groups and settings
- Inform the development of improved healthcare monitoring tools to measure the success of prevention activities by tracking and monitoring trends in HA-VTE occurrence over time

The CDC has worked with Emory University to evaluate an electronic tool for accurately identifying VTE events reported in electronic medical records.

The CDC has brought together experts on VTE to inform, promote, and guide their activities around CDC's monitoring and prevention of healthcare-associated VTE.

The CDC has worked with partners to develop and share information for patients, healthcare providers, and the public at large to improve both awareness of VTE and methods of preventing or managing blood clots.

- In 2015, the National Blood Clot Alliance was funded to develop a national digital media campaign that promotes the awareness of the signs, symptoms, and factors that increase the risk for blood clots.

- The CDC also funded Duke University to develop the This Is Serious campaign. This campaign addresses how to prevent blood clots if you are a hospitalized patient, particularly if you are undergoing surgery, being treated for trauma, receiving cancer treatment, or hospitalized due to pregnancy, since all these can increase the risk of developing a blood clot.

WHAT IS VENOUS THROMBOEMBOLISM?

Deep vein thrombosis and pulmonary embolism (DVT/PE) are often underdiagnosed and serious, but preventable medical conditions.

DVT is a medical condition that occurs when a blood clot forms in a deep vein. These clots usually develop in the lower leg, thigh, or pelvis, but they can also occur in the arm.

It is important to know about DVT because it can happen to anybody and can cause serious illness, disability, and in some cases, death. The good news is that DVT is preventable and treatable if discovered early.

COMPLICATIONS OF DEEP VEIN THROMBOSIS

The most serious complication of DVT happens when a part of the clot breaks off and travels through the bloodstream to the lungs, causing a blockage called pulmonary embolism (PE). If the clot is small, and with appropriate treatment, people can recover from PE. However, there could be some damage to the lungs. If the clot is large, it can stop blood from reaching the lungs and is fatal.

In addition, one-third to one-half of people who have a DVT will have long-term complications caused by the damage the clot does to the valves in the vein called post-thrombotic syndrome (PTS). People with PTS have symptoms such as swelling, pain, discoloration, and in severe cases, scaling or ulcers in the affected part of the body. In some cases, the symptoms can be so severe that a person becomes disabled.

For some people, DVT and PE can become a chronic illness; about 30% of people who have had a DVT or PE are at risk for another episode.

RISK FACTORS OF DEEP VEIN THROMBOSIS

Almost anyone can have a DVT. However, certain factors can increase the chance of having this condition. The chance increases even more for someone who has more than one of these factors at the same time.

Following is a list of factors that increase the risk of developing DVT:

- Injury to a vein, often caused by:
  - Fractures,
  - Severe muscle injury, or
  - Major surgery (particularly involving the abdomen, pelvis, hip, or legs).
- Slow blood flow, often caused by:
  - Confinement to bed (e.g., due to a medical condition or after surgery)
  - Limited movement (e.g., a cast on a leg to help heal an injured bone)
  - Sitting for a long time, especially with crossed legs; or
  - Paralysis.
- Increased estrogen, often caused by:
  - Birth control pills
  - Hormone replacement therapy, sometimes used after menopause
  - Pregnancy, for up to three months after giving birth
- Certain chronic medical illnesses, such as:
  - Heart disease
  - Lung disease
  - Cancer and its treatment
  - Inflammatory bowel disease (Crohn disease or ulcerative colitis)
- Other factors that increase the risk of DVT include:
  - Previous DVT or PE
  - Family history of DVT or PE
  - Age (risk increases as age increases)
  - Obesity
  - A catheter located in a central vein
  - Inherited clotting disorders

900,000
EACH YEAR

VTE affects as many
as 900,000 Americans
each year.

3 IN 10 3 in 10 people who
have a blood clot will
have another episode
within 10 years.

Figure 48.1. Blood Clots Affect Many People

100,000
PEOPLE DIE EACH YEAR

As many as 100,000 people die
of blood clots each year.

PE is a leading cause of
death in a woman during
pregnancy or just after
having a baby.

**SUDDEN
DEATH**

1 of 4 people who have
a PE die without warning.

Blood clots are a leading
cause of death in people
with cancer after the
cancer itself.

Figure 48.2. Blood Clots Can Be Deadly

**10 BILLION
DOLLARS**

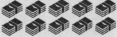

Blood clots cost our nation
up to $10 billion each year.

**+ $15K TO
$20K**

Treatment can be as much as
$15,000 to $20,000 per person
and often results in readmission
to the hospital.

Figure 48.3. Blood Clots Are Costly

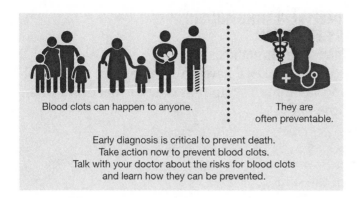

Blood clots can happen to anyone.

They are
often preventable.

Early diagnosis is critical to prevent death.
Take action now to prevent blood clots.
Talk with your doctor about the risks for blood clots
and learn how they can be prevented.

Figure 48.4. Things to Know

PREVENTING DEEP VEIN THROMBOSIS

The following tips can help prevent DVT:

- Move around as soon as possible after having been confined to bed, such as after surgery, illness, or injury.
- If you are at risk for DVT, talk to your doctor about:
  - Graduated compression stockings (sometimes called "medical compression stockings")
  - Medication (anticoagulants) to prevent DVT
- When sitting for long periods of time, such as when traveling for more than four hours:
  - Get up and walk around every 2 to 3 hours.
  - Exercise your legs while you are sitting by:
  - Raising and lowering your heels while keeping your toes on the floor
  - Raising and lowering your toes while keeping your heels on the floor
  - Tightening and releasing your leg muscles
  - Wear loose-fitting clothes.
- You can reduce your risk by maintaining a healthy weight, avoiding a sedentary lifestyle, and following your doctor's recommendations based on your individual risk factors.

SYMPTOMS OF DEEP VEIN THROMBOSIS AND PULMONARY EMBOLISM
Symptoms of Deep Vein Thrombosis

About half of people with DVT have no symptoms at all. The following are the most common symptoms of DVT that occur in the affected part of the body:

- Swelling
- Pain
- Tenderness
- Redness of the skin

If you have any of these symptoms, you should see your doctor as soon as possible.

Symptoms of Pulmonary Embolism

You can have a PE without any symptoms of a DVT.
Signs and symptoms of PE can include:

- Difficulty breathing
- Faster than normal or irregular heartbeat
- Chest pain or discomfort, which usually worsens with a deep breath or coughing
- Coughing up blood
- Very low blood pressure, lightheadedness, or fainting

If you have any of these symptoms, you should seek medical help immediately.

DIAGNOSIS OF DEEP VEIN THROMBOSIS AND PULMONARY EMBOLISM

There are other conditions with signs and symptoms similar to those of DVT. For example, muscle injury, cellulitis (a bacterial skin infection), and inflammation (swelling) of veins that are just under the skin can mimic the signs and symptoms of DVT. Therefore, special tests that can look for clots in the veins or in the lungs (imaging tests) are needed to diagnose DVT.

Diagnosis of Deep Vein Thrombosis

- **Duplex ultrasonography** is an imaging test that uses sound waves to look at the flow of blood in the veins. It can detect blockages or blood clots in the deep veins. It is the standard imaging test to diagnose DVT.
- A **D-dimer blood test** measures a substance in the blood that is released when a clot breaks up. If the D-dimer test is negative, it means that the patient probably does not have a blood clot.
- **Contrast venography** is a special type of x-ray where contrast material (dye) is injected into a large vein in the foot or ankle so that the doctor can see the deep veins in the legs and hip. It is the most accurate test for diagnosing blood clots but it is an invasive procedure, which means it is a medical test that requires doctors to use instruments to enter the body. Therefore, this test has been largely replaced by duplex ultrasonography, and it is used only in certain patients.
- **Magnetic resonance imaging (MRI)**—a test that uses radio waves and a magnetic field to provide images of the body—and **computed tomography (CT)** scan—a special x-ray test—are imaging tests that help doctors diagnose and treat a variety of medical conditions. These tests can provide images of veins and clots, but they are not generally used to diagnose DVT.

Diagnosis of Pulmonary Embolism

- **Computed tomographic pulmonary angiography (CTPA)** is a special type of x-ray test that includes injection of contrast material (dye) into a vein. This test can provide images of the blood vessels in the lungs. It is the standard imaging test to diagnose PE.
- **Ventilation-perfusion (V/Q) scan** is a specialized test that uses a radioactive substance to show the parts of the lungs that are getting oxygen (ventilation scan) and

getting blood flow (perfusion scan) to see if there are portions of the lungs with differences between ventilation and perfusion. For example, if there are clots in some of the blood vessels in the lungs, the V/Q scan might show normal amounts of oxygen, but low blood flow to the portions of the lungs served by the clotted blood vessels. This test is used when CTPA is not available or when the CPTA test should not be done because it might be harmful to the particular patient.

- **Pulmonary angiography** is a special type of X-ray test that requires insertion of a large catheter (a long, thin hollow tube) into a large vein (usually in the groin) and into the arteries within the lung, followed by injection of contrast material (dye) through the catheter. It provides images of the blood vessels in the lung and it is the most accurate test to diagnose PE. However, it is an invasive test so it is used only in certain patients.
- **Magnetic resonance imaging (MRI)** uses radio waves and a magnetic field to provide images of the lung, but this test is usually reserved for certain patients, such as for pregnant women or in patients where the use of contrast material could be harmful.

TREATMENTS OF DEEP VEIN THROMBOSIS AND PULMONARY EMBOLISM
Anticoagulants

- Anticoagulants (commonly referred to as "blood thinners") are the medications most commonly used to treat DVT or PE. Although called "blood thinners," these medications do not actually thin the blood. They reduce the ability of the blood to clot, preventing the clot from becoming larger while the body slowly reabsorbs it, and reducing the risk of further clots developing.
- The most frequently used injectable anticoagulants are:
  - Unfractionated heparin (injected into a vein),
  - Low molecular weight heparin (LMWH) (injected under the skin), and

- Fondaparinux (injected under the skin).
- Anticoagulants that are taken orally (swallowed) include:
  - Warfarin,
  - Dabigatran,
  - Rivaroxaban,
  - Apixaban, and
  - Edoxaban.

All of the anticoagulants can cause bleeding, so people taking them have to be monitored to prevent unusual bleeding.

Thrombolytics
- Thrombolytics (commonly referred to as "clot busters") work by dissolving the clot. They have a higher risk of causing bleeding compared to the anticoagulants, so they are reserved for severe cases.

Inferior Vena Cava Filter
- When anticoagulants cannot be used or do not work well enough, a filter can be inserted inside the inferior vena cava (a large vein that brings blood back to the heart) to capture or trap an embolus (a clot that is moving through the vein) before it reaches the lungs.

Thrombectomy or Embolectomy
In rare cases, a surgical procedure to remove the clot may be necessary. Thrombectomy involves removal of the clot in a patient with DVT. Embolectomy involves removal of the blockage in the lungs caused by the clot in a patient with PE.

Chapter 49 | Surgical Adverse Events: An Overview

Chapter Contents

Section 49.1 | Wrong-Site, Wrong-Procedure, and Wrong-Patient Surgery

This section includes text excerpted from "Wrong-Site, Wrong-Procedure, and Wrong-Patient Surgery," Agency for Healthcare Research and Quality (AHRQ), U.S. Department of Health and Human Services (HHS), September 2019.

Few medical errors are as vivid and terrifying as those that involve patients who have undergone surgery on the wrong body part, undergone the incorrect procedure, or had a procedure intended for another patient. These "wrong-site, wrong-procedure, wrong-patient errors" (WSPEs) are rightly termed "never events"—errors that should never occur and indicate serious underlying safety problems.

Wrong-site surgery may involve operating on the wrong side, as in the case of a patient who had the right side of her vulva removed when the cancerous lesion was on the left, or the incorrect body site. One example of surgery on the incorrect site is operating on the wrong level of the spine, a surprisingly common issue for neurosurgeons. A classic case of wrong-patient surgery involved a patient who underwent a cardiac procedure intended for another patient with a similar last name.

While much publicity has been given to these high-profile cases of WSPEs, these errors are in fact relatively rare. A seminal study estimated that such errors occur in approximately 1 of 112,000 surgical procedures, infrequent enough that an individual hospital would only experience one such error every 5 to 10 years. However, this estimate only included procedures performed in the operating room; if procedures performed in other settings (for example, ambulatory surgery or interventional radiology) are included, the rate of such errors may be significantly higher. One study using Veterans Affairs data found that fully half of WSPEs occurred during procedures outside of the operating room.

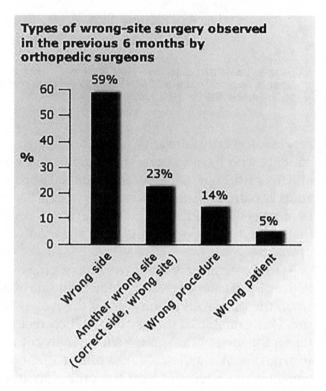

Figure 49.1. Wrong-Site Surgery in Last Six Months

PREVENTING WRONG-SITE, WRONG-PROCEDURE, AND WRONG-PATIENT SURGERY

Early efforts to prevent WSPEs focused on developing redundant mechanisms for identifying the correct site, procedure, and patient, such as "sign your site" initiatives, that instructed surgeons to mark the operative site in an unambiguous fashion. However, it soon became clear that even this seemingly simple intervention was problematic. An analysis of the United Kingdom's efforts to prevent WSPEs found that, although dissemination of a site-marking protocol did increase use of preoperative site marking, implementation and adherence to the protocol differed significantly across surgical specialties and hospitals, and many clinicians voiced concerns about unintended consequences of the protocol. In some cases, there was even confusion over whether the marked site indicates the area to be operated on, or the area to be avoided. Site marking remains a core component of The Joint Commission's Universal Protocol to prevent WSPEs.

Root cause analyses of WSPEs consistently reveal communication issues as a prominent underlying factor. The concept of the surgical timeout—a planned pause before beginning the procedure in order to review important aspects of the procedure with all involved personnel—was developed to improve communication in the operating room and prevent WSPEs. The Universal Protocol also specifies use of a timeout prior to all procedures. Although initially designed for operating room procedures, timeouts are now required before any invasive procedure. Comprehensive efforts to improve surgical safety have incorporated timeout principles into surgical safety checklists; while these checklists have been proven to improve surgical and postoperative safety, the low baseline incidence of WSPEs makes it difficult to establish that a single intervention can reduce or eliminate WSPEs.

It is worth noting, however, that many cases of WSPEs would still occur despite full adherence to the Universal Protocol. Errors may happen well before the patient reaches the operating room, a timeout may be rushed or otherwise ineffective, and production pressures may contribute to errors during the procedure itself. Ultimately, preventing WSPEs depends on the combination of system solutions, strong teamwork and safety culture, and individual vigilance.

CURRENT CONTEXT

Wrong-patient, wrong-site, and wrong-procedure errors are all considered never events by the National Quality Forum, and are considered sentinel events by The Joint Commission. In February 2009, the Centers for Medicare and Medicaid Services (CMS) announced that hospitals will not be reimbursed for any costs associated with WSPEs. (CMS has not reimbursed hospitals for additional costs associated with many preventable errors since 2007.)

695

Section 49.2 | "Never Events" in Surgery

This section contains text excerpted from the following sources: Text in this section begins with excerpts from "Never Events," Agency for Healthcare Research and Quality (AHRQ), U.S. Department of Health and Human Services (HHS), September 2019; Text beginning with the heading "Medical Harm" is excerpted from "Adverse Events, Near Misses, and Errors," Agency for Healthcare Research and Quality (AHRQ), U.S. Department of Health and Human Services (HHS), September 2019.

The term "Never Event" was first introduced in 2001 by Ken Kizer, MD, former CEO of the National Quality Forum (NQF), in reference to particularly shocking medical errors—such as wrong-site surgery—that should never occur. Over time, the term's use has expanded to signify adverse events that are unambiguous (clearly identifiable and measurable), serious (resulting in death or significant disability), and usually preventable. Since the initial never event list was developed in 2002, it has been revised multiple times, and now consists of 29 "serious reportable events" grouped into 7 categories:

- Surgical or procedural events
- Product or device events
- Patient protection events
- Care management events
- Environmental events
- Radiologic events
- Criminal events

SURGICAL EVENTS

- Surgery or other invasive procedure performed on the wrong body part
- Surgery or other invasive procedure performed on the wrong patient
- Wrong surgical or other invasive procedure performed on a patient
- Unintended retention of a foreign object in a patient after surgery or other procedure
- Intraoperative or immediately postoperative/postprocedure death in an American Society of Anesthesiologists (ASA) Class I patient

Most Never Events are very rare. For example, a 2006 study estimated that a typical hospital might experience a case of wrong-site surgery once every 5 to 10 years. However, when Never Events occur, they are devastating to patients—71 percent of events reported to the Joint Commission over the past 12 years were fatal—and may indicate a fundamental safety problem within an organization. Although individual events are uncommon, on a population basis, many patients still experience these serious errors. A 2013 study estimated that more than 4000 surgical never events occur yearly in the United States.

INCREASING ACCOUNTABILITY AND IMPROVING THE QUALITY OF CARE

Because Never Events are devastating and preventable, healthcare organizations are under increasing pressure to eliminate them completely. The Centers for Medicare & Medicaid Services (CMS) announced in August 2007 that Medicare would no longer pay for additional costs associated with many preventable errors, including those considered Never Events. Since then, many states and private insurers have adopted similar policies. Since February 2009, CMS has not paid for any costs associated with wrong-site surgeries.

Never Events are also being publicly reported, with the goal of increasing accountability and improving the quality of care. Since the NQF disseminated its original Never Events list in 2002, 11 states have mandated reporting of these incidents whenever they occur, and an additional 16 states mandate reporting of serious adverse events (including many of the NQF Never Events). Healthcare facilities are accountable for correcting systematic problems that contributed to the event, with some states (such as Minnesota) mandating performance of a root cause analysis and reporting its results.

MEDICAL HARM

The concept of medical harm has existed since antiquity, famously discussed by Hippocrates and passed on in the word iatrogenesis, from the Greek for originating from a physician. Since then, the topic has received attention from notable physicians. A paper in the *New England Journal of Medicine* (*NEJM*) in 1956 discussed the topic of diseases of medical progress, and this paper evolved into a book that used the phrase "iatrogenic disease" in its title.

ADVERSE EVENTS

Adverse events refer to harm from medical care rather than an underlying disease. Important subcategories of adverse events include:

- **Preventable adverse events.** Those that occurred due to error or failure to apply an accepted strategy for prevention;
- **Ameliorable adverse events.** Events that, while not preventable, could have been less harmful if care had been different;
- **Adverse events due to negligence.** Those that occurred due to care that falls below the standards expected of clinicians in the community.

Two other terms that define hazards to patients but do not result in harm:

- **Near miss.** An unsafe situation that is indistinguishable from a preventable adverse event except for the outcome. A patient is exposed to a hazardous situation, but does not experience harm either through luck or early detection.
- **Error.** A broader term referring to any act of commission (doing something wrong) or omission (failing to do the right thing) that exposes patients to a potentially hazardous situation.

Part 5 | **Recovery and Rehabilitation after Surgery**

Chapter 50 | **What to Expect after Surgery**

Chapter Contents

The postanesthesia care unit (PACU) is a recovery room where patients who have had surgery or diagnostic procedures requiring anesthesia or sedation are monitored. This area allows patients to regain consciousness and fully recover from the effects of anesthesia under the supervision of experienced nurses. The patient may be disoriented after a procedure, so the recovery room nursing staff will try to ease their anxiety and ensure physical and emotional comfort. They also monitor the surgical site, dressings, drains, and tubes and help with the patient's feeling of nausea by medicating them accordingly. The patients are carefully observed and continually assessed until the doctor or nurse determines that they are stable and ready to be discharged.

POSTANESTHESIA CARE

The postanesthesia period allows a monitored transition from the intraoperative period to evaluate and manage the patient's vitals for a fast and optimal recovery. The PACU or a separate postanesthesia recovery area, such as the surgical intensive care unit (SICU), provides resources appropriate for patients who receive sedation, regional anesthesia, or general anesthesia.

Before the administration of anesthesia or during the intraoperative period, the decision to admit the patient to the PACU or intensive care area is decided by the surgeon and anesthesia professional. The postanesthesia care unit (PACU) is made up of a team of nurses who have extensive training in critical care. Under the direct supervision of an anesthesiologist, they attend to the patients, by providing services such as:

Monitoring Vital Signs

Patients will not be discharged from the PACU until their vital signs are stable.

The patient will be closely monitored by a nurse who will assess the vital signs that include:

- Temperature
- Blood pressure
- Heart rate
- Respiratory rate
- Oxygen levels

Pain Management

Pain management in the PACU may be in the form of pills, injections, or a "pain pump." A pain pump is a form of patient-controlled analgesia (PCA) and gives patients a role in administering the medication. It works by allowing the patient to press a button to administer the pain medication via the pain pump, which delivers the medication directly to the spinal cord or the veins.

Administering Blood Products

Patients who have lost blood during their surgery may be given blood products such as red cells, platelets, or plasma in the PACU.

Discharging from the PACU

The patient will stay in the PACU before they are discharged home or to an inpatient unit until:

- They have recovered from the anesthetic.
- They can feel and move their legs if an epidural or spinal anesthetic was given.
- Their vital signs are stable.
- They have reached a level of pain that is manageable.

The length of stay in the PACU is different for each patient, since it is based on the type of surgery, overall health of the patient, and type of anesthetic involved.

When patients have long or complex operations, or if they have preexisting medical problems, they may be required to stay in the PACU for a longer period of time after the operation. These patients benefit from the specialized care and monitoring provided in the PACU.

SPECIALIZED MONITORING EQUIPMENT

Depending on the type of surgery, the patient may require specialized monitoring equipment. An oxygen mask may be changed to either oxygen through a tube in the nose, or in some cases, an alternate form of oxygen may be required, such as a respirator—a machine that helps breath by moving air in and out of the lungs. A heart monitor may be used by connecting wires to the top of the chest to monitor heart rate and rhythm. A probe is usually placed in the armpit to monitor body temperature. If the body temperature is low, the patient will be placed under a warming blanket.

The patient is monitored in the PACU for one or more hours after the vital signs are determined to be normal. Once it is normal, the patient will be transferred to a room in the hospital or to the outpatient surgery unit, where they will be prepared for discharge.

References

1. "Postanesthesia Care," American Association of Nurse Anesthetists (AANA), August 24, 2019.
2. "Post Anesthesia Care Unit (PACU)," MaineHealth, January 24, 2019.
3. "About the Post Anesthesia Care Unit (PACU)," University Health Network, November 29, 2019.
4. "Post Anesthesia Care Unit (PACU)," St. Thomas Elgin General Hospital (STEGH), July 12, 2019.

Section 50.2 | What to Expect If You Are Going Home the Day of Surgery

"What to Expect If You Are Going Home the Day of Surgery," © 2020 Omnigraphics. Reviewed April 2020.

Once a patient has been moved from the postanesthesia care unit (PACU) after an outpatient surgery, the nurses will get them ready to go home.

The discharge criteria are strict for outpatient/same-day surgery, and the patient must meet certain guidelines before the surgeon decides to get them discharged. The patient should:

- Be able to urinate before discharge
- Have controlled nausea
- Be treated with painkillers instead of an intravenous (IV) sedation to ease their pain
- Have normal breathing and blood pressure
- Be able to think and respond well
- Be able to walk unassisted
- Be able to tolerate food and drink

HOW LONG IT WILL TAKE FOR A PATIENT TO FEEL NORMAL AGAIN

The patients may feel minor changes or discomfort postsurgery due to the effect of anesthesia. This includes:

- Feeling tired
- Muscle aches
- Sore throat
- Dizziness
- Headaches

Patients may sometimes throw up or feel sick to their stomach. These effects usually go away in a few hours postsurgery, but it might take several days for the patient to feel normal and for these effects to be completely gone.

FIRST 24 HOURS POSTSURGERY

Outpatient surgery patients must bring a person along with them to drive them home and to stay with the patient for 24 hours postsurgery. The medications that were given during the surgery might affect their memory and mental judgment for the next 24 hours.

The other thing that one should remember postsurgery is to avoid alcohol and tobacco products.

The patients are advised not to use machinery, electrical equipment, or make any personal or important business decisions for 24 hours postsurgery.

WHAT YOU NEED TO KNOW ABOUT MEDICATIONS

The patient should understand their medicines and know when to take them. If the surgeon has advised to stop certain medications, such as blood thinners before surgery, inquire when it is safe to resume them. Get the doctor's contact information in case of an emergency.

OUTPATIENT POSTSURGERY EXPECTATIONS FOR CHILDREN

Outpatient surgery has significant benefits in children as it decreases their separation from their family and home. When the child is discharged within 24 hours postsurgery, the parent might notice that the child:

- Sleeps for a longer duration on the first few days
- Has some nausea and vomiting
- Maybe a little unsteady while walking

These symptoms are usually due to anesthesia or pain medications and will decrease in 24 to 48 hours at home postsurgery. Call the doctor right away if the symptoms persist beyond 48 hours. Make sure to understand the following before the child's discharge. Ask the doctor if:

- There are any additional care that has to be given at home. For instance, breathing exercises or changing wound dressings.
- There are any restrictions of activity for the child
- The child can take a shower or bath and when they can return to school or day care
- They have to return for a review or a follow-up treatment

References

1. "What to Expect If You Are Going Home on the Day of Surgery," American Society of PeriAnesthesia Nurses (ASPAN), July 2017.
2. "Going Home after Your Child's Surgery," The Children's Hospital of Philadelphia, September 2, 2014.
3. "What to Expect When You're Sent Home after Surgery," Webmd, September 13, 2017.

Chapter 51 | Artificial Airways and Assisted Ventilation

Chapter Contents

Section 51.1 | Intubation and Extubation

WHAT IS INTUBATION?

The medical procedure of inserting a tube into the mouth and the airway of a patient to assist in breathing is known as "intubation." The tube is known as "endotracheal tube" (ET) and is used when a patient is placed on a ventilator during anesthesia, severe illness, or sedation. It is then connected to a ventilator, which pushes air into the lungs of the patient.

The process is usually done when the anesthesia paralyzes the muscles of the body, including the diaphragm, making it impossible for the patient to breathe without a ventilator.

THE PROCEDURE

The patient is sedated and made unconscious prior to the intubation, allowing the muscles in the mouth and airway to relax. She or he is made to lie flat on their back and the mouth is opened to guide the tube into it, keeping the tongue out of the way. It is then gently guided through the throat and into the airway.

A small balloon-shaped instrument around the tube holds it in place to keep oxygen from escaping. Once inflated, the tube is securely positioned in the airway and is taped in place at the mouth. The lungs are checked using a stethoscope to ensure successful placement of the tube.

WHAT IS NASAL INTUBATION?

Some medical cases require the mouth or throat to be operated upon and, under such circumstances, the breathing tube is inserted through the nose instead of the mouth. This process is called "nasal intubation."

The nasotracheal tube (NT) is inserted into the nose, down the back of the throat, and into the upper airway. This procedure allows the mouth to be kept free and helps in the surgery to be performed. Intubation is preferred over nasal intubation as the insertion of the tube through an open mouth is much easier than nasal insertion.

RISKS OF INTUBATION

While intubation risk after surgery is practically low, a few potential threats that can arise when a patient remains on the ventilator for longer periods are:

- Trauma to the teeth, mouth, tongue, trachea, and/or larynx
- Tube being accidentally inserted into the esophagus (food tube) instead of the trachea (air tube)
- Bleeding due to improper insertion
- Drawing in fluids such as vomit, saliva, or other fluids while being intubated
- Pneumonia, if aspiration occurs
- Sore throat
- Hoarseness

WHAT IS EXTUBATION?

The final step in liberating a patient from a mechanical ventilator is by removing the endotracheal tube, which is called "extubation." The extubation procedure involves other processes known as "weaning" and "liberation."

The gradual transition from full invasive ventilatory support to spontaneous ventilation with minimal support is "weaning." On the other hand, the complete discontinuation of mechanical ventilation is "liberation." The current trend involves liberating patients as soon as possible, whereas weaning is more common in long-term, acute care settings.

The extubation procedure will not be carried out until the patient's medical situation is confirmed to be safe. A weaning trial has to be completed and any possible reintubation complications have to be eliminated. Many patients are extubated during daytime hours, but under limited cases, nocturnal extubation is carried out.

Most people in the intensive care unit (ICU) will not be extubated until the patient has undergone a successful weaning trial. Exceptions involve postoperative patients who are recovering in ICU for a brief time (e.g., 24 hours) and terminally extubated patients. A decrease in the rate of reintubation has been shown by studies when patients were asked to rest back on the ventilator for an hour before extubation and after the completion of a spontaneous breathing trial.

References

1. Whitlock, Jennifer, "What Is Intubation and Why Is It Done?" Verwell Health, April 13, 2020.
2. Saeed, Faisel; Lasrado, Savita; "Extubation," National Center for Biotechnology Information (NCBI), March 24, 2020.
3. "Extubation Management in the Adult Intensive Care Unit," UpToDate, October 12, 2019.

Section 51.2 | Mechanical Ventilator

This section includes text excerpted from "Ventilator/Ventilator Support," National Heart, Lung, and Blood Institute (NHLBI), December 26, 2012. Reviewed April 2020.

WHAT IS A VENTILATOR?

A ventilator is a machine that supports breathing. These machines mainly are used in hospitals. Ventilators:

- Deliver oxygen into the lungs
- Remove carbon dioxide from the body (Carbon dioxide is a waste gas that can be toxic)
- Help people breathe easier
- Provide life support for people who have lost all ability to breathe on their own

A ventilator often is used for short periods, such as during surgery when you were under general anesthesia. The term "anesthesia" refers to a loss of feeling and awareness. General anesthesia temporarily puts you to sleep.

The medicines used to induce anesthesia can disrupt normal breathing. A ventilator helps make sure that you continue breathing during surgery.

A ventilator also may be used during treatment for a serious lung disease or other conditions that affects normal breathing.

Some people may need to use ventilators long term or for the rest of their lives. In these cases, the machines can be used outside of the hospital—in long-term care facilities or at home.

A ventilator does not treat a disease or condition. It is used only for life support.

Other Names for Ventilator

- Mechanical ventilator
- Respirator
- Breathing machine

WHO NEEDS A VENTILATOR

Ventilators most often are used:
- During surgery if you are under anesthesia (that is, if you are given medicine that makes you sleep and/or causes a loss of feeling)
- If a disease or condition impairs your lung function

DURING SURGERY

If you have general anesthesia during surgery, you will likely be connected to a ventilator. The medicines used to induce anesthesia can disrupt normal breathing. A ventilator helps make sure that you continue breathing during surgery.

After surgery, you may not even know you were connected to a ventilator. The only sign may be a slight sore throat for a short time. The sore throat is caused by the tube that connects the ventilator to your airway.

Once the anesthesia wears off and you begin breathing on your own, the ventilator is disconnected. The tube in your throat also is taken out. This usually happens before you completely wake up from surgery.

However, depending on the type of surgery you have, you could stay on a ventilator for a few hours to several days after your surgery. Most people who have anesthesia during surgery only need a ventilator for a short time, though.

FOR IMPAIRED LUNG FUNCTION

You may need a ventilator if a disease, condition, or other factor has impaired your breathing. Although you might be able to breathe on your own, it is very hard work. You may feel short of breath and uncomfortable. A ventilator can help ease the work of breathing. People who cannot breathe on their own also use ventilators.

Many diseases, conditions, and factors can affect lung function. Examples include:

- Pneumonia and other infections
- Chronic obstructive pulmonary disease (COPD) or other lung diseases
- Upper spinal cord injuries, polio, amyotrophic lateral sclerosis (ALS), myasthenia gravis, and other diseases or factors that affect the nerves and muscles involved in breathing.
- Brain injury or stroke
- Drug overdose

A ventilator helps you breathe until you recover. If you cannot recover enough to breathe on your own, you may need a ventilator for the rest of your life.

HOW DOES A VENTILATOR WORK?

Ventilators blow air—or air with extra oxygen—into the airways and then the lungs. The airways are pipes that carry oxygen-rich air to your lungs. They also carry carbon dioxide, a waste gas, out of your lungs.

715

The airways include your:
- Nose and linked air passages, called "nasal cavities"
- Mouth
- Larynx or voice box
- Trachea or windpipe
- Tubes called "bronchial tubes or bronchi," and their branches

THE BREATHING TUBE

A ventilator blows air into your airways through a breathing tube. One end of the tube is inserted into your windpipe and the other end is attached to the ventilator. The breathing tube serves as an airway by letting air and oxygen from the ventilator flow into the lungs.

The process of inserting the tube into your windpipe is called "intubation." Usually, the breathing tube is put into your windpipe through your nose or mouth. The tube is then moved down into your throat. A tube placed like this is known as an "endotracheal tube."

In an emergency, you are given medicine to make you sleepy and ease the pain of the breathing tube being put into your windpipe. If it is not an emergency, the procedure is done in an operating room using anesthesia. (That is, you are given medicine that makes you sleep and/or causes a loss of feeling.)

An endotracheal tube is held in place by tape or with an endotracheal tube holder. This holder often is a strap that fits around the head.

Sometimes the breathing tube is placed through a surgically made hole known as a "tracheostomy." The hole goes through the front of your neck and into your windpipe. The tube put into the hole sometimes is called a "trach tube."

The procedure to make a tracheostomy usually is done in an operating room. Anesthesia is used, so you would not be awake or feel any pain. Specially made ties or bands that go around the neck hold the trach tube in place.

Both types of breathing tubes pass through your vocal cords and affect your ability to talk.

For the most part, endotracheal tubes are used for people who are on ventilators for shorter periods. The advantage of this tube is that it can be placed in an airway without surgery.

Trach tubes are used for people who need ventilators for longer periods. For people who are awake, this tube is more comfortable than the endotracheal tube. Under certain conditions, a person who has a trach tube may be able to talk.

THE VENTILATOR

A ventilator uses pressure to blow air or a mixture of gases (like oxygen and air) into the lungs. This pressure is known as "positive pressure." You usually exhale (breathe out) the air on your own, but sometimes the ventilator does this for you too.

A ventilator can be set to "breathe" a set number of times a minute. Sometimes it is set so that you can trigger the machine to blow air into your lungs. But, if you fail to trigger it within a certain amount of time, the machine automatically blows air to keep you breathing.

Rarely, doctors recommend a ventilator called a "chest shell." This type of ventilator works like an iron lung—an early ventilator used by many polio patients in the last century. However, the chest shell is not as bulky and confining as the iron lung.

The chest shell fits snugly to the outside of your chest. A machine creates a vacuum between the shell and the chest wall. This causes your chest to expand, and air is sucked into your lungs. No breathing tube is used with a chest shell.

When the vacuum is released, your chest falls back into place and the air in your lungs comes out. This cycle of vacuum and release is set at a normal breathing rate.

WHAT TO EXPECT WHILE ON A VENTILATOR

Ventilators normally do not cause pain. The breathing tube in your airway may cause some discomfort. It also affects your ability to talk and eat.

If your breathing tube is a trach tube, you may be able to talk. (A trach tube is put directly into your windpipe through a hole in the front of your neck.)

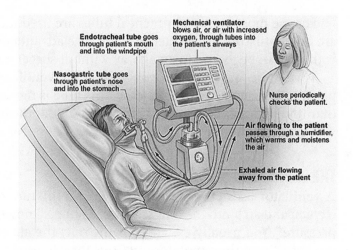

Figure 51.1. Patient on a Ventilator

Figure 51.1 shows a standard setup for a ventilator in a hospital room. The ventilator pushes warm, moist air (or air with increased oxygen) to the patient. Exhaled air flows away from the patient.

Instead of food, your healthcare team may give you nutrients through a tube inserted into a vein. If you were on a ventilator for a long time, you will likely get food through a nasogastric, or feeding, tube. The tube goes through your nose or mouth, or directly into your stomach or small intestine, through a surgically made hole.

A ventilator greatly restricts your activity and also limits your movement. You may be able to sit up in bed or in a chair, but you usually cannot move around much.

If you need to use a ventilator long term, you may be given a portable machine. This machine allows you to move around and even go outside, although you need to bring your ventilator with you.

Sometimes the ventilator is set so that you can trigger the machine to blow air into your lungs. But, if you fail to trigger it within a certain amount of time, the machine automatically blows air to keep you breathing.

ONGOING CARE

While you are on a ventilator, your healthcare team will closely watch you. The team may include doctors, nurses, and respiratory therapists. You may need periodic chest x-rays and blood tests to check the levels of oxygen and carbon dioxide (blood gases) in your body.

These tests help your healthcare team find out how well the ventilator is working for you. Based on the test results, they may adjust the ventilator's airflow and other settings as needed.

Also, a nurse or respiratory therapist will suction your breathing tube from time to time. This helps remove mucus from your lungs. Suctioning will cause you to cough, and you may feel short of breath for several seconds. You may get extra oxygen during suctioning to relieve shortness of breath.

WHAT ARE THE RISKS OF BEING ON A VENTILATOR?
Infections

One of the most serious and common risks of being on a ventilator is pneumonia. The breathing tube that is put in your airway can allow bacteria to enter your lungs. As a result, you may develop ventilator-associated pneumonia (VAP).

The breathing tube also makes it hard for you to cough. Coughing helps clear your airways of lung irritants that can cause infections.

The VAP is a major concern for people using ventilators because they were often already very sick. Pneumonia may make it harder to treat their other disease or condition.

The VAP is treated with antibiotics. You may need special antibiotics if the VAP is caused by bacteria that are resistant to standard treatment.

Another risk of being on a ventilator is a sinus infection. This type of infection is more common in people who have endotracheal tubes. (An endotracheal tube is put into your windpipe through your mouth or nose.) Sinus infections are treated with antibiotics.

Other Risks

Using a ventilator also can put you at risk for other problems, such as:

- **Pneumothorax.** This is a condition in which air leaks out of the lungs and into the space between the lungs and the chest wall. This can cause pain and shortness of breath, and it may cause one or both lungs to collapse.

- **Lung damage.** Pushing air into the lungs with too much pressure can harm the lungs.
- **Oxygen toxicity.** High levels of oxygen can damage the lungs.

These problems may occur because of the forced airflow or high levels of oxygen from the ventilator.

Using a ventilator also can put you at risk for blood clots and serious skin infections. These problems tend to occur in people who have certain diseases, and/or who are confined to bed or a wheelchair, and must remain in one position for long periods.

Another possible problem is damage to the vocal cords from the breathing tube. If you find it hard to speak or breathe after your breathing tube is removed, let your doctor know.

WHAT TO EXPECT WHEN YOU ARE TAKEN OFF OF A VENTILATOR

"Weaning" is the process of taking you off of a ventilator so that you can start to breathe on your own. People usually are weaned after they have recovered enough from the problem that caused them to need the ventilator.

Weaning usually begins with a short trial. You stay connected to the ventilator, but you will be given a chance to breathe on your own. Most people are able to breathe on their own the first time weaning is tried. Once you can successfully breathe on your own, the ventilator is stopped.

If you cannot breathe on your own during the short trial, weaning will be tried at a later time. If repeated weaning attempts over a long time do not work, you may need to use the ventilator long term.

After you are weaned, the breathing tube is removed. You may cough while this is happening. Your voice may be hoarse for a short time after the tube is removed.

Chapter 52 | **Tube Feeding**

Chapter Contents

Section 52.1 | Basics of Enteral Feeding

This section includes text excerpted from "Home Pump Tube Feeding Instructions," U.S. Department of Veterans Affairs (VA), May 2012. Reviewed April 2020.

WHAT IS TUBE FEEDING?

For some people, eating, drinking, and swallowing become impossible. They cannot eat enough, or at all, so they get their nutrition through a feeding tube. Unlike regular eating, the mouth and esophagus are bypassed.

Tube feeding through the stomach is accomplished by using a gastrostomy (also called a "G-tube").

Tube feeding can also be done through the jejunum (a section of the small intestine) using a jejunostomy (J-tube).

TUBE FEEDING METHODS

Your medical team will determine the delivery method for your tube feeding, as well as your feeding schedule. The most common tube feeding methods are:

Bolus Feedings

The formula is placed in a syringe and flows slowly into the feeding tube. 1 to 2 cans of formula are given a few times during the day.

Gravity Feeding

The formula is placed in a feeding bag and bag is hung from IV pole. Formula flows slowly into the feeding tube. Rate is controlled by roller clamp. 1 to 2 cans of formula are given a few times during the day.

Pump Feeding

The formula is placed in a feeding bag and is pumped through the tubing into the patient. Your tube feeding will run all day or just at night with the pump.

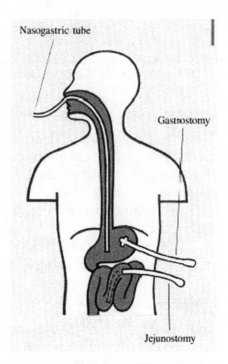

Nasogastric tube

Gastrostomy

Jejunostomy

Figure 52.1. Home Pump Tube Feeding

Section 52.2 | Feeding Tube Complications

This section includes text excerpted from "Home Pump Tube Feeding Instructions," U.S. Department of Veterans Affairs (VA), May 2012. Reviewed April 2020.

MANAGING DIARRHEA

Diarrhea means many loose and watery bowel movements (stools). Loose stools may be normal with tube feeding. A few loose stools in 24 hours is not a problem. Five or more loose stools per day for more than two days can be a problem.

Prevention of Dehydration

- Relax.
- Do not give the tube feeding any faster than the ordered rate.

- Make sure all tube feeding equipment is clean.
- Cover and refrigerate any opened feeding not being used.
- Throw away any feeding that has been opened for more than two days.
- Take medications as ordered. Do not mix them with the formula unless approved by your healthcare professional.
- Make sure you give the amount of water ordered by the doctor.

Treatment
- Give the tube feeding more slowly.
- Give more water after feedings (2 to 4 cups per day) to replace any water loss.

DEHYDRATION
Dehydration means that the body needs more water.

Causes of Dehydration
- Not enough water in the tube feeding
- Fever
- Medication
- Diarrhea or vomiting

Signs of Dehydration
- Dry or cracked lips
- Dry Mouth
- Less urination
- Steady weight loss week after week

Prevention
- After each feeding, give the right amount of water.
- Check weight twice a week.
- Know if your medication can cause dehydration.
- If you have fever or diarrhea, give more water than usual.

PERSONAL CARE
Care of the Mouth

It is important to have good oral health. The following steps are helpful to keep your mouth as clean as possible:

- Brush your teeth, gums, and tongue at least two times a day using a soft toothbrush and toothpaste.
- Use mouthwash or mild salt water (1 tsp salt in 1 quart of water) to freshen mouth and breath.
- To moisten lips, use lip balm or petroleum jelly.
- To moisten your mouth, use ice chips or sugar-free chewing gum.
- To avoid chapping, do not lick lips.

STOMACH UPSET

An upset stomach is a feeling of nausea, bloating, heartburn, or gas pain. Belching or vomiting may also occur.

Prevention or Treatment of Stomach Upset

- Give the tube feeding slowly.
- Never force a feeding. If you feel full, wait an hour before giving more feeding. Restart feeding at a slower rate.
- Do not start feeding or continue feeding if your stomach is upset or if you vomit.
- Sit upright or at a 30-degree angle when lying in bed during the feeding and for at least one hour after.

Chapter 53 | **Hospital Discharge Planning**

A patient is discharged from the hospital when they no longer require inpatient care and can go home or to a different type of facility, such as a rehab center or nursing home.

Discharge planning is a process that helps determine the requirements of a patient for transition from one level of care to another. A doctor authorizes a patient's release from the hospital, but the process of discharge is completed either by a social worker, nurse, or a case manager. Discharge planning is usually done as a team approach for a patient with complicated medical conditions.

WHAT IS HOSPITAL DISCHARGE PLANNING?

Hospital discharge planning determines the kind of care required after an individual leaves the hospital. Discharge plans are intended to provide patients with adequate information and necessary resources to improve or maintain their health during the posthospital period and to prevent adverse events and unnecessary rehospitalization.

A discharge plan should include information about where the patient will be discharged to, the types of care required, and who will provide that care. It should be written in simple language and include a complete list of medications with dosages and usage information.

The basics of a hospital discharge plan include:

- Evaluation of the patient by qualified personnel

"Hospital Discharge Planning," © 2020 Omnigraphics. Reviewed April 2020.

- Discussion with the patient or their representative about posthospital care
- Planning for posthospital discharge destination
- Determining if caregiver training or other assistance is necessary
- Referral to home care agencies and suitable support organizations in the community
- Arranging for follow-up appointments or tests

Many hospitals have a dedicated discharge planner who helps coordinate the information and care required by a patient after leaving the hospital.

STEPS INVOLVED IN EFFECTIVE DISCHARGE PLANNING

Getting discharged from the hospital is a positive step for the patient, but transitioning from 24-hour care in a hospital ward to the community can be challenging. Careful assessment, planning, and communication can ensure the flow of care and help the patient recover and adjust to the new environment. Many patients who are discharged from the hospital will have ongoing care needs that must be met in the community, including the use of specialized equipment at home such as a hospital-type bed, support from caregivers to fulfill their daily activities, or regular visits from district nurses to administer medication.

The following steps can be taken for effective discharge planning, acknowledging a patient's individual needs.

Step 1: Early Planning

An ideal discharge planning begins on the day of admission or prior to admission if a patient has an elective procedure. Rushed or unplanned discharges may lead to problems at home and rehospitalization. Detailed and accurate patient information should be gathered from the patient's family, general practitioner (GP), the primary healthcare team, and caregivers, if any.

An expected discharge date should ideally be set within 48 hours of admission and will need to be revised based on the patient's health, progress, and any evolving care needs. This can be very difficult to implement, but an estimated discharge date can be useful since it can help predict hospital capacity, track the progress of the clinical plan, and allow patients to understand expectations. A discharge checklist is to be completed 48 hours before the scheduled time of transfer to ensure that essential aspects of discharge planning are being carried out.

Step 2: Identifying the Patient's Needs

It is important to know whether the patient has simple or complex health needs. A simple discharge can be organized by the ward, the multidisciplinary team, the individual, and their family. Discharges that involve funding issues, a change of residence to a nursing home or sheltered accommodation, or significant health and social care needs are considered complex, and hence require more planning. Patients who require end-of-life care should also be identified so that their requirements can be met by the caregiver or by the facility to which they are being transferred.

Step 3: Developing a Clinical Management Plan

A clinical management plan is to be developed during the first 24 hours after admission. An abstract plan will usually be created by the junior medical or surgical staff while admitting the patient. This should be reviewed so that the plan engages the whole multidisciplinary team, and all aspects of care needed prior to discharge are identified in the plan.

The clinical management plan should be reviewed on a daily basis to track progress, and the plan should be updated along with the patient and the multidisciplinary team in response to their health and well-being.

Step 4: Involving Patients and Caregivers

Depending on the patient's care needs and home circumstances, the ability to provide care should be discussed among the patient, family, the multidisciplinary team, and any social care providers. This helps them comprehend the challenges involved and to manage their expectations. The patient's involvement in their discharge and their right to choose the care they prefer is equally essential. The caregiver must also get trained in special tasks depending on the patient's condition such as wound caring, using a feeding tube or a catheter, procedures for a ventilator, transferring someone from a bed to a chair, and dealing with incontinence and dementia.

Step 5: Care Provided after a Hospital Discharge

Each patient will have individual needs and preferences about how and where they would like to live after the discharge. A nursing home may offer support for a period of rehabilitation, allowing the patient to regain strength and mobility.

Alternatively, most people prefer to recuperate in their own homes, in which case, the discharge planner can help the caregivers get in touch with the community support available in their region. Some organizations can provide services such as transportation, meals, support groups, counseling, and possibly a break from care responsibilities that allows a caregiver to rest.

Discharge planning is complicated, especially in those who are frail, elderly, or have complex care needs. However, effective discharge planning can ensure that a patient leaves the hospital promptly, has continuity of care, and remains safe and healthy without the need of readmission.

References

1. "Hospital Discharge Planning," MATRIX Neurological, August 1, 2017.
2. Dr. Gilbert, Jane, "Hospital discharge planning," December 12, 2018.
3. "Hospital Discharge Guide," NurseRegistry, April 2, 2018.
4. "Hospital Discharge," The Johns Hopkins University, January 22, 2017.

Chapter 54 | **Moving to a Nursing Home or Rehab Facility**

HOW DO YOU CHOOSE A NURSING HOME?

After you choose a nursing home, you will need to make arrangements to be admitted. Have this information ready when you contact the nursing home:

Information for the Nursing Home Office Staff

Insurance information. Provide information about any health coverage and long-term care insurance you have that pays for nursing home care, healthcare, or both. This includes the name of the insurance company and the policy number.

If Medicare or Medicaid will cover your nursing home care, the nursing home cannot require you to pay a cash deposit. They may ask that you pay your Medicare coinsurance and other charges you would normally have to pay. The nursing home cannot require you to pay more than the rates allowed by Medicare or Medicaid for covered services. There may be charges for items or services that Medicare or Medicaid do not cover, but the nursing home cannot

This chapter contains text excerpted from the following sources: Text beginning with the heading "How Do You Choose a Nursing Home?" is excerpted from "Your Guide to Choosing a Nursing Home or Other Long-Term Services and Supports" Centers for Medicare & Medicaid Services (CMS), October 2019; Text under the heading "Resident of a Rehabilitation Facility" is excerpted from "Skilled Nursing Facility Rights," Centers for Medicare & Medicaid Services (CMS), August 18, 2012. Reviewed April 2020.

require that you accept services that Medicare or Medicaid do not cover as a condition of your continued stay.

It is best to pay charges once they are billed to you—not in advance. You may have to pay a cash deposit before you are admitted to a nursing home, if your care would not be covered by either Medicare or Medicaid, and the nursing home is not limited to the rates allowed by Medicare or Medicaid.

Information for the Nursing Home Medical Staff

- **Your medical history.** Your doctor may give the staff some of this information. This includes a list of past health problems, any past surgeries or treatments, any vaccination shots you have had, and allergies you may have to food or medicine.
- **Your current health status.** Your doctor should give the staff this information, including a list of your current health problems, recent diagnostic test results, and information about any activities of daily living that might be difficult for you to do by yourself.
- **Your current medications.** Include the dose, how often you take it, and when and why you take it.
- **Your healthcare providers.** Include their names, addresses, and phone numbers.
- **Your family members to call in case of an emergency.** Include their names, addresses, and phone numbers.

Other Important Information to Have Ready
HEALTHCARE ADVANCE DIRECTIVES

You may be asked if you have a healthcare advance directive, which is a written legal document that says how you want medical decisions to be made if you become unable to make decisions for yourself. There are 2 common types of healthcare advance directives:

- **A living will.** A living will is a written legal document that shows what type of treatments you want or do not want in case you cannot speak for yourself, like whether you want life support. Usually, this document only comes into effect if you were unconscious.

- **A durable power of attorney for healthcare.** A durable power of attorney for healthcare is a legal document that names someone else to make healthcare decisions for you. This is helpful if you become unable to make your own decisions. If you do not have a healthcare advance directive and need help preparing one, or you need more information, talk to a social worker, discharge planner, your doctor, or the nursing home staff. You can use the Eldercare Locator to find out if your state has any legal services that can help you prepare these forms.

ONCE YOU ARE A RESIDENT
Information the Nursing Home Must Give You

Once you choose a nursing home, they must give you information about how to apply for and use Medicare and Medicaid benefits in a language and format you understand. They must also give you information on how to get refunds for previous payments you may have made that are covered by these benefits.

Personal Needs Accounts

You may want to open an account managed by the nursing home, although the nursing home cannot require this. You can deposit money into the account for personal use. Check with the nursing home to find out what expenses you can use the account for and how they manage the accounts.

Your Assessment and Care Plan

Once you have selected a nursing home and are a resident, the nursing home staff will get your health information and review your health condition to prepare your care plan. You (if you are able), your family (with your permission), or someone acting on your behalf has the right to take part in planning your care with the nursing home staff. Your assessment begins on the day you are admitted and must be completed within 14 days. Staff will gather information about how well you function, your care needs, and your general well-being. The nursing home staff will review your assessment at least every 90 days, and possibly more often if your medical status changes. Once your assessment is complete, the nursing home staff will develop your care plan. Your care plan is a strategy for how the staff will help you with everyday needs—both medical and nonmedical.

Depending on your needs, your care plan may include:
- What kind of personal or healthcare services you need?
- What type of staff should give you these services?
- How often do you need the services?
- What kind of equipment or supplies you need (like a wheelchair or feeding tube)?
- Activity preferences
- Your food preferences and dietary needs
- How will your care plan help you reach your goals?
- Information on whether you plan to return to the community and, if so, a plan to help you meet that goal

Your Resident Rights and Protections

As a resident in a Medicare- and/or Medicaid-certified nursing home, you have certain rights and protections under federal and state law to make sure you get the care and services you need. You have the right to be informed, make your own decisions, and have your personal information kept private.

The nursing home must communicate these rights to you in a format and language you understand. They must also explain in writing your rights and responsibilities while you were in the nursing home. This must be done before or at the time you were admitted, as well as during your stay. You must acknowledge in writing that you got this information. Here is a list of some of your rights:
- Be free from discrimination.
- Be free from abuse and neglect.
- Exercise your rights as a U.S. citizen.
- Have your representative notified about your care.
- Get proper medical care.

- Be treated with respect.
- Be free from restraints.
- Have protections against involuntary transfer or discharge.
- Participate in activities.
- Spend time with visitors.
- Form or participate in resident groups.
- Manage your money.
- Get information on services and fees.
- Get proper privacy, property, and living arrangements.
- Make complaints.

Reporting and Resolving Problems

If you have a problem at the nursing home, talk to the staff involved. For example, if you have a problem with your surgical care, talk to the nurse or Certified Nurse Assistant (CNA). The staff may not know there is a problem unless you tell them. If the problem is not resolved, ask the nursing staff to talk with the supervisor, social worker, director of nursing, administrator, or your doctor.

If your problem continues, follow the facility's grievance procedure for complaints. The Medicare- and/or Medicaid-certified nursing home must have a grievance procedure. You may also want to bring the problem to the resident or family group.

A Medicare- and/or Medicaid-certified nursing home must post the name, address, and phone number of groups that may be helpful to you, like the State Survey Agency, State Licensure Office, State Long-Term Care Ombudsman Program, Protection and Advocacy Agency, and the Medicaid Fraud Control Unit. If you feel you need outside help to resolve your problem, call the Long-Term Care Ombudsman, State Survey Agency, or the Protection and Advocacy Agency for your area.

What If You Do Not Like a Nursing Home You Are Currently In?

If you do not like the nursing home you are currently living in, you can move to another facility with an available bed. Moving can be difficult, but an extra move may be better for you than choosing to stay at a facility that is not right for you.

The nursing home you leave may require that you let them know ahead of time that you are planning to leave. Talk to the nursing home staff about their rules for leaving. If you do not follow the rules for leaving, you may have to pay extra fees.

If you want information about living in the community, nursing homes are required to reach out to a local agency that can give you more information. Talk to the nursing home social worker about your plan to transition to the community.

RESIDENT OF A REHABILITATION FACILITY

As a resident of a rehabilitation facility, you have certain rights and protections under federal and state law. These laws can vary by state.

The rehabilitation facility must provide you with a written description of your legal rights. Keep the information you get about your rights, admission and transfer policies, and any other information you get from the rehabilitation facility in case you need to look at them later.

As a person with Medicare, you have certain guaranteed rights and protections. By federal law, rehabilitation facility residents also have these rights:

Freedom from Discrimination

Rehabilitation facility do not have to accept all applicants, but they must comply with Civil Rights laws that do not allow discrimination based on these:

- Race
- Color
- National origin
- Disability
- Age
- Religion under certain conditions

If you believe you have been discriminated against, contact the U.S. Department of Health and Human Services (HHS), Office for Civil Rights (OCR).

Respect

You have the right to be treated with dignity and respect. You have the right to choose the activities you want to go to. As long as it fits your care plan, you have the right to make your own schedule, including when you:

- Go to bed
- Rise in the morning
- Eat your meals

Freedom from Abuse and Neglect

You have the right to be free from verbal, sexual, physical, and mental abuse, involuntary seclusion, and misappropriation of your property by anyone. This includes, but is not limited to, rehabilitation facility staff, other residents, consultants, volunteers, staff from other agencies, family members, legal guardians, friends, or other individuals. If you feel you have been abused or neglected (your needs are not met), report this to the rehabilitation facility, your family, your local Long-Term Care Ombudsman, or your State Survey Agency.

It may be appropriate to report the abuse to local law enforcement or the Medicaid Fraud Control Unit (their phone number should be posted in the rehabilitation facility).

Freedom from Restraints

Physical restraints are any manual method or physical or mechanical device, material, or equipment attached to or near your body so that you cannot remove the restraint easily. Physical restraints prevent freedom of movement or normal access to one's own body. A chemical restraint is a drug that is used for discipline or convenience and is not needed to treat your medical symptoms.

It is against the law for a rehabilitation facility to use physical or chemical restraints, unless it is necessary to treat your medical symptoms. Restraints may not be used to punish or for the convenience of the rehabilitation facility staff. You have the right to refuse restraint use except if you are at risk of harming yourself or others.

Information on Services and Fees

You must be informed in writing about services and fees before you move into the rehabilitation facility. The rehabilitation facility cannot require a minimum entrance fee as a condition of residence.

Money

You have the right to manage your own money or choose someone you trust to do this for you. If you ask the rehabilitation facility to manage your personal funds, you must sign a written statement that allows the rehabilitation facility to do this for you. However, the rehabilitation facility must allow you access to your bank accounts, cash, and other financial records. The rehabilitation facility must place your money (over $50) in an account that provides interest, and they must give you quarterly statements. The rehabilitation facility must protect your funds from any loss by buying a bond or providing other similar protections.

Privacy, Property, and Living Arrangements

You have the right to privacy, and to keep and use your personal belongings and property as long as they do not interfere with the rights, health, or safety of others. The rehabilitation facility staff should never open your mail unless you allow it. You have the right to use a phone and talk privately. The rehabilitation facility must protect your property from theft. This may include a safe in the facility or cabinets with locked doors in resident rooms. If you and your spouse live in the same rehabilitation facility, you are entitled to share a room (if you both agree to do so).

Medical Care

You have the right to be informed about your medical condition, medications, and to see your own doctor. You also have the right to refuse medications and treatments (but this could be harmful to your health). You have the right to take part in developing your care plan. You also have the right to look at your medical records and reports when you ask.

Visitors

You have the right to spend private time with visitors at any reasonable hour. The rehabilitation facility must permit your family to visit you at any time, as long as you want to see them. You do not have to see any visitor you do not want to see. Any person who gives you help with your health or legal services may see you at any reasonable time. This includes your doctor, representative from the health department, and your Long-Term Care Ombudsman, among others.

Social Services

The rehabilitation facility must provide you with any needed medically-related social services, including counseling, help solving problems with other residents, help in contacting legal and financial professionals, and discharge planning.

Complaints

You have the right to make a complaint to the staff of the rehabilitation facility, or any other person, without fear of punishment. The rehabilitation facility must resolve the issue promptly.

Protection against Unfair Transfer or Discharge

You cannot be sent to another rehabilitation facility or made to leave the rehabilitation facility, except in these situations:

- It is necessary for the welfare, health, or safety of you or others.
- Your health has declined to the point that the rehabilitation facility cannot meet your care needs.
- Your health has improved to the point that rehabilitation facility care is no longer necessary.
- You do not pay for the services you are responsible for.
- The rehabilitation facility closes down.
- A rehabilitation facility cannot make you leave if you are waiting to get Medicaid. The rehabilitation facility should work with other state agencies to get payment if a family member or other individual is holding your money.

Your Family and Friends

Family members and legal guardians may meet with the families of other residents and may participate in family councils. Family and friends can help make sure you get good quality care. They can visit and get to know the staff and the rehabilitation facility rules.

By law, rehabilitation facilities must develop a plan of care (care plan) for each resident. You have the right to take part in this process and family members can help with your care plan with your permission. If your relative is your legal guardian, she or he has the right to look at all medical records about you. She or he also has the right to make important decisions on your behalf.

Chapter 55 | Reducing Health Disparity in Surgical Outcomes

Chapter Contents

Section 55.1 | Disparities in Surgical Care

This section includes text excerpted from "NIH Launches Research Program to Reduce Health Disparities in Surgical Outcomes," National Institutes of Health (NIH), April 18, 2016. Reviewed April 2020.

The National Institute on Minority Health and Health Disparities (NIMHD), part of the National Institutes of Health (NIH), has launched an initiative to support research to better understand and address disparities in surgical care and outcomes for disadvantaged populations. The surgical disparities research program will involve collaborations among several institutes and centers, along with the Agency for Healthcare Research and Quality (AHRQ). Full funding levels will be determined by the number of meritorious grant applications received.

Health disparities are the differences in health status and outcomes that are most often observed across different racial and ethnic populations, as well as across differing socioeconomic status. These disparities can include higher rates of chronic disabling conditions, greater comorbidity, and greater risk of premature death, as well as poorer quality of life (QOL), worse functioning, and prolonged recovery from disease.

Research has demonstrated that the benefits of surgical procedures are not equal across the population. For example, a study of surgical disparities in the United States showed an increase in surgical mortality rates among patients with lower socioeconomic status independent of race, age, access to surgical care, hospital facility, or insurance status.

"Disparities in surgical care can result in poorer functional outcomes, prolonged rehabilitation, recovery and lower quality of life, particularly for disadvantaged population groups," said NIMHD Director Eliseo J. Pérez-Stable, M.D. "Racial and ethnic minority and low-income population groups are oftentimes disproportionately affected by access, availability, and affordability to the most advanced healthcare services."

Research suggests that as much as 11 to 30 percent of the global burden of disease requires surgical care or anesthesia management or both—a figure that underscores the fundamental role of surgery as part of essential healthcare. According to the Centers for Disease Control and Prevention (CDC), approximately 51 million inpatient and 53 million outpatient surgical cases are performed in the United States each year. These numbers account for an appreciable share of the healthcare costs and resources.

"We need to better understand the integral role of optimal access to safe surgical care and medical management, which has not been well studied in health services or health disparities research," said Dr. Pérez-Stable.

Section 55.2 | Surgical Disparities

This section includes text excerpted from "Minority Health: Recent Findings," Agency for Healthcare Research and Quality (AHRQ), U.S. Department of Health and Human Services (HHS), February 2013. Reviewed April 2020.

LESS EFFECTIVE TREATMENT AND LOWER SOCIOECONOMIC STATUS MAY ACCOUNT FOR DISPARITIES IN BREAST CANCER SURVIVAL

Researchers studied more than 35,000 Medicare-insured women with early-stage breast cancer for as long as 11 years and found that black women were more likely than white women to live in the poorest census tract quartiles. Also, more black women (15.7%) received breast-conserving surgery without follow-up radiation therapy than white women (12.4%), Hispanic women (11%), and Asian women (7.9%). Since the recommended therapy for early-stage breast cancer is breast-conserving surgery plus radiation, these treatment differences could have contributed to disparities in survival, suggest the researchers.

STUDY FINDS DISPARITIES IN RECEIPT OF CHEMOTHERAPY FOLLOWING OVARIAN CANCER SURGERY

Clinical guidelines have recommended since 1994 that all women diagnosed with ovarian cancer stage IC-IV or higher receive chemotherapy following surgery to remove the cancer. This study of more than 4,000 black and white women 65 years of age or older who were diagnosed with stage IC-IV ovarian cancer found that white women were more likely than black women to receive chemotherapy after surgery (65 percent versus 50 percent, respectively), although survival rates did not differ between the two groups of women. Women with higher socioeconomic status (SES) had increased use of both surgery and chemotherapy, and women in the lowest quartile of SES were more likely to die than those in the highest quartile of SES. The study finds disparities in receipt of chemotherapy following ovarian cancer surgery.

BLACKS ARE LESS LIKELY THAN WHITES TO HAVE SURGERY PERFORMED BY HIGH VOLUME SURGEONS AND HOSPITALS

Researchers examined data from New York city hospitals for surgical procedures that have shown a direct relationship between volume and reduced short-term mortality. Examples include heart bypass surgery, total hip replacement, and certain cancer surgeries. For procedures, black patients were significantly less likely than whites to have their surgery performed by a high-volume surgeon or in a high-volume hospital. Asian and Hispanic patients also were more likely to have a less-experienced surgeon perform the procedure at a low-volume hospital.

BLACK AND HISPANIC MEDICARE PATIENTS OFTEN WAIT LONGER THAN WHITE PATIENTS FOR SURGERY AFTER HIP FRACTURE

According to this study, black and Hispanic Medicare patients with hip fractures had approximately a half-day delay in receiving hip stabilization surgery compared with white patients. Most often, the delay in surgery was due to the need to evaluate and stabilize other medical problems, such as chest pain. Other possible explanations include the higher prevalence in blacks and Hispanics of undiagnosed and uncontrolled medical conditions such as diabetes and hypertension, or delayed transportation to the hospital leading to an afternoon admission and surgery deferral until the next day.

RACE INFLUENCES PARTICIPATION OF COMPANIONS IN CANCER CONSULTATIONS

Companions can play an important role in meetings between newly diagnosed cancer patients and their clinicians. For this study involving newly diagnosed lung cancer patients, researchers recorded and analyzed conversations between clinicians from a medical center's oncology or thoracic surgery clinic and the patients and their companions (if applicable). They found that the companions of black patients were less active participants in the conversation compared with the companions of white patients. Companions were more likely to be active participants when the physician's communication emphasized partnership-building and supportive talk and when the lung cancer diagnosis had been made before the visit.

Part 6 | **Additional Help and Information**

Chapter 56 | **Glossary of Terms Related to Surgery**

amputation: Removal of part or all of a body part, except for organs in the body. It usually takes place during surgery in a hospital operating room.

aneurysm: A thin or weak spot in an artery that balloons out and can burst.

antibiotic: Drugs used to fight bacteria in the body.

atherosclerosis: A disease in which fatty material is deposited on the wall of the arteries. This fatty material causes the arteries to become narrow and it eventually restricts blood flow.

bacteria: Microorganisms that can cause infections.

benign: A tumor or cells that are not cancerous.

biopsy: The removal of body tissues for examination under a microscope or for other tests on the tissue.

bladder: The organ in the human body that stores urine. It is found in the lower part of the abdomen.

blood transfusion: A procedure in which a person is given an infusion of whole blood or parts of blood. The blood may be donated by another person, or it may have been taken from the patient earlier and stored until needed.

body mass index (BMI): A measure of body weight relative to height. The BMI tool uses a formula that produces a score often used to determine if a person is underweight, at a normal weight, overweight, or obese.

carbohydrate: A major source of energy for your body. Your digestive system changes carbohydrates into blood glucose (sugar).

cataracts: Cloudy or thick areas in the lens of the eye.

This glossary contains terms excerpted from documents produced by several sources deemed reliable.

cholesterol: A fat-like substance that is made by your body and found naturally in animal foods such as dairy products, eggs, meat, poultry, and seafood.

chronic illness: An illness that persists over a long period of time.

colonoscopy: A colonoscopy is a procedure that allows your doctor to look inside your large intestine using an instrument with a tiny camera called a "scope."

critical care: A subspecialty of medicine concerned with the diagnosis, treatment, and support of patients with multiple organ dysfunction (i.e., critically ill) during a medical emergency or crisis.

Crohn disease: An ongoing condition that causes inflammation of the digestive tract, also called the "gastrointestinal (GI) tract." It can affect any part of the GI tract from the mouth to the anus.

elective surgery: A surgery that is optional and not required.

endoscope: A thin illuminated flexible or rigid tubelike optical system used to examine the interior of a hollow organ or body cavity by direct insertion. Instruments can be attached for biopsy and surgery.

episiotomy: This is a procedure where an incision is made in the perineum (area between the vagina and the anus) to make the vaginal opening larger in order to prevent the area from tearing during delivery.

estrogen: A type of hormone made by the body that helps develop and maintain female sex characteristics and the growth of long bones.

exercise: A type of physical activity that is planned and structured. Exercise is done on purpose to improve or maintain health, physical fitness, and/or physical performance.

fat: A major source of energy in the diet, fat helps the body absorb fat-soluble vitamins such as vitamins A, D, E, and K.

fatigue: A feeling of lack of energy, weariness or tiredness.

gallbladder: A sac that stores a fluid called "bile," which is produced by the liver. After eating, bile is secreted into the small intestine, where it helps digest fats.

gastrointestinal: A term that refers to the stomach and the intestines or bowels.

general surgery: The branch of surgery that covers the main areas of surgical treatment. General surgeons treat diseases of the abdomen, breast, head and neck, blood vessels, and digestive tract. They also manage care of patients who have been injured or who have deformities or other conditions that need surgery.

glucose: A major source of energy for our body and a building block for many carbohydrates. The food digestion process breaks down carbohydrates in foods and drinks into glucose.

heart attack: Also called an "acute myocardial infarction" (AMI), happens when one of the heart's arteries becomes blocked and the supply of blood and oxygen to part of the heart muscle is slowed or stopped. When the heart muscle does not get the oxygen and nutrients it needs, the affected heart tissue may die.

hormone: Substance produced by one tissue and conveyed by the bloodstream to another to effect a function of the body, such as growth or metabolism.

hypnosis: A focused state of concentration used to reduce pain. With self-hypnosis, you repeat a positive statement over and over. With guided imagery, you create relaxing images in your mind.

hysterectomy: Surgery to remove the uterus and, sometimes, the cervix. When the uterus and the cervix are removed, it is called a "total hysterectomy." When only the uterus is removed, it is called a partial hysterectomy.

immune system: The body's natural defense system against getting an infection and disease. White blood cells are the main part of your immune system that fight infections.

incision: A cut made in the body to perform surgery.

infection: A condition when germs enter a person's body and multiply, causing disease. The germs may be bacteria, viruses, yeast, or fungi. When the body's natural defense system is strong, it can often fight the germs and prevent infection. Some cancer treatments can weaken the natural defense system.

kidney stones: Hard mass developed from crystals that separate from the urine and build up on the inner surfaces of the kidney.

larynx: Valve structure between the trachea (windpipe) and the pharynx (the upper throat) that is the primary organ of voice production.

long-term care: Services that help meet the medical and nonmedical needs of people with a chronic illness or disability.

malignant: A tumor or cell that is cancerous.

medical error: An unintended but preventable adverse effect of care, whether or not it is evident or harmful to the patient.

medical record: Documentation of a patient's medical history and care.

mortality: Mortality refers to the death rate, or the number of deaths in a certain group of people in a certain period of time.

nonsteroidal anti-inflammatory drugs (NSAIDs): Pain relievers such as aspirin, ibuprofen, and naproxen. These medicines are safe and effective when taken as directed, but they can cause stomach bleeding or kidney problems in some people.

nutrition: The clinical practice concerned with nutrients and other substances contained in food and their action, interaction, and balance in relation to health and disease.

pharmacist: A person licensed to prepare and give out (dispense) prescription drugs and medicines and who has been taught how they work, how to use them, and their side effects.

prescription: A direction written by the physician to the pharmacist for the preparation and use of a medicine or remedy.

radiation: The emission of energy as electromagnetic waves or as moving subatomic particles, especially high-energy particles that cause ionization.

radiologist: Doctors who specialize in diagnosing and treating diseases and injuries using medical imaging techniques such as x-rays, computed tomography (CT), magnetic resonance imaging (MRI), nuclear medicine, positron emission tomography (PET), and ultrasound.

rehabilitation: In medicine, a process to restore mental and/or physical abilities lost to injury or disease, in order to function in a normal or near-normal way.

side effect: An effect of a drug, chemical, or other medicine that is in addition to its intended effect, especially an effect that is harmful or unpleasant.

spinal block: A small dose of medicine given as a shot into the spinal fluid in the lower back.

surgical site infection: An infection that occurs after surgery in the part of the body where the surgery took place. Surgical site infections can sometimes be superficial infections involving the skin only. Other surgical site infections are more serious and can involve tissues under the skin, organs, or implanted material.

Glossary of Terms Related to Surgery

tracheostomy: Surgical opening into the trachea (windpipe) to help some-one breathe who has an obstruction or swelling in the larynx (voice box) or upper throat or who has had the larynx surgically removed.

tumor: An abnormal growth of body tissue. Tumors can be cancerous (malignant) or noncancerous (benign). Cancerous tumors can have uncon-trolled growth and may spread to other parts of the body. Noncancerous tumors do not grow or spread.

ventilator: In medicine, a machine used to help a patient breathe. Also called a "respirator."

viruses: Small microscopic organisms that often cause disease.

x-ray: A type of high-energy radiation. In low doses, x-rays are used to diagnose diseases by making pictures of the inside of the body.

Chapter 57 | **Directory of Organizations That Provide Information about Surgery**

GOVERNMENT AGENCIES THAT PROVIDE INFORMATION ABOUT SURGERY

Agency for Healthcare Research and Quality (AHRQ)
Office of Communications and
Knowledge Transfer (OCKT)
5600 Fishers Ln., Seventh Fl.
Rockville, MD 20857
Phone: 301-427-1364
Website: www.ahrq.gov

Centers for Medicare & Medicaid Services (CMS)
7500 Security Blvd.
Baltimore, MD 21244
Toll-Free: 800-MEDICARE
(800-633-4227)
Phone: 410-786-3000
Toll-Free TTY: 877-486-2048
Website: www.cms.gov

Centers for Disease Control and Prevention (CDC)
1600 Clifton Rd., N.E.
Atlanta, GA 30333
Toll-Free: 800-CDC-INFO
(800-232-4636)
Phone: 404-639-3311
Toll-Free TTY: 888-232-6348
Website: www.cdc.gov

Federal Trade Commission (FTC)
600 Pennsylvania Ave., N.W.
Washington, DC 20580
Toll-Free: 877-FTC-HELP
(877-382-4357)
Phone: 202-326-2222
Website: www.ftc.gov

Resources in this chapter were compiled from several sources deemed reliable; all contact information was verified and updated in April 2019.

Healthfinder®

National Health Information
Center (NHIC)
200 Independence Ave., S.W.
Washington, DC 20201
Website: healthfinder.gov
E-mail: healthfinder@hhs.gov

National Cancer Institute (NCI)

9609 Medical Center Dr.
Bethesda, MD 20892-9760
Toll-Free: 800-4-CANCER
(800-422-6237)
Website: www.cancer.gov
E-mail: NCIinfo@nih.gov

National Center for Health Statistics (NCHS)

3311 Toledo Rd.
Hyattsville, MD 20782-2064
Phone: 301-458-4000
Website: www.cdc.gov/nchs

National Eye Institute (NEI)

Information Office
31 Center Dr., MSC 2510
Bethesda, MD 20892-2510
Phone: 301-496-5248
Website: www.nei.nih.gov
E-mail: 2020@nei.nih.gov

National Heart, Lung, and Blood Institute (NHLBI)

P.O. Box 30105
Bethesda, MD 20824-0105
Phone: 301-592-8573
TTY: 240-629-3255
Website: www.nhlbi.nih.gov
E-mail: nhlbiinfo@nhlbi.nih.gov

National Institute of Neurological Disorders and Stroke (NINDS)

NIH Neurological Institute
P.O. Box 5801
Bethesda, MD 20824
Toll-Free: 800-352-9424
Phone: 301-496-5751
Website: www.ninds.nih.gov

National Institute on Aging (NIA)

31 Center Dr., MSC 2292
Bldg. 31, Rm. 5C27
Bethesda, MD 20892
Toll-Free: 800-222-2225
Phone: 301-496-1752
Toll-Free TTY: 800-222-4225
Website: www.nia.nih.gov
E-mail: niaic@nia.nih.gov

National Institute of Arthritis and Musculoskeletal and Skin Diseases (NIAMS)

1 AMS Cir.
Bethesda, MD 20892-3675
Toll-Free: 877-22-NIAMS
(877-226-4267)
Phone: 301-495-4484
TTY: 301-565-2966
Fax: 301-718-6366
Website: www.niams.nih.gov
E-mail: NIAMSinfo@mail.nih.gov

National Institute of Diabetes and Digestive and Kidney Diseases (NIDDK)
National Institutes of Health (NIH)
9000 Rockville Pike
Bethesda, MD 20892
Toll-Free: 800-860-8747
Toll-Free TTY: 866-569-1162
Website: www.niddk.nih.gov
E-mail: healthinfo@niddk.nih.gov

National Institutes of Health (NIH)
9000 Rockville Pike
Bethesda, MD 20892
Phone: 301-496-4000
TTY: 301-402-9612
Website: www.nih.gov

National Women's Health Information Center (NWHIC)
Office on Women's Health (OWH)
200 Independence Ave., S.W.
Rm. 712E
Washington, DC 20201
Toll-Free: 800-994-9662
Phone: 202-690-7650
Toll-Free TDD: 888-220-5446
Fax: 202-205-2631
Website: www.womenshealth.gov

U.S. Department of Health and Human Services (HHS)
200 Independence Ave., S.W.
Washington, DC 20201
Toll-Free: 877-696-6775
Website: www.hhs.gov

U.S. Food and Drug Administration (FDA)
10903 New Hampshire Ave.
Silver Spring, MD 20993
Toll-Free: 888-INFO-FDA
(888-463-6332)
Phone: 301-796-8240
Website: www.fda.gov

U.S. National Library of Medicine (NLM)
8600 Rockville Pike
Bethesda, MD 20894
Toll-Free: 888-FIND-NLM
(888-346-3656)
Phone: 301-594-5983
Website: www.nlm.nih.gov
E-mail: custserv@nlm.nih.gov

PRIVATE AGENCIES THAT PROVIDE INFORMATION ABOUT SURGERY

Accreditation Association for Ambulatory Health Care (AAAHC)
5250 Old Orchard Rd., Ste. 200
Skokie, IL 60077
Phone: 847-853-6060
Fax: 847-853-9028
Website: www.aaahc.org
E-mail: info@aaahc.org

Ambulatory Surgery Center Association (ASCA)
1012 Cameron St.
Alexandria VA 22314-2427
Phone: 703-836-8808
Fax: 703-549-0976
Website: www.ascassociation.org

American Academy of Cosmetic Surgery (AACS)

225 W. Wacker Dr.
Ste. 650
Chicago, Illinois 60606
Phone: 312-981-6760
Fax: 312-265-2908
Website: www.cosmeticsurgery.org
E-mail: info@cosmeticsurgery.org

American Academy of Dermatology (AAD)

P.O. Box 1968
Des Plaines, IL 60017
Toll-Free: 866-503-SKIN
(866-503-7546)
Phone: 847-240-1280
Fax: 847-240-1859
Website: www.aad.org

American Academy of Facial Plastic and Reconstructive Surgery (AAFPRS)

310 S. Henry St.
Alexandria, VA 22314
Phone: 703-299-9291
Fax: 703-299-8898
Website: www.aafprs.org
E-mail: info@aafprs.org

American Academy of Family Physicians (AAFP)

11400 Tomahawk Creek Pkwy
Leawood, KS 66211-2680
Toll-Free: 800-274-2237
Phone: 913-906-6000
Fax: 913-906-6075
Website: www.aafp.org

American Academy of Neurological and Orthopaedic Surgeons

1516 N. Lake Shore Dr.
Chicago, IL 60610
Phone: 312-787-1608
Fax: 312-787-9289
Website: aanos.org

American Academy of Ophthalmology (AAO)

655 Beach St.
San Francisco, CA 94109
Phone: 415-561-8500
Fax: 415-561-8533
Website: www.aao.org
E-mail: customer_service@aao.org

American Academy of Orthopaedic Surgeons (AAOS)

9400 W. Higgins Rd.
Rosemont, IL 60018
Phone: 847-823-7186
Fax: 847-823-8125
Website: www.aaos.org

American Academy of Otolaryngology—Head and Neck Surgery (AAO—HNS)

1650 Diagonal Rd.
Alexandria, VA 22314
Phone: 703-836-4444
Website: www.entnet.org

The American Association for the Surgery of Trauma

633 N. Saint Clair St., Ste. 2600
Chicago, IL 60611
Toll-Free: 800-789-4006
Fax: 312-202-5064
Website: www.aast.org/Default.aspx
Email: aast@aast.org

American Association of Endodontists (AAE)

180 N. Stetson Ave.
Ste. 1500
Chicago, IL 60601
Toll-Free: 800-872-3636
Phone: 312-266-7255
Fax: 312-266-9867
Toll-Free Fax: 866-451-9020
Website: www.aae.org
E-mail: info@aae.org

American Association of Hip and Knee Surgeons (AAHKS)

9400 W. Higgins Rd.
Ste. 230
Rosemont, IL 60018-4976
Phone: 847-698-1200
Fax: 847-698-0704
Website: www.aahks.org
E-mail: helpdesk@aahks.org

American Association of Nurse Anesthetists (AANA)

222 S. Prospect Ave.
Park Ridge, IL 60068-4001
Toll-Free: 855-526-2262
Phone: 847-692-7050
Fax: 847-692-6968
Website: www.aana.com

American Association of Surgical Physician Assistants (AASPA)

121 W. State
Geneva, IL 60134
Website: www.aaspa.com

American Board of Cosmetic Surgery (ABCS)

8840 Calumet Ave.
Ste. 205
Munster, IN 46321
Phone: 219-203-1551
Fax: 219-836-552
Website: www.americanboardcos-meticsurgery.org

American Board of Plastic Surgery (ABPS)

1635 Market St., 7 Penn Ctr.
Ste. 400
Philadelphia, PA 19103-2204
Phone: 215-587-9322
Fax: 215-587-9622
Website: www.abplasticsurgery.org
E-mail: info@ABplasticsurgery.org

American Board of Surgery (ABS)

1617 John F. Kennedy Blvd.
Ste. 860
Philadelphia, PA 19103
Phone: 215-568-4000
Fax: 215-563-5718
Website: www.absurgery.org

American Cancer Society (ACS)

250 Williams St., N.W.
Atlanta, GA 30303
Toll-Free: 800-227-2345
Website: www.cancer.org

American College of Chest Physicians (CHEST)
2595 Patriot Blvd.
Glenview, IL 60026
Toll-Free: 800-343-2227
Phone: 224-521-9800
Fax: 224-521-9801
Website: www.chestnet.org

American College of Obstetricians and Gynecologists (ACOG)
409 12th St., S.W.
Washington, DC 20024-2188
Toll-Free: 800-673-8444
Phone: 202-638-5577
Website: www.acog.org
E-mail: resources@acog.org

American College of Radiology (ACR)
1891 Preston White Dr.
Reston, VA 20191
Toll-Free: 800-227-5463
Phone: 703-648-8900
Website: www.acr.org
E-mail: info@acr.org

American College of Surgeons (ACS)
633 N. Saint Clair St.
Chicago, IL 60611-3295
Toll-Free: 800-621-4111
Phone: 312-202-5000
Fax: 312-202-5001
Website: www.facs.org
E-mail: postmaster@facs.org

American Dental Association (ADA)
211 E. Chicago Ave.
Chicago, IL 60611-2678
Phone: 312-440-2500
Website: www.ada.org
E-mail: International-Member@ada.org

American Heart Association (AHA)
7272 Greenville Ave.
Dallas, TX 75231
Toll-Free: 800-AHA-USA-1
(800-242-8721)
Website: www.heart.org

American Medical Association (AMA)
AMA Plaza 330 N., Wabash Ave.
Ste. 39300
Chicago, IL 60611-5885
Toll-Free: 800-621-8335
Website: www.ama-assn.org

American Optometric Association (AOA)
243 N. Lindbergh Blvd., First Fl.
St. Louis, MO 63141-7881
Toll-Free: 800-365-2219
Phone: 314-597-1939
Website: www.aoa.org

American Pediatric Surgical Association (APSA)
1 Parkview Plaza, Ste. 800
Oakbrook Terrace, IL 60181
Phone: 847-686-2237
Fax: 847-686-2253
Website: eapsa.org
E-mail: eapsa@eapsa.org

American Pregnancy Association

3007 Skyway Cir., N.
Ste. 800
Irving, TX 75038
Toll-Free: 800-672-2296
Website: americanpregnancy.org
E-mail: info@americanpregnancy.org

American Psychological Association (APA)

750 First St., N.E.
Washington, DC 20002-4242
Toll-Free: 800-374-2721
Phone: 202-336-5500
TDD/TTY: 202-336-6123
Website: www.apa.org

American Rhinologic Society (ARS)

P.O. Box 269
Oak Ridge, NJ 07438
Phone: 973-545-2735
Website: www.american-rhino-logic.org

American Society for Dermatologic Surgery (ASDS)

5550 Meadowbrook Dr.
Ste. 120
Rolling Meadows, IL 60008
Phone: 847-956-0900
Fax: 847-956-0999
Website: www.asds.net

American Society for Laser Medicine and Surgery (ASLMS)

2100 Stewart Ave.
Ste. 240
Wausau, WI 54401
Toll-Free: 877-258-6028
Phone: 715-845-9283
Fax: 715-848-2493
Website: www.aslms.org
E-mail: information@aslms.org

American Society for Metabolic and Bariatric Surgery (ASMBS)

14407 S.W. Second Pl.
Ste. F-3
Newberry, FL, 32669
Phone: 352-331-4900
Fax: 352-331-4975
Website: asmbs.org
E-mail: info@asmbs.org

American Society for Radiation Oncology (ASTRO)

251 18th St., S.
Eighth Fl.
Arlington, VA 22202
Toll-Free: 800-962-7876
Phone: 703-502-1550
Fax: 703-502-7852
Website: www.astro.org

American Society for Reproductive Medicine (ASRM)

1209 Montgomery Hwy
Birmingham, AL 35216-2809
Phone: 205-978-5000
Fax: 205-978-5005
Website: www.reproductivefacts.org
E-mail: asrm@asrm.org

American Society for Surgery of the Hand (ASSH)
822 W. Washington Blvd.
Fl. 2
Chicago, IL 60607
Phone: 312-880-1900
Website: www.assh.org
E-mail: info@assh.org

American Society of Anesthesiologists (ASA)
1061 American Ln.
Schaumburg, IL 60173-4973
Phone: 847-825-5586
Fax: 847-825-1692
Website: www.asahq.org
E-mail: info@asahq.org

American Society of Colon and Rectal Surgeons (ASCRS)
2549 Waukegan Rd.
Ste. 210
Bannockburn, IL 60015
Phone: 847-607-6410
Website: fascrs.org
E-mail: ascrs@fascrs.org

American Society of Ophthalmic Plastic and Reconstructive Surgery (ASOPRS)
1041 Grand Ave.
Ste. 132
St Paul, MN 55105
Phone: 612-601-3168
Website: www.asoprs.org
E-mail: info@asoprs.org

American Society of PeriAnesthesia Nurses (ASPAN)
90 Frontage Rd.
Cherry Hill, NJ 08034-1424
Toll-Free: 877-737-9696
Fax: 856-616-9601
Website: www.aspan.org
E-mail: aspan@aspan.org

American Society of Plastic Surgeons (ASPS)
444 E. Algonquin Rd.
Arlington Heights, IL 60005
Phone: 847-228-9900
Website: www.plasticsurgery.org
E-mail: memserv@plasticsurgery.org

American Society of Transplantation (AST)
1120 Rt. 73
Ste. 200
Mt. Laurel, NJ 08054
Phone: 856-439-9986
Fax: 856-581-9604
Website: www.myast.org

American Thoracic Society (ATS)
25 Bdwy.
New York, NY 10004
Phone: 212-315-8600
Fax: 212-315-6498
Website: www.thoracic.org
E-mail: atsinfo@thoracic.org

American Thyroid Association (ATA)

6066 Leesburg Pike
Ste. 550
Falls Church, VA 22041
Phone: 703-998-8890
Fax: 703-998-8893
Website: www.thyroid.org
E-mail: thyroid@thyroid.org

Amputee Coalition of America (ACA)

900 E. Hill Ave.
Ste. 390
Knoxville, TN 37915
Website: www.amputee-coalition.org

Arthritis Foundation® (AF)

1355 Peachtree St., N.E.
Ste. 600
Atlanta, GA 30309
Toll-Free: 844-571-4357
Phone: 404-872-7100
Website: www.arthritis.org

Association for Academic Surgery (AAS)

11300 W. Olympic Blvd.
Suite 600
Los Angeles, CA 90064
Phone: 310-437-1606
Fax: 310-437-0585
Website: www.aasurg.org
E-mail: jj@aasurg.org

Association of American Physicians and Surgeons (AAPS)

1601 N. Tucson Blvd.
Ste. 9
Tucson, AZ 85716
Toll-Free: 800-635-1196
Fax: 520-325-4230
Website: aapsonline.org
Email: aaps@aapsonline.org

Cleveland Clinic

9500 Euclid Ave.
Cleveland, OH 44195
Toll-Free: 800-223-2273
TTY: 216-444-0261
Website: my.clevelandclinic.org

Eastern Association for the Surgery of Trauma

633 N. Saint Clair St.
Suite 2400
Chicago, IL 60611-3295
Phone: 312-202-5508
Fax: 312-202-5064
Website: www.east.org
E-mail: managementoffice@east.org

General Surgery News

McMahon Publishing
545 W. 45th St.
Eighth Fl.
New York, NY 10036
Phone: 212-957-5300; ext. 262
Website: www.generalsurgerynews.com

The Joint Commission
One Renaissance Blvd.
Oakbrook Terrace, IL 60181
Phone: 630-792-5800
Fax: 630-792-5005
Website: www.jointcommission.org

Mayo Foundation for Medical Education and Research (MFMER)
Mayo Clinic
200 First St., S.W.
Rochester, MN 55905
Phone: 507-284-0274
Fax: 507-266-4743
Website: www.mayoclinic.org

National Hospice and Palliative Care Organization (NHPCO)
1731 King St.
Alexandria, VA 22314
Toll-Free: 800-658-8898
Phone: 703-837-1500
Fax: 703-837-1233
Website: www.nhpco.org

Planned Parenthood Federation of America (PPFA)
123 William St.
10th Fl.
New York, NY 10038
Toll-Free: 800-230-PLAN
(800-230-7526)
Phone: 212-541-7800
Website: www.plannedparenthood.org

The Plastic Surgery Foundation (PSF)
444 E. Algonquin Rd.
Arlington Heights, IL 60005-4664
Toll-Free: 800-766-4955
Phone: 847-228-9900
Website: www.thepsf.org

Society of Critical Care Medicine (SCCM)
500 Midway Dr.
Mount Prospect, IL 60056
Phone: 847-827-6888
Fax: 847-439-7226
Website: www.sccm.org
E-mail: support@sccm.org

Society of Interventional Radiology (SIR)
3975 Fair Ridge Dr.
Ste. 400 N.
Fairfax, VA 22033
Toll-Free: 800-488-7284
Phone: 703-691-1805
Fax: 703-691-1855
Website: www.sirweb.org

Society of Nuclear Medicine and Molecular Imaging (SNMMI)
1850 Samuel Morse Dr.
Reston, VA 20190
Phone: 703-708-9000
Fax: 703-708-9015
Website: www.snmmi.org

Society of Thoracic Surgeons (STS)

633 N. Saint Clair St.
Ste. 2100
Chicago, IL 60611
Phone: 312-202-5800
Fax: 312-202-5801
Website: www.sts.org

Surgery Specialty Hospitals of America (SSHA)

4301 Vista Rd.
Pasadena, TX 77504
Phone: 713-378-3000
Website: ssha.us.com/services

Texas Heart Institute (THI)

6770 Bertner Ave.
Houston, TX 77030
Phone: 832-355-3792
Website: www.texasheart.org

United Network for Organ Sharing (UNOS)

700 N. Fourth St.
Richmond, VA 23219
Toll-Free: 800-292-9548
Phone: 804-782-4800
Fax: 804-782-4817
Website: www.unos.org
E-mail: patientservices@unos.org

United Ostomy Associations of America, Inc. (UOAA)

P.O. Box 525
Kennebunk, ME 04043-0525
Toll-Free: 800-826-0826
Website: www.ostomy.org
E-mail: info@ostomy.org

INDEX

INDEX

Page numbers followed by 'n' indicate a footnote. Page numbers in *italics* indicate a table or illustration.

Index

American Society of Transplantation
(AST), contact 762
American Thoracic Society (ATS),
contact 762
American Thyroid Association (ATA),
contact 763
amputation
defined 749
inpatient surgery 81
overview 579–89
surgery types 22
"Amputation System of Care Traumatic
Amputation" (VA) 587n
Amputee Coalition of America (ACA),
contact 763
amyotrophic lateral sclerosis (ALS),
mechanical ventilator 715
anaphylactic shock, elective surgery 16
anemia
bariatric surgery 492
bowel diversion surgeries 456
hemorrhoid surgery 471
lower limb amputation 585
postoperative complications 363
anesthesia
accidental injuries 164
ambulatory surgery 61
angioplasty and stent
placement 348
cesarean section (C-section) 503
cochlear implant surgery 242
cosmetic surgery 20
disparities in surgical care 743
emergency surgery 13
hemorrhoids 472
mechanical ventilator 714
middle ear infections 238
overview 145–54
plastic surgery 597
postanesthesia care unit
(PACU) 703
postoperative complications 635

anesthesia, *continued*
reducing anxiety before
surgery 184
surgery 119
"Anesthesia" (NIGMS) 145n
anesthesia awareness, plastic
surgery 597
anesthesiologists
ambulatory surgical centers 132
anxiety before surgery 184
breast biopsy 305
cosmetic surgery 20
described 146
emergency surgery 13
heart transplantation and artificial
heart 554
postanesthesia care unit
(PACU) 703
prehabilitation in surgery 142
preparing for surgery 138
surgery 119
aneurysm
angioplasty and stent
placement 349
defined 749
emergency surgery 11
heart surgery 344
second opinion 124
aneurysm repair
angioplasty and stent
placement 354
heart surgery 344
overview 378–83
angiotensin-converting
enzyme (ACE) inhibitors,
coronary artery bypass grafting
surgery 370
angiotensin receptor blockers (ARBs),
coronary artery bypass grafting
surgery 371
ankle block, regional anesthesia for
postsurgical pain 152

Index

Index

Index

CDC *see* Centers for Disease Control
and Prevention
cemented replacement, hip
replacement surgery 415
Centers for Disease Control and
Prevention (CDC)
contact 755
publications
Acinetobacter in healthcare
settings 653n
aortic aneurysm 378n
avoiding infection 205n
blood safety 175n
carbapenem-resistant
Enterobacteriaceae 663n
catheter-associated urinary tract
infections (CAUTIs) 641n
central line-associated
bloodstream infections 643n
gram-negative bacteria
infections 653n
medical tourism 223n
methicillin-resistant
Staphylococcus aureus
(MRSA) 661n
National Health Statistics
Reports 61n
Pseudomonas aeruginosa 655n
septicemia or sepsis 649n
surgical site infections
(SSIs) 639n
total hip replacement 89n, 94n
venous thromboembolism
(blood clots) 679n
ventilator-associated
pneumonia 665n
Centers for Medicare & Medicaid
Services (CMS)
contact 755
publications
choosing a nursing home or
other long-term services and
supports 731n

Centers for Medicare & Medicaid
Services (CMS)
publications, *continued*
getting a second opinion before
surgery 123n
guide to choosing a
hospital 127n
Medicare 209n
skilled nursing facility
rights 731n
central line-associated bloodstream
infections (CLABSIs),
overview 643–6
"Central Line-Associated Bloodstream
Infections: Resources for Patients
and Healthcare Providers"
(CDC) 643n
central line catheter, healthcare-
associated infections 206
central vision, macular degeneration
surgery 271
cerebrospinal fluid
head and neck surgery 233
surgical implant procedure 245
certification
ambulatory surgical centers 134
breast implant surgery 318
healthcare providers 36
certified nurse assistant (CNS),
nursing home or rehab facility 735
certified registered nurse anesthetist
(CRNA)
anesthesia complications 157
surgery preparation 138
cervical intraepithelial neoplasia,
cryosurgery 28
cervix
cancer 496
dilation and curettage 497
gynecologic and obstetric
surgery 511
pelvic exenteration 466
resection 23
urological surgery 565

Index

Index

Index

Index

Index

Index

Index

Index

Index

Index

Index

Index

Index

Index

U.S. Department of Veterans Affairs
(VA)
  publications, *continued*
    thyroidectomy 255n
    tonsillectomy 253n
U.S. Food and Drug Administration
(FDA)
  contact 757
  publications
    before, during, and after
      implant surgery 240n
    before, during, and after
      surgery 273n, 282n
    benefits and risks of cochlear
      implants 240n
    breast implant surgery 316n
    computer-assisted surgical
      systems 35n
    delivery of ear tubes under
      local anesthesia to treat ear
      infection 236n
    hernia surgical mesh
      implants 472n
    LASIK 273n
    medical lasers 47n
    phakic intraocular lens
      implantation surgery 282n
    stress urinary incontinence
      (SUI) 568n
    working to reduce medication
      errors 201n
U.S. National Library of Medicine
(NLM), contact 757
uterine fibroid embolization (UFE),
uterine fibroid surgery 512
uterine fibroid surgery,
  overview 510–2
uterine fibroids
  hysterectomy 495
  uterine fibroid surgery 511
"Uterine Fibroids" (OWH) 510n
uterine prolapse, hysterectomy 495

uterus
  abdominal adhesions 670
  birth control sterilization 508
  cesarean section (C-section) 504
  dilation and curettage 499
  exploratory surgery 18
  hysterectomy 495
  uterine fibroid surgery 511

V

"VA/DoD Clinical Practice Guideline
  for Rehabilitation of Individuals
  with Lower Limb Amputation"
  (VA) 582n
"VA/DoD Clinical Practice Guideline
  for Rehabilitation of Lower Limb
  Amputation" (VA) 582n
"VA/DoD Clinical Practice
  Guideline for the Management
  of Upper Extremity Amputation
  Rehabilitation" (VA) 579n
vaginal birth after cesarean (VBAC),
  described 503
vaginal hysterectomy,
  hysterectomy 496
valve-in-valve procedure, valve repair
  and replacement 377
VAP *see* ventilator-associated
  pneumonia
vascular surgery
  heart, overview 339–84
  lower limb amputation 586
  surgical specialties 8
vascularized composite allograft
  transplantation, overview 547–9
vasectomy, overview 509–10
vasopressors, cardiogenic shock 676
vein bypass, heart surgery 339
"Venous Thromboembolism
  (Blood Clots)—Learn about
  Healthcare Associated Venous
  Thromboembolism" (CDC) 679n

Index